THE THERAPEUTIC ALLIANCE

THE THERAPEUTIC ALLIANCE
■ ■ ■ ■ ■

An Evidence-Based Guide to Practice

Edited by
J. CHRISTOPHER MURAN
JACQUES P. BARBER

THE GUILFORD PRESS
New York   London

Library of Congress Cataloging-in-Publication Data

The therapeutic alliance : an evidence-based guide to practice / edited by
J. Christopher Muran, Jacques P. Barber.
    p. ; cm.
 Includes bibliographical references and index.
 ISBN 978-1-60623-873-8 (hardcover : alk. paper)
 1. Therapeutic alliance. 2. Evidence-based psychotherapy. I. Muran,
J. Christopher. II. Barber, Jacques P.
 [DNLM: 1. Psychotherapy—methods. 2. Evidence-Based Practice.
3. Professional–Patient Relations. 4. Treatment Outcome.
 WM 420 T39685 2010]
 RC489.T66T469 2010
 616.89′14—dc22
                                                              2010020256

To Arnold Winston
—J. C. M.

To Lester Luborsky
—J. P. B.

About the Editors

J. Christopher Muran, PhD, is Associate Dean and Professor at the Derner Institute for Advanced Psychological Studies, and Director of the Psychotherapy Research Program at Beth Israel Medical Center. His research, which has been supported in part by the National Institute of Mental Health and presented at national and international forums, has concentrated on developing intervention and training models relating to the therapeutic alliance. His many publications include such books as *The Therapeutic Alliance in Brief Psychotherapy*, *Negotiating the Therapeutic Alliance: A Relational Treatment Guide*, *Self-Relations in the Psychotherapy Process*, and *Dialogues on Difference: Studies of Diversity in the Therapeutic Relationship*. Dr. Muran is also a fellow of the American Psychological Association and coeditor of the journal *Psychotherapy Research*.

Jacques P. Barber, PhD, ABPP, is Professor of Psychology in the Department of Psychiatry at the University of Pennsylvania School of Medicine and the Philadelphia VA Medical Center. He conducts research on the outcome and process of dynamic and cognitive therapies for depression, panic disorder, posttraumatic stress disorder, substance dependence, and personality disorders. Dr. Barber has also written extensively on the impact of the therapeutic alliance and therapists' use of theoretically relevant interventions on the outcomes of various therapies. He is the coauthor (with Richard F. Summers) of *Psychodynamic Therapy: A Guide to Evidence-Based Practice* and (with Hadas Wiseman) of *Echoes of the Trauma: Relational Themes and Emotions in Children of Holocaust Survivors*. He is also a recent past president of the Society for Psychotherapy Research.

Contributors

Jacques P. Barber, PhD, ABPP, Department of Psychiatry, University of Pennsylvania School of Medicine and Philadelphia VA Medical Center, Philadelphia, Pennsylvania

Lorna Smith Benjamin, PhD, Department of Psychology, University of Utah, Salt Lake City, Utah

Jeffrey L. Binder, PhD, American School of Professional Psychology, Argosy University, Atlanta, Georgia

Louis G. Castonguay, PhD, Department of Psychology, Pennsylvania State University, University Park, Pennsylvania

Kenneth L. Critchfield, PhD, Neuropsychiatric Institute and Department of Psychology, University of Utah, Salt Lake City, Utah

Katherine Crits-Christoph, PhD, Center for Psychotherapy Research, Department of Psychiatry, University of Pennsylvania School of Medicine, Philadelphia, Pennsylvania

Paul Crits-Christoph, PhD, Center for Psychotherapy Research, Department of Psychiatry, University of Pennsylvania School of Medicine, Philadelphia, Pennsylvania

Mary Beth Connolly Gibbons, PhD, Center for Psychotherapy Research, Department of Psychiatry, University of Pennsylvania School of Medicine, Philadelphia, Pennsylvania

Michael J. Constantino, PhD, Department of Psychology, University of Massachusetts, Amherst, Massachusetts

Valentín Escudero, PhD, Department of Psychology, Faculty of Education, University of La Coruña, La Coruña, Spain

Catherine Eubanks-Carter, PhD, Psychotherapy Research Program, Beth Israel Medical Center, New York, New York

Myrna L. Friedlander, PhD, Department of Educational and Counseling Psychology, University at Albany/State University of New York, Albany, New York

Marvin R. Goldfried, PhD, Department of Psychology, Stony Brook University, Stony Brook, New York

Jacob Z. Goldsmith, MA, Department of Psychology, Miami University, Oxford, Ohio

Robert L. Hatcher, PhD, Wellness Center, The Graduate Center, The City University of New York, New York, New York

Laurie Heatherington, PhD, Psychology Department, Williams College, Williamstown, Massachusetts

William P. Henry, PhD, private practice, Tampa, Florida

Clara E. Hill, PhD, Department of Psychology, University of Maryland, College Park, Maryland

Adam O. Horvath, EdD, Faculty of Education and Department of Psychology, Simon Fraser University, Vancouver, British Columbia, Canada

Freda Kalogerakos, PhD, Department of Adult Education and Counselling Psychology, Ontario Institute for Studies in Education, University of Toronto, Toronto, Ontario, Canada

Jonathan W. Kanter, PhD, Psychology Department, University of Wisconsin–Milwaukee, Milwaukee, Wisconsin

Shabad-Ratan Khalsa, BA, Department of Psychiatry, University of Pennsylvania School of Medicine, Philadelphia, Pennsylvania

Robert J. Kohlenberg, PhD, ABPP, Department of Psychology, University of Washington, Seattle, Washington

Andrew A. McAleavey, BA, Department of Psychology, Pennsylvania State University, University Park, Pennsylvania

Stanley B. Messer, PhD, Graduate School of Applied and Professional Psychology, Rutgers University, Piscataway, New Jersey

J. Christopher Muran, PhD, Derner Institute of Advanced Psychological Studies, Adelphi University, Garden City, New York, and Psychotherapy Research Program, Beth Israel Medical Center, New York, New York

John S. Ogrodniczuk, PhD, Department of Psychiatry, University of British Columbia, Vancouver, British Columbia, Canada

William E. Piper, PhD, Department of Psychiatry, University of British Columbia, Vancouver, British Columbia, Canada

Jeremy D. Safran, PhD, Psychology Department, New School for Social Research, New York, New York

Brian A. Sharpless, PhD, Center for Psychotherapy Research, Department of Psychiatry, University of Pennsylvania School of Medicine, Philadelphia, Pennsylvania

William B. Stiles, PhD, Department of Psychology, Miami University, Oxford, Ohio

Dianne Symonds, PhD, Community and Health Studies, Kwantien Polytechnic University, Surrey, British Columbia, Canada

Luis Tapia, MD, Couples Therapy Unit, School of Psychology, University of Development, Las Condes, Santiago, Chile

Mavis Tsai, PhD, private practice and Functional Analytic Psychotherapy Specialty Clinic, Psychological Services and Training Center, University of Washington, Seattle, Washington

Jeanne C. Watson, PhD, Department of Adult Education and Counselling Psychology, Ontario Institute for Studies in Education, University of Toronto, Toronto, Ontario, Canada

David L. Wolitzky, PhD, Department of Psychology, New York University, New York, New York

Contents

II. PRACTICE AND THE THERAPEUTIC ALLIANCE

III. TRAINING PROGRAMS
ON THE THERAPEUTIC ALLIANCE

An Introduction

Establishing the
Context and Rationale

J. Christopher Muran
Jacques P. Barber

Once described as "the quintessential integrative variable" (Wolfe & Gold-fried, 1988) and probably the most often cited "common factor" in psycho-therapy (Wampold, 2001), the therapeutic alliance has received a great deal of empirical attention over the past 40 years or so. Much of the research has focused on the predictive validity of the construct, and there have been now two well-cited meta-analyses demonstrating that it is one of the most con-sistent and strongest predictors of treatment success (Horvath & Symonds, 1991; Martin, Garske, & Davis, 2000). There have recently been some noteworthy challenges to the causal interpretation of the alliance-outcome correlation (Barber, Connolly, Crits-Christoph, Gladis, & Siqueland, 2000; Crits-Christoph, Connolly Gibbons, & Hearon, 2006; DeRubeis, Broth-man, & Gibbons, 2005). These studies have specifically examined the rela-tionship between early treatment gains and alliance, with some finding that the former carries the predictive load.

In addition, there have also been a good number of efforts to go beyond demonstrating the predictive validity of the alliance and to understand its function in the change process. These include studies of how the alliance develops over time, specifically investigations of shifts in the alliance over time; of overall U-shaped patterns, suggesting a strain in the alliance during the middle phase of treatment; and of localized V-patterns, suggesting rupture and repair events (e.g., Stevens, Muran, Safran, Gorman, & Winston, 2007; Stiles et al., 2004; Strauss et al., 2006). There have been more intensive studies that attempted to define rupture events and resolution processes, which have included qualitative research efforts examining negative experiences and essential interventions (see Safran, Muran, Samstag, & Stevens, 2002 for a review).

Finally, there have been a few studies that have examined the impact of therapist training specifically designed to enhance the therapeutic alliance and address negative transactions between patients and therapists (Bambling, King, Raue, Schweittzer, & Lambert, 2006; Crits-Christoph, Connolly Gibbons, Crits-Christoph, et al., 2006; Hilsenroth, Ackerman, Clemence, Strassle, & Handler, 2002; Muran, Safran, Samstag, & Winston, 2005; Safran, Muran, Samstag, & Winston, 2005; Strupp, 1993). The results of these studies have ranged from mixed to very promising, from highlighting the complexities of conducting such training to demonstrating significant benefits.

As result, there is much that can now be said about the therapeutic alliance with empirical support. The stage is set for a discussion of the alliance that is practical in focus and stays close to the empirical data. The aim of this book is to provide an evidence-based approach to the therapeutic alliance—specifying practice and training guidelines from various psychotherapy orientations that can be supported by the research literature. It was written primarily for therapists and supervisors, but also for students from the various disciplines, at all levels of experience, and from diverse orientations. With the increasing emphasis on evidenced-based practice from apparently all quarters, the field seems ready for such a treatment of this widely recognized and studied concept.

The volume was organized into three sections: The first concerns critical studies of the empirical literature, focusing on what can be said about the topics of measuring the alliance, its predictive validity, rupture and repair. It includes a careful reconsideration of the alliance construct and its measurement, the predictive relationship of the alliance to overall outcome, the research looking at changes in the alliance over time, qualitative studies of patient and therapist negative experiences in psychotherapy, and the empirical literature on alliance ruptures and resolution processes. All these chapters discuss the implications of their research reviews for practice and training. They are written in summary fashion and aim to "cut to the chase" in their analysis of the research literature.

The second section concentrates on the therapeutic alliance from the standpoint of various psychotherapy orientations and modalities, including psychodynamic/psychoanalytic, interpersonal, cognitive-behavioral, behavioral, humanistic, couples, family, and group. The authors were advised to discuss the alliance from their respective orientations and research (or relevant research from others) and then to present clinical material and practice recommendations based on the research evidence. These chapters are unique in their emphasis on practice in their orientation and justification with research. They each provide a conceptualization of the alliance based on their theoretical orientation, what are essential considerations of the alliance from their perspective, and then discuss how the alliance is developed and maintained, specific alliance-building strategies or principles, and how poor alliances or breaches in the alliance are considered and redressed.

The third section concentrates on describing three large-scale research programs—at Vanderbilt University, University of Pennsylvania, and Beth Israel Medical Center—that aimed to train therapists to improve their abilities to negotiate interpersonal process and the therapeutic alliance. These chapters provide details regarding their various training methods and recommendations based on their results—a level of presentation that has yet to be published. These chapters begin with a brief history of their training program, contextualizing their approach and its rationale and providing summary findings regarding its effect. They describe basic technical principles and essential therapist skills targeted in their training, providing details about training strategies, the structure of their training regimen, and including a sense of a typical training session. These chapters read to some extent like brief manuals for trainers.

The volume closes with a concluding chapter that attempts to define guidelines and standards for practice and training relating to the therapeutic alliance, including future considerations, as suggested by the preceding sections and chapters. Although there has been a proliferation of research on the alliance over the past few decades, we have no illusions about how much can be definitively said about the alliance based on the empirical evidence. We do hope, however, that with this book we can at once distill what we know and stir further research to extend this knowledge.

REFERENCES

Bambling, M., King, R., Raue, P., Schweittzer, R., & Lambert, W. (2006). Clinical supervision: Its influence on client-rated working alliance and client symptom reduction in the brief treatment of major depression. *Psychotherapy Research, 16*, 317–331.

Barber, J. P., Connolly, M. B., Crits-Christoph, P., Gladis, M., & Siqueland, L. (2000). Alliance predicts patients' outcome beyond in-treatment change in symptoms. *Journal of Consulting and Clinical Psychology, 68*, 1027–1032.

Crits-Christoph, P., Connolly Gibbons, M. B., Crits-Christoph, K., Narducci, J., Schamberger, M., & Gallop, R. (2006). Can therapists be trained to improve their alliances?: A preliminary study of alliance-fostering psychotherapy. *Psychotherapy Research, 16*, 268–281.

Crits-Christoph, P., Connolly Gibbons, M. B., & Hearon, B. (2006). Does the alliance cause good outcome?: Recommendations for future research on the alliance. *Psychotherapy, 43*, 280–285.

DeRubeis, R. J., Brothman, M. A., & Gibbons, C. J. (2005). A conceptual and methodological analysis of the nonspecifics argument. *Clinical Psychology: Science and Practice, 12*, 174–183.

Hilsenroth, M. J., Ackerman, S. J., Clemence, A. J., Strassle, C. G., & Handler, L. (2002). Effects of structured clinician training on patient and therapist perspectives of alliance early in psychotherapy. *Psychotherapy, 39*, 309–323.

Horvath, A. O., & Symonds, B. D. (1991). Relation between working alliance and outcome in psychotherapy: A meta-analysis. *Journal of Counseling Psychology, 38*, 139–149.

Martin, D. J., Garske, J. P., & Davis, M. K. (2000). Relation of the therapeutic alliance with outcome and other variables: A meta-analytic review. *Journal of Consulting and Clinical Psychology, 68*, 438–450.

Muran, J. C., Safran, J. D., Samstag, L. W., & Winston, A. (2005). Evaluating an alliance-focused treatment for personality disorders. *Psychotherapy.*

Safran, J. D., & Muran, J. C. (2000). *Negotiating the therapeutic alliance: A relational treatment guide.* New York: Guilford Press.

Safran, J. D., Muran, J. C., Samstag, L. W., & Stevens, C. (2002). Repairing alliance ruptures. In J. C. Norcross (Ed.), *Psychotherapy relationships that work: Therapist contributions and responsiveness to patients* (pp. 235–254). New York: Oxford University Press.

Safran, J. D., Muran, J. C., Samstag, L. W., & Winston, A. (2005). Evaluating an alliance-focused treatment for potential treatment failures. *Psychotherapy, 46*, 233–248.

Stiles, W. B., Glick, M. J., Osatuke, K., Hardy, G. E., Shapiro, D. A., Agnew-Davies, R., et al. (2004). Patterns of alliance development and the rupture–repair hypothesis: Are productive relationships U-shaped or V-shaped? *Journal of Counseling Psychology, 51*, 81–92.

Strauss, J. L., Hayes, A. M., Johnson, S. L., Newman, C. F., Brown, G. K., Barber, J. P., et al. (2006). Early alliance, alliance ruptures, and symptom change in a nonrandomized trial of cognitive therapy for avoidant and obsessive–compulsive personality disorders. *Journal of Consulting and Clinical Psychology, 74*, 337–345.

Stevens, C. L., Muran, J. C., Safran, J. D., Gorman, B. S., & Winston, A. (2007). Levels and patterns of the therapeutic alliance in brief psychotherapy. *American Journal of Psychotherapy, 61*, 109–129.

Strupp, H. H. (1993). The Vanderbilt Psychotherapy Studies: Synopsis. *Journal of Consulting and Clinical Psychology, 61*, 431–433.

Wampold, B. E. (2001). *The great psychotherapy debate: Models, methods, and findings.* Mahwah, NJ: Erlbaum.

Wolfe, B. E., & Goldfried, M. R. (1988). Research on psychotherapy integration: Recommendations and conclusions from an NIMH workshop. *Journal of Consulting and Clinical Psychology, 56*, 448–451.

PART I
■ ■ ■ ■ ■
CRITICAL STUDIES
OF THE
THERAPEUTIC ALLIANCE

CHAPTER 1

■　■　■　■　■

Alliance Theory
and Measurement

Robert L. Hatcher

Alliance issues confront therapists in their practices every day. When things go as expected and the patient is engaged and responsive, we know we are working well together. Our patients blossom, making the approach we have offered them their own, moving forward with confidence and satisfaction. Our work is on track. And we know the work is off-course when our patient seems to be losing interest, becomes silent or angry with us, or seems to feel misunderstood. At these times, we look to our technique, or to our creativity in the moment, to find ways to help the patient reengage in the work of therapy. Alliance theory, and its precursors in early psychoanalysis, emerged as a way to think about and address these important issues in clinical work. Along the way, researchers developed ways to measure alliance, with valuable applications for research and practice.

The aim of this chapter is to develop a broad perspective on alliance theory and measurement, tracing its development over the years as therapists wrestled with issues like these. We will sift out the key features of alliance to help understand its place in our theories of therapy and in research, and to see how these features have been measured. Here is an outline of these key features. When conducting therapy, therapists bring their expectations for how the work should go, based primarily on the treatment method they choose to apply. Patients have their own goals and bring their own expectations for how therapy should go. Differences are continually negotiated

7

between the two. Across different therapeutic approaches, a good alliance means that patients and therapists are working well together toward the goals of therapy. Good work is expected to be purposeful and collaborative. Thus, alliance is a way to think about how the patient and therapist are working together. Alliance measures assess this working relationship. Over the years, therapists have expanded their techniques to address the problems that interfere with effective collaborative work. Often these new approaches have themselves become central to clinical work. In this chapter we will find how the recognition and use of these key alliance concepts help clarify some nagging issues in clinical theory and research, such as whether alliance is part of the relationship in therapy, how alliance is related to technique, and, more broadly, whether it is still useful to think in alliance terms.

THE ORIGINS OF ALLIANCE
THEORY IN PSYCHOANALYSIS

Freud encountered alliance issues as soon as he began to use psychological methods to treat his patients. He expected his patients to submit to hypnosis, but they resisted his efforts to hypnotize them. After he abandoned hypnosis in favor of free association, they resisted free association. Later Freud recognized that the patient's transference to him interfered with the work of analysis, which included the task of remembering rather than repeating old pathogenic relationships and experiences. All of these phenomena he called "resistance," which meant that his patients were not participating in the work as expected; at worst, they left treatment. In current alliance terms, these were strains or ruptures in the alliance. Freud did not think in alliance terms and used the concept late, in 1937 (Freud, 1937/1964). Nevertheless, we can identify as alliance issues his struggles to engage and keep his patients in treatment. We can see that many of the techniques of analysis were designed to help patients become or remain engaged in the work of treatment. Analysis of resistance was designed to help patients get back to facing their conflicts more directly. Analysis of transference began when patients' feelings toward Freud as a helpful physician were eclipsed by other strong feelings toward him, interfering with the work of analysis.

The picture of the patient as a partner in the work of treatment is implicit in Freud's writing (1912/1958a, p. 104). His vision is of a person with a reasonable understanding of the goals and tasks of the therapy but whose participation is susceptible to interferences that lead to breaches in the working relationship. In response Freud modified his technique to help steer the patient back. This pattern is a recurring theme in the development of theories of treatment and alliance.

Freud was especially concerned about dealing with the obstacles to sustaining engagement and commitment, and gave relatively little attention to how patients become engaged in therapy and to what sustains their commitment when things are difficult. His few early comments on these issues, however, are cited by contemporary authors as the origin of alliance thinking (see Freud, 1913/1958b, pp. 139–140). Freud emphasized the personal tie—the bond—between patient and therapist, based on an "unobjectionable" positive (but not excessively positive) transference derived from earlier experiences of care from benevolent others (1912/1958a, p. 99). This bond keeps the patient in treatment, helps overcome doubt, and promotes cooperativeness. It is maintained by careful work on interfering interpersonal patterns (transferences) and on other avoidance moves (defenses/resistances). In Freud's early focus on the bond, there is less emphasis on the "reasonable" patient. But the purpose of the bond is clear: to help the patient participate effectively in the work of treatment.

As psychoanalysts took more interest in the ego, the rational, reality-oriented aspect of the person, Freud's picture of the patient as ally came more clearly into view. Sterba (1934) introduced the term "alliance" and expanded the idea that the patient has a rational, observing capacity with which the analyst can ally against the irrational forces of the patient's transference and defenses. In one of his last publications, Freud (1937/1964) discussed what he called the analytic "pact," noting that "the analytic situation consists in our allying ourselves with the ego of the person under treatment" (p. 235) and considering at length the limits placed on this pact by various features of the patient's personality and by the particular demands of psychoanalytic treatment on the patient. Over time, the idea of collaborative work became more prominent as compared to Freud's early emphasis on the emotional tie.

A number of important elements in our picture of the alliance came from this early work. The key issues are these: as clinicians, we want our patients to be engaged in and committed to the work of therapy as we and our theory define it, whether we are psychoanalysts or behavioral therapists. This engagement is a product of an alliance between the therapist and the patient's reasonable, realistic self around the goals of treatment and the particular therapeutic activities that are prescribed by our theories of therapy and technique. Patients make this commitment based on their determination that this therapist, and this therapy, can provide a treatment that will lead to desired changes. The patient's commitment and engagement in the work are also supported by an overall positive feeling toward the therapist, a sense of trust that enhances good will and suppresses doubt and hostility. When the patient's engagement and commitment falter, techniques need to be developed to help bring the patient back on track.

The discussion of alliance was relatively dormant in psychoanalysis from the 1940s to the mid-1960s, when Greenson's (1965, 1967) contributions appeared. In an extensively documented clinical discussion, Greenson used the term "working alliance" to emphasize what he called the "outstanding function" of the alliance, which is "the patient's ability to work in the analytic situation" (1965, p. 202). Greenson focused strongly on the collaborative aspect of the alliance, which he felt, following Sterba (1934) and Freud (1937/1964), was gradually achieved through interpretation of interfering transferences and the patient's identification with the analyst's ways of working in the treatment. He tried to separate the working alliance proper from its roots in transference and attachment, recognizing though that the alliance is sustained by a base of trust and goodwill. An innovative part of Greenson's approach was to talk directly with his patients about alliance issues, seen as more than manifestations of transference or defense. When needed, Greenson discussed the goals, methods, and purposes of the psychoanalytic work with his patients (1965, 1967). He explored their ideas about and reactions to the expectations that psychoanalysis sets for patients and analysts. It is true that Greenson's definition of the working alliance refers only to the patient's ability to work in treatment. But his technical advice and his many examples of analysts' failed efforts to work effectively with patients, point to the therapist's as well as the patient's ability to work together. As we shall see, Greenson's contributions evoked strong reactions from many different quarters within psychoanalysis.

Up to this point, alliance was mostly of interest to psychoanalysts. In the mid-1970s they were joined by several major psychotherapy researchers. Of these, Bordin developed the most comprehensive theory with his innovative (1979, 1980, 1994) working alliance theory. This work stimulated a vast array of research studies on the alliance that continue to this day. Bordin (1979) saw the alliance concept as a unifying theoretical framework for all types of interpersonal change processes, including the psychotherapies that were then proliferating at an alarming rate. His core idea was this: Every form of therapy has a set of expectations or demands for the patient and therapist and how they will work together. These are the rules of treatment that follow from the clinical theory, and they vary in degree and kind, depending on the approach.

Bordin recognized that clinical theories demand specific work from patients and therapists, which he called "embedded working alliances" (1979, p. 253). We might better call these "embedded working alliance expectations." In any case, Bordin's alliance theory is a theory of therapy as work, which is why he called it the working alliance. His alliance theory was designed to account for how clinical theory (e.g., psychoanalysis, gestalt therapy, cognitive-behavioral therapy) gets translated into a clinical change process: theory prescribes the work expected of patient and therapist to effect change; to the extent they work together as expected, change will occur. This broad theory is accompanied by a set of hypotheses about the work. These hypotheses are that the alliance is strong to the extent that patient and therapist can jointly negotiate and carry out the expected work, as negotiation of expectations is required for effective engagement in the work; that the stronger the alliance, the better the result of treatment; and that strong alliances result from good matches between the treatment's alliance expectations and the personal characteristics of the patient and therapist (1979, p. 253).

The negotiation of the alliance between patient and therapist begins at the start of therapy and continues throughout. This negotiation is between the expectations of the therapist, as guided by clinical theory, and those of the patient, reflecting the patient's understanding of the problems and the best means to solve them, conditioned by the patient's level of trust, and so on (Bordin, 1979, p. 255; see also Safran & Muran, 2006). Bordin saw three elements of this negotiation: agreement on goals, collaboration on tasks, and establishment of the bond. These categories are compelling, and many clinicians and researchers take them to be Bordin's alliance theory. But these are simply operational parts of his broader theory of alliance, which concerns the work required by the type of therapy being engaged in. Bordin's alliance theory gives us more than a way to think about how alliance is built and maintained through negotiation of goals, tasks, and bonds. It opens a broader perspective, enabling us to raise questions about therapy as collaborative, purposeful work. The full theory begins with the idea that work is an activity directed toward a goal—it is purposeful. Two people working together toward a goal requires collaboration. Thus, this work is anchored in agreement on goals, collaboration on tasks, and supported by an appropriate bond. If, however, we think only in terms of implementing the alliance through agreement on goals and tasks, and the supporting bond, we can lose sight of the broader perspective that Bordin's theory offers of alliance as collaborative, purposeful work.

Bordin's work has been enhanced by later contributors. His view of alliance as negotiated and dyadic was a significant contribution, ahead of its time. However, Bordin underplayed the client's active contribution to the negotiation process, stressing instead the role of the therapist in creating consensus and collaboration (e.g., Bordin, 1979, p. 254). His valuable concept of alliances embedded within therapeutic approaches underemphasizes the fact that patients have their own ideas about how therapy should work and these ideas play a significant role in the negotiation of work in therapy. In a series of important contributions, Safran and Muran (e.g., 2000, 2006) and colleagues have highlighted the negotiation process in forming and maintaining the alliance, paying particular attention to the issue of openly and effectively countering the client's disagreement or doubt about the treatment.

INTERNAL WORKING ALLIANCE MODELS

The concept of an internal working alliance model can help anchor these ideas. Patients and therapists both come to therapy with their own ideas about what good work consists in. This is the starting point for their negotiation of the alliance. The patient judges his or her experience of the work with the therapist based on this initial model. If the experience does not meet expectations, the patient will withdraw temporarily or permanently (or perhaps endure submissively); a mismatch for the therapist leads to a search for methods to address the problem. These working models, reflecting the cumulative and ongoing evaluation of the quality of the work in therapy, are an important part of the working alliance. In this sense, the working alliance model is an active ingredient in therapy—it provides a sustaining rationale and basis for participating in the work of treatment. It is also, in this sense, the glue of therapy, holding things together, providing an organizing, motivating perspective for the patient. Because the patient can see where the therapy is going and what the value of therapy is even when the going gets tough, the model keeps the patient from abandoning the project. Bordin's ideas would suggest that direct negotiation directed toward these models would help advance therapy. But since the models are the result of the patient's evaluation of the work, the quality of the work will have a significant effect on the model as well, as we shall see.

In the remainder of this chapter, we discuss the relationship between alliance and the therapeutic bond. We examine how alliance is measured and discuss several key conceptual issues in alliance from this working alliance point of view, including some of the major objections to the use of alliance as a concept. We review how the working alliance viewpoint relates to technique and to the overall relationship between patient and therapist. And finally we discuss the issue of the alliance as a curative agent in its own right. During the course of this discussion we suggest some modifications to alliance theory.

THE THERAPEUTIC BOND

Looking back at Freud's early reports (1910/1957, 1912/1958a, 1913/1958b), we see him struggling with what keeps patients in treatment and how to deal with interferences in the alliance. One positive force he identified was the patient's "unobjectionable" positive transference—the bond in alliance terms. The important feature of this bond is that it facilitates the working alliance. Alliance-facilitating bonds are bonds that support the work of treatment. They are not bonds for bonds' sake, but rather they facilitate the work. In the "unobjectionable" positive transference, Freud identified what he saw as an optimal alliance-facilitating bond for psychoanalysis. Bordin generalized this point by asking, what level or type of bond is required by a given treatment approach in order for it to work properly? (1979, p. 254). He suggested that psychoanalysis requires a very different level of trust and attachment than a brief symptom-oriented therapy (p. 254). Many interesting points about the role of the bond follow from this approach. A patient's positive idealizing bond, which might well support a cognitive-behavioral treatment, may interfere with a process–experiential treatment's efforts to explore angry feelings toward the therapist. Similarly, a high level of care and concern from a therapist may facilitate some types of treatment or be suitable to some kinds of patients but not to others. Overall, there may be an optimal level of liking and trust for a given therapy, where too little may inhibit effective engagement while too much may as well (Hatcher & Barends, 2006).

These considerations point to a "work-supporting" bond that is distinct from the overall level of liking, respect, and concern (Hatcher & Barends, 2006). It would be valuable to take a closer look at the components of the work-supporting bond. To help build collaboration on the tasks of therapy, Bordin (1979, p. 254) recommended building the patient's confidence that the therapeutic method will lead to the desired outcome. Providing the patient with good evidence-based information aids in this task, but conveying the therapist's engagement and optimism in the work helps too. This emotional appeal may lead to what Hatcher and Barends called the "potentiating bond." These authors also identified an "appreciating bond" that is fostered by the therapist's genuine interest and appreciation for the patient as a person, showing empathy and a desire to understand the patient's experience. These two aspects of the work-supporting bond may be important to the early remoralization stage of therapy, promoting confidence, optimism, and commitment to the treatment (Howard, Lueger, Maling, & Martinovich, 1993). Of course, Rogers's extensive work on therapist-facilitating conditions (e.g., 1957) overlaps especially with the "appreciating bond." However, Rogers's idea was that providing these conditions was what brought desired change to the patient; the idea presented here is that these conditions contribute to making collaborative, purposeful work possible. These are not incompatible views, but they can easily be confused with each other.

Bordin (1979) did not consistently distinguish between the overall bond as mutual liking, respect, etc., and the work-supporting bond that is linked to purposeful work. This delinking has persisted in contemporary accounts of the alliance. For example, in their meta-analysis of alliance outcome research, Martin, Garske, and Davis (2000) described "the affective bond between patient and therapist" (p. 438) as a common feature across current alliance theories. This very broad definition of the bond is problematic because it embraces a wide range of relationship features such as respect, liking, appreciation, attachment, and warmth without linking them to the work of treatment. In most circumstances, the bond is likely to facilitate the therapeutic work, but it cannot be assumed that this is always so. As noted, some types of positive bonds may interfere with treatment, and some may be unrelated to effective work, as one can like and respect another person despite being unable to work productively together (Hatcher & Barends, 1996).

ALLIANCE MEASUREMENT

As interest in the alliance grew during the 1970s and '80s, researchers worked to translate the years of accumulated clinical indicators of alliance into reliable and valid alliance measures. Important advantages come to researchers and practicing clinicians from standardized alliance measurement. Standard measures allow researchers to compare alliance across therapist–client pairs and over time, and thus to investigate the role of alliance in therapy process and outcome. Clinicians can objectify their own clinical sense of the alliance and add to it the perspective of the client, whose views of the alliance may at times be quite divergent. Lambert and colleagues have demonstrated that use of routine client ratings of the alliance, along with other variables, can significantly reduce the rather large percentage of clients who deteriorate during treatment (Harmon et al., 2007).

The precursors of alliance measurement first appeared during the 1960s, and alliance measures multiplied extensively following Bordin's call for a research focus on alliance (Bordin, 1979). Important early developments included scales created by Luborsky (Alexander & Luborsky, 1986), Horvath (Horvath & Greenberg, 1989), and the Vanderbilt group (Hartley & Strupp, 1983; see Elvins & Green, 2008, for a comprehensive history and catalog of alliance scales). Many scales were designed for use with adult psychotherapy outpatients. More recently, others were developed for use with children, adolescents, inpatients, groups, couples, and families and in such diverse settings as medical offices and inpatient centers. Nevertheless, the bulk of alliance-related research is conducted with a few core measures: the Working Alliance Inventory (WAI; Horvath & Greenberg, 1989); the California Psychotherapy Alliance Scales (CALPAS; Gaston & Marmar, 1994), which have therapist-, patient-, and observer-rated versions; and the observer-rated Vanderbilt Therapy Alliance Scale (VTAS; Hartley & Strupp, 1983). These scales, with the exception of the WAI, were developed on the basis of an eclectic conceptualization of the alliance. However, for the most part they contain items that refer to issues that have a fairly clear link to the state of the collaborative, purposeful working alliance. For example, the VTAS includes the item "Patient and therapist relate in honest, straight-forward way." It can be argued that this item reflects an "embedded alliance" requirement present in virtually every form of psychotherapy. Most other VTAS items are very clearly related to the expected work of therapy, such as "Patient makes effort to carry out therapeutic procedures." Thus, available alliance questionnaires do a creditable job in assessing patient, therapist, and observer perceptions of the quality of the working collaboration—with the exception of a few overly general bond items (e.g., WAI: "I believe my therapist likes me") and questions that reflect tasks of specific types of therapy (e.g., CALPAS: "When your therapist commented about one situation, did it bring to mind other related situations in your life?"). The WAI has the clearest conceptual footing, as it was developed on the basis of Bordin's (1979) conceptualization of the alliance as constituted by agreement on goals and tasks and supported by the bond. The WAI includes no items referring to specific treatment methods, although as mentioned it has a number of bond items not linked to the work of treatment. This clear theoretical link may account for the commanding popularity of the WAI in alliance studies (Martin et al., 2000). Short forms for many of these measures have been developed, exhibiting good psychometric properties and validities (e.g., VTAS—Shelef & Diamond, 2008; WAI—Hatcher & Gillaspy, 2006). These measures give a general overall reading of the state of the working alliance at the session level. Although there is some evidence that these measures tap discernible dimensions of alliance (e.g., Hatcher & Gillaspy, 2006), a compelling argument can be made that these measures are like room thermometers in that they give an overall reading of the quality of the working alliance without being very localized or specific about it.

Measurement of specific alliance features can be guided by examining the "embedded alliances" that exist in particular therapies. Different treatments demand different alliances, as Bordin (1979) pointed out. This aspect of alliance measurement remains largely unexplored. It appears likely that for particular treatment approaches some components of the collaborative work will have greater influence on the outcome or may even be critical to success. For example, a study of depressed patients in cognitive therapy by Brotman (2004) showed that "patients who facilitated therapists' adherence to concrete techniques demonstrated significantly more improvements in the following session," citing as an example "patients who were able, interested and/or willing to provide specific examples of events or cognitions" (p. 33). Brotman suggested that therapists' "encouraging active involvement in their patients will improve patient adherence" (p. 35). Although encouraging active involvement is a general alliance-enhancing technique, here the focus is quite specific: patients should facilitate therapist adherence to concrete techniques, and therapists should do whatever they can to encourage patients to participate in this way. This approach demonstrates the close link between productive work and alliance and may be a rich and rewarding area of growth in alliance research and clinical work. A good alliance measure for this therapy would include items related to this specific treatment feature. Further, we can see research potential in determining exactly which work requirements are critical to a given treatment's success. This line of investigation would bridge "unpacking" research that determines which components are most critical to success (e.g., exposure vs. cognitive restructuring for anxiety) with research aimed at determining what the work requirements are for the participants so as to maximize implementation of these components.

THE RELATIONSHIP BETWEEN TECHNIQUE AND ALLIANCE

Differentiating Alliance and Technique

The relationship between technique and alliance has been much discussed. We define technique as the therapist's deliberate planful tactics to effect desired changes in the patient. Technique is based on and guided by clinical theory. For example, the technique of exposure to anxiety-provoking situations is based on the theory that anxiety is extinguished by blocking avoidance processes and permitting graded exposure to the anxiety-provoking situation. Technique is the therapist's effort to structure what the patient and therapist do together in the treatment so as to achieve desired change. Alliance deals with how the patient and therapist are working together. Good alliance is good collaborative work. If the therapist, using technique, effectively engages the patient in the work, there is a good alliance. (We recognize that there are times when it is the patient who, taking the initiative, engages the therapist in good work.) When patients are actively, collaboratively engaged with the therapist's techniques in pursuit of shared goals, a good alliance exists, and in fact the alliance is seamless. When there is a disruption in the work, alliance issues appear, as we have seen with Freud and Greenson and, in fact, as we see in our daily work with patients. When alliances falter, a treatment approach should have additional techniques available to restore the collaborative work. If these methods are absent or if they fail, the technique is incomplete and should lead to the development of new technique, designed to deal with the problems in the collaborative work. We recognized this process in Freud's (1912/1958a) developing his technique of transference analysis. Patterson and Forgatch (1985) gave an example of alliance problems in behavioral therapy at a time when it had not yet developed alliance-repairing techniques, due largely to the fact that its clinical theory of resistance and alliance was quite sketchy. In this instance, the practitioners in their study simply stuck to the same techniques that first led to the alliance problems, making the problems worse. Issues of this sort have led cognitive and cognitive-behavioral clinicians to develop additional techniques based on expanded clinical theory (e.g., Leahy, 2001; Safran & Segal, 1990).

These observations point to the fact that technique and alliance are not at the same conceptual level. Technique is part of the work, and alliance considers how the work is going. Some researchers (e.g., Bedi, Davis, & Williams, 2005) have blurred the distinction between techniques designed to address alliance issues, such as building an alliance-supporting bond, and alliance itself, reserving the term "technique" for interventions aimed at distal treatment outcomes. This approach divides therapist actions into alliance actions and technical actions, placing alliance and technique on equal conceptual levels. As noted earlier, it is important to distinguish between the method of forming an alliance and alliance itself, which refers to the nature and quality of the collaborative work. In Bedi et al.'s (2005) study, patients were asked what therapist actions contributed most to their engagement in treatment. Bedi et al. were surprised when patients reported that techniques addressing symptoms played a more important role in enhancing their commitment to therapy than actions specifically aimed at developing the alliance (p. 320). The major point here is that any activity, including technique, that enhances the collaborative work will contribute positively to the quality of the alliance. Therapists are responsive (Stiles, Honos-Webb, & Surko, 1998) to the particular clinical situation, shaping their technique to maximize productive, purposeful work with their client. In this way, as we saw with Freud early on, therapists are attentive to maximizing the alliance with their patients.

These observations imply that although alliance and technique are on different conceptual planes, they are not independent variables. We would expect effective use of technique to correlate highly with good alliance, because a technique that engages the patient in therapeutic work already has alliance considerations built into it, while technique that does not engage the patient has failed to incorporate alliance considerations. Furthermore, if the therapy is seen to be effective, both patient and therapist will (usually) become or remain more deeply engaged in the work. Thus good outcome (or progress) will promote good alliance, and deeper or continuing engagement in work that has been productive so far is likely to continue to be productive.

Goldfried and Davila (2005) have proposed viewing alliance as a principle of change, grouped with other principles including facilitation of expectations, offering feedback, encouragement of corrective experience, and emphasis on reality testing. These latter principles are composed of technical interventions. Alliance as described in this chapter is not a set of technical activities but rather a way of looking at these activities. Thus, working alliance theory places alliance one conceptual level above Gold-fried and Davila's grouping of techniques into principles of change, asking of each of them, "Are the patient and therapist actively and collaboratively engaged in these activities?"

The Interplay between Alliance, Technique, and Clinical Theory

When Freud altered his technique to include analysis of transference, he also modified his clinical theory to include the value of transference analysis in helping the patient change. This change in theory and technique in turn led to new expectations for what patients and therapists should be doing in analysis. Thus, analysts should be alert to transferences, and patients should be able to understand and work with a transference way of thinking. Some years later, Gill (1982) extended psychoanalytic clinical theory to include these expectations, describing "resistance to the transference," where patients resist becoming aware of their transference feelings toward their therapists, and adding the corresponding technique, analysis of transference resistance. From this sequence we can recognize an ongoing dialectic between technique, theory, and alliance, where difficulties in working collaboratively with the therapist lead to new clinical theories and associated techniques to deal with these difficulties, which then lead to new difficulties when patients have problems working with these new techniques. We will see more how this progression plays out when we discuss the links between alliance and the relationship in therapy.

Techniques to Address Alliance Issues

We have seen that techniques have evolved over the years to deal with alliance difficulties. In recent years explicit attention has been given to alliance-addressing techniques, with the expectation that this emphasis would lead to better alliances and better outcomes. Crits-Christoph et al. (2006) trained clinicians to be more aware of signs of alliance strains and to implement specific alliance-enhancing techniques to address them. This approach resulted in patients reporting increased alliance scores and possibly better outcomes (the number of respondents was too small to be certain). Summers and Barber (2003) demonstrated how building alliances is a measurable clinical skill. These efforts are valuable expansions of technique for the treatments involved and seek to engage more directly what we have called the patient's internal working alliance model. But perhaps this effort would be better framed in the broader recognition that alliance is always being addressed in treatment through good use of technique designed to help patients with their problems, which, since Freud, have included problems in working with the therapist. Safran and Muran (2000) have taken this process a step farther, proposing a relational treatment that is centered on addressing alliance issues. But the working alliance point of view still remains: we would still ask whether the patient and therapist are working well together as they address alliance issues in treatment. Is the patient resisting the therapist's effort to work on the alliance?

CRITIQUES OF ALLIANCE THEORY: TWO WAYS TO SEE ALLIANCE AS IRRELEVANT

Working alliance is centered on a powerful fault line within psychoanalysis, and Greenson's contribution has been attacked and misunderstood by both classical psychoanalysts and contemporary relational analysts. This fault line parallels a similar one in contemporary psychotherapy practice and research. It will be helpful in understanding the current theoretical status of the alliance concept to elaborate on this point.

Alliance and Technique as Rival Concepts: Alliance Loses

Classical analysts objected strongly to the alliance concept (e.g., Brenner, 1979), believing that accepting any interpersonal connection with the patient as real fails to examine its transference features, considered at that time to be the core curative activity in analysis. These critics followed Freud's early assertion (1912/1958a) that analysis of transference will deal with any problems in the relationship. They thought that alliance repair is an unneeded concept, because it is just another way to describe the major technical activity of psychoanalysis, transference analysis. These critics saw this as an either–or situation, where alliance competes with other concepts for primacy as a way of understanding the clinical situation. Further, classical analysts such as Brenner tended to think that any disagreement about the therapy on the patient's part was due to irrational transference-based ideas. Contemporary analysts (e.g., Gill, 1982) apply both perspectives, honoring the patient's objections in their own right while remaining alert to possible transference influences. These analysts do not see an either–or choice, leaving room to think of alliance as an assessment of the quality of the collaborative work. A parallel to the classical analysts' objection is expressed by some contemporary cognitive therapists, who, like the classical analysts, stress the primacy of their core techniques in effecting change and see the alliance with the therapist as a sidelight that diverts attention from true curative processes (e.g., DeRubeis, Brotman, & Gibbons, 2005).

Alliance as Relationship: Alliance Annexed

Relational analysts have tended to dismiss the value of thinking in alliance terms. Their focus is on the relationship between patient and therapist, with full acknowledgment of the real mutual effects each has on the other (Greenberg & Mitchell, 1983; Safran & Muran, 2006). Mainstream American psychoanalysis was slow to embrace a fully dyadic view of treatment. Until the 1990s its emphasis was chiefly on the patient's internal dynamics of conflict and defense, consistently viewing as transference the patient's interpersonal reach toward the analyst and emphasizing the analyst's neutrality or anonymity. Any needs that the analyst had for the patient were understood as (unwelcome) countertransference. Relational analysts point out (e.g., Greenberg & Mitchell, 1983) that the alliance concept was a beachhead for a relational viewpoint in psychoanalysis, because it at least implicitly acknowledged an ongoing set of interacting reality-based needs between analyst and patient, which required the analyst's attention in their own right, above and beyond analyzing the patient's transference. Once this acknowledgment was fully made, however, analysts believed that the special place Greenson gave the working alliance was no longer relevant—for relational analysts, all analysis is interpersonal work, so the alliance concept was no longer needed (Greenberg & Mitchell, 1983; Safran & Muran, 2000, 2006).

The view held by relational analysts is shared by a number of psychotherapy researchers as well. For example, Henry and Strupp (1994), using a detailed measure of the nature of the relationship in therapy, identified a critical role for hostile therapist responses in reducing (or even preventing) treatment success. They believed that this broad assessment of relationship quality was superior to alliance measures and recommended abandoning the alliance concept. Safran and Muran (2006) make the same point about contemporary psychotherapy that Greenberg and Mitchell (1983) made about psychoanalysis in the 1980s, suggesting that alliance had been important in keeping the relationship in focus at a time when cognitive and behavioral therapies gave it little attention. However, with increasing recognition of the importance of the relationship in contemporary theory and practice, they say, the need for thinking in alliance terms has passed. Safran and Muran (2006) noted that they had earlier stressed that alliance "highlights the fact that at a fundamental level the patient's ability to trust, hope and have faith in the therapist's ability to help always plays a central role in the change process" (Safran & Muran, 2000, p. 13) and that the alliance negotiation process is important to change more generally. But, overall, they feel that the alliance concept is not that useful.

The problem with the relational approach is similar to the problem we found when technique and alliance are equated. Alliance is a way of looking at the relationship, not the relationship itself. Alliance asks, in what way and to what degree does this relationship demonstrate a working collaboration between the patient and the therapist directed toward therapy goals? Or, put another way, alliance is a feature or property of relationship, as characterized by its collaborative effort towards therapy goals. Therapists continually scan the relationship for indicators of their patients' level of collaboration and participation in the ongoing work. A frown at a question, a smile of relief at being understood—anything at all about the relationship might give an indication about the state of the alliance. Of course, the work of therapy is implicit in each of these researchers' clinical theories, and, like all working clinicians, they monitor whether patient and therapist are working together as expected. Thus, cognitive therapists, some of whom see alliance as an epiphenomenon (e.g., DeRubeis et al., 2005), still are actively concerned about engaging and sustaining their patients' participation in the techniques of cognitive therapy. Their focus on technique, like the relationalists' focus on relationships, eclipses the link between collaborative work and outcome, and they lose sight of their ongoing evaluation of the alliance. Along these lines, we can see how Henry and Strupp's (1994) focus on relationship deprives us of an alliance theory account of how therapist hostility leads to a poor outcome. Alliance theory would see therapist hostility as toxic to collaborative work. Therapist hostility undermines the client's collaboration in the work by criticizing the patient's effort to work in therapy. It betrays the therapist's implicit or explicit promise that the therapeutic work will help to open the patient to new positive self-views. It corrodes the levels of trust needed to sustain openness and depletes the client's sense of optimism that good things can result from therapy (Hatcher & Barends, 2006).

ALLIANCE AS A RELATIONSHIP COMPONENT

Some clinicians and researchers divide the relationship between the patient and the therapist into components, with alliance among them. The chief source for this way of thinking is likely Greenson's (1965, 1967) proposal to divide the relationship into the transference, the alliance, and the real relationship. This point of view has been taken up by many authorities, particularly by Gelso and his colleagues (e.g., Gelso & Hayes, 1998). As we have seen above, this stand got Greenson into trouble with his analytic colleagues, who complained that considering any portion of the patient's relationship with the analyst as "not transference" can lead to missing important transferences that are "hiding" behind apparently reasonable behavior. In fact, however, Greenson himself arrived at the working alliance concept as a result of numerous experiences of finding that behavior that appeared at first to be analytically appropriate and cooperative was actually based on strong disruptive transferences, experiences that he described in detail in his writings on the subject (1965, 1967). Rather than taking patient behavior as raw data that can be evaluated from multiple points of view—examined in turn as transference features; as realistic sensible qualities; or as efforts to work analytically with the analyst—Greenson chose to divide up behavior in a way that was unstable from the very start. Efforts to draw these kinds of boundaries within the broad domain of the relationship are doomed to failure because the concepts used to draw the boundaries are not exclusive. If we persist anyway, the lesson from this encounter is parallel to that of the transference noted above; that is, if we restrict the domain of alliance to specific types of actions in or features of the relationship, we lose our grip on the ways that alliance plays out in all aspects of the therapy relationship. Putting it another way, anything that happens in the relationship can be evaluated from the alliance point of view, suggesting such questions as: In what way does this behavior, attitude, etc., indicate the quality of the work in therapy? Does this behavior, attitude, etc., promote or detract from the work?

ALLIANCE AS CURATIVE: RELATIONSHIP IN THERAPY

Bordin's (1979) hypothesis that "the effectiveness of a therapy is a function in part, if not entirely, of the strength of the working alliance" (p. 253) basically claims that therapy will be effective to the extent that the patient and therapist are working collaboratively according to the expectations of the treatment method being employed. It is important to differentiate this idea from the idea that the process of developing, maintaining, and repairing the alliance is helpful in itself. Clinicians and researchers who use the concept "therapeutic alliance," as opposed to "working alliance," tend to mix these ideas. Generally speaking, those who focus on the helpfulness of the alliance also blur the distinction between alliance and the relationship as discussed above. Building an alliance is not the same as the alliance itself, any more than building or maintaining a car is the same as driving a car. This distinction does not mean that building and maintaining an alliance is not helpful. For example, the patient's relationship with an empathic, nonjudgmental, and perhaps affirming therapist can be seen as part of the work-supporting bond to the extent that it in fact supports the work. But the therapist's support can serve as a curative factor in its own right, as has been recognized for many years (Bibring, 1937; Rosenzweig, 1936; Wampold, 2001). The therapist's empathy, affirmation, and nonjudgmentalness can thus be considered to be curative techniques, although they are often seen as "common factors" (e.g., by Rosenzweig and Wampold) rather than theorized as techniques.

Many helpful aspects of the relationship are not well theorized in particular therapies. Some researchers have used the concept of "common factors" to describe these features, and others have simply mystified them as generic interpersonal processes. Both approaches have complicated thinking about alliance theory, because these researchers have identified certain relational activities as the alliance, which is then seen as a common factor or as murky "interpersonal processes" that are curative in their own right. However, there is no logical reason that common factors could not be effectively incorporated into clinical theory, thus shifting these factors from an untheorized state into deliberately applied techniques or evaluative criteria. An example would be therapist empathy, which is widely regarded as a common factor (Wampold, 2001). But empathy can be theorized as a helpful curative technique, applied and modulated responsively in any given case. This approach is one thrust of Safran and Muran's (2000) relational treatment approach. A similar problem is posed by Elvins and Green's (2008) definition of "treatment alliance" as "a summary term referring to a number of interpersonal processes at play in psychological treatment which can generally be considered to act in parallel to (and theoretically independently of) specific manualized treatment techniques" (p. 1168). On the one hand, it is not clear how these authors think that techniques can be theoretically independent of interpersonal processes, since application of technique is an interpersonal process. On the other hand, they equate helpful interpersonal process with the alliance rather than with technique. This muddle can be effectively resolved by recognizing that building, maintaining, and repairing the alliance all involve technical activity, which is separate from evaluating the nature and quality of the work involved.

Closely related to the idea of alliance as helpful in itself is the idea that work on difficulties in the alliance is curative. Proposed in his 1979 article, this idea became an increasing focus for Bordin in his later work (1994) and is the core idea in Safran and Muran's relational treatment approach (2000). Bordin noted that the patient's interpersonal problems often interfere with forming and maintaining the alliance and that the firsthand encounter with these problems in the therapeutic relationship brings these problems to life in a setting uniquely suitable to addressing them. This idea is a theory of therapy that joins the large set of theories of therapy. It is not a theory of alliance. It is basically a modern development of Freud's (1912/1958a) point about transference that has been transformed into the contemporary conceptual frame of relationship issues.

THE THERAPIST'S RELATIONSHIP
TO THE EMBEDDED ALLIANCE

Bordin (1979) pointed out that alliances embedded in a treatment approach make demands on therapists as well as patients. In a given therapy, the therapist works from within this treatment approach, and in that sense the alliance is embedded in the therapist. This situation leads to therapists' enjoying good work and feeling frustrated when the patient resists the treatment. However, therapists struggle to one degree or another with the expectations placed on them by their treatment method. Therapists may not fully embrace the theory or its related techniques. Adherence to the expected work can become difficult for the therapist, for example, when a patient evokes strong personal reactions, as often happens when working with child or spousal abuse cases. More generally, we can consider the therapist's alliance with his or her treatment method, which, like the alliance between patient and therapist, requires a productive collaboration, and is subject to negotiation of a sort, as the therapist shapes the particular demands of the treatment method to his or her own personality and ideas about what is helpful. Adherence and competence could be considered as indicators of this extended view of alliance.

THE PATIENT'S EXPERIENCE OF ALLIANCE

The alliance is built and sustained by ongoing negotiation between patient and therapist. Accordingly, the patient's experience of the alliance, organized into the patient's internal working alliance model, is an important focus for clinicians and researchers alike. Special attention has been paid to the patient's experience of being helped or cared for and of his or her growing trust in the therapist. This experience is emotional, but it is also an appraisal of the intentions of the therapist and of the value of the therapist's method. It is a reaction to the therapist's interest, concern, thoughtfulness, dedication, etc., and to the experienced value of the therapist's efforts to address the patient's problems. Thus the bond is an aspect of an evaluative process, based on the patient's ideas of what therapy should achieve and how the therapist should behave. How does this affect the "embedded alliance," the expectations of the therapist's clinical theory for the work to be done? Depending on the flexibility of the clinical theory and its associated technique, the therapist may be able to incorporate the patient's input as to how the therapy should be conducted into the larger framework of the treatment approach. If, for example, the phobic patient is uncomfortable with the generally expected *in vivo* exposure, imaginal exposure may be brought in as the first task for therapy.

CONCLUSION

For years, therapists and researchers have talked about "the alliance," conveying a sense of its being a demonstrable "thing"—distinct from other components of therapy—like technique or transference. In this chapter, we have worked to establish a clearer understanding of the nature of the alliance, beginning with our everyday clinical experience of the patient's struggle to work with us as we hope and expect, together with our efforts to deal with these struggles with technique. We have argued that alliance is a way of talking about the quality of the collaborative work between patient and therapist. Thus alliance is an evaluative concept that can be and is applied by both patient and therapist to the moment-by-moment interaction in therapy, to a single session, to a week's worth of work, to the therapy as a whole—asking, "How well are we working together toward the goals of therapy?" The cumulative results of this evaluation lead to ongoing, continually updated internal working alliance models held separately by the patient and the therapist. Everything that happens in therapy can affect this cumulative working model, insofar as these things reflect or affect the quality of the work toward the goals of therapy. A good interpretation will contribute positively if the patient finds it helpful; a warm smile will contribute to the patient's evaluation of the quality of the work together. Thus good technique promotes good alliance. It may be that specific efforts to address the patient's internal working alliance model will be beneficial through, for example, explaining how a technique can be helpful or reassuring the patient of our respect. But it is most likely that good technique, technique that engages the patient in work that feels meaningful and goal-directed, is the best promoter of good alliance. Such technique includes that designed to address problems in the patient's efforts to work with us. We have discussed how alliance is not the same thing as the relationship. Rather, it is a way of looking at the relationship through the lens of effective goal-directed work. So we ask, does this or that element of the relationship promote and reflect good, collaborative work, or does it detract from it?

Measurement of the patient's and the therapist's perception of the quality of the work can be accomplished with current alliance measures and can be helpful to the treatment by identifying areas of strain and disagreement about the therapeutic work. Further advances in measurement and theory may come through identifying more specific kinds of work that are critical to good outcomes in specific types of therapies (e.g., concrete examples in cognitive therapy for depression) and assessing whether the patient and therapist are working well together in these specific areas. It may also prove useful to examine the patient's internal working alliance model more extensively—how these are formed, what it consists in for the given patient, and how best to modify or influence it, beyond simply doing good therapeutic work with the person.

REFERENCES

Alexander, L. B., & Luborsky, L. (1986). The Penn Helping Alliance Scales. In L. S. Greenberg & W. M. Pinsof (Eds.), *The psychotherapeutic process: A research handbook* (pp. 325–366). New York: Guilford Press.

Bedi, R. P., Davis, M. D., & Williams, M. (2005). Critical incidents in the formation of the therapeutic alliance from the client's perspective. *Psychotherapy: Theory, Research, Practice, Training, 42,* 311–323.

Bibring, E. (1937). Symposium on the theory of the therapeutic results of psycho-analysis. *International Journal of Psychoanalysis, 18,* 125–189.

Bordin, E. S. (1979). The generalizability of the psychoanalytic concept of the working alliance. *Psychotherapy: Theory, Research, and Practice, 16,* 252–260.

Bordin, E. S. (1980, June). *Of human bonds that bind or free.* Presidential address to 10th annual meeting of the Society for Psychotherapy Research, Pacific Grove, CA.

Bordin, E. S. (1994). Theory and research on the therapeutic working alliance: New directions. In A. O. Horvath & L. S. Greenberg (Eds.), *The working alliance: Theory, research and practice* (pp. 13–37). New York: Wiley.

Brenner, C. (1979). Working alliance, therapeutic alliance, and transference. *Journal of the American Psychoanalytic Association, 27S,* 137–157.

Brotman, M. A. (2004). Therapeutic alliance and adherence in cognitive therapy for depression. *Dissertation Abstracts International, 65*(3146), 6B. (UMI No. 3169565)

Crits-Christoph, P., Connolly Gibbons, M. B., Crits-Christoph, K., Narducci, J., Schamberger, M., & Gallop, R. (2006). Can therapists be trained to improve their alliances?: A preliminary study of alliance-fostering psychotherapy. *Psychotherapy Research, 16,* 268–281.

DeRubeis, R. J., Brotman, M. A., & Gibbons, C. J. (2005). A conceptual and methodological analysis of the nonspecifics argument. *Clinical Psychology: Science and Practice, 12,* 174–183.

Elvins, R., & Green, J. (2008). The conceptualization and measurement of therapeutic alliance: An empirical review. *Clinical Psychology Review, 28,* 1167–1187.

Freud, S. (1957). 'Wild' psycho-analysis. In J. Strachey (Ed. & Trans.), *The standard edition of the complete psychological works of Sigmund Freud* (Vol. 11, pp. 219–228). London: Hogarth Press. (Original work published 1910)

Freud, S. (1958a). The dynamics of transference. In J. Strachey (Ed. & Trans.), *The standard edition of the complete psychological works of Sigmund Freud* (Vol. 12, pp. 99–108). London: Hogarth Press. (Original work published 1912)

Freud, S. (1958b). Further recommendations on the technique of psychoanalysis: On beginning the treatment. In J. Strachey (Ed. & Trans.), *The standard edition of the complete psychological works of Sigmund Freud* (Vol. 12, pp. 122–144). London: Hogarth Press. (Original work published 1913)

Freud, S. (1964). Analysis terminable and interminable. In J. Strachey (Ed. & Trans.), *The standard edition of the complete psychological works of Sigmund Freud* (Vol. 23, pp. 209–254). London: Hogarth Press. (Original work published 1937)

Gaston, L., & Marmar, C. (1994). The California Psychotherapy Alliance Scales. In A. O. Horvath & L. S. Greenberg (Eds.), *The working alliance: Theory, research and practice* (pp. 85–108). New York: Wiley.

Gelso, C. J., & Hayes, J. A. (1998). *The psychotherapy relationship: Theory, research, and practice.* Hoboken, NJ: Wiley.

Gill, M. M. (1982). *Analysis of transference: Vol. 1. Theory and technique.* New York: International Universities Press.

Goldfried, M. R., & Davila, J. (2005). The role of relationship and technique in therapeutic change. *Psychotherapy: Theory, Research, Practice, 42,* 421–430.

Greenberg, J. R., & Mitchell, S. A. (1983). *Object relations in psychoanalytic theory.* Cambridge, MA: Harvard University Press.

Greenson, R. R. (1965). The working alliance and the transference neurosis. In Greenson, *Explorations in psychoanalysis* (pp. 199–224). New York: International Universities Press.

Greenson, R. R. (1967). *The technique and practice of psychoanalysis.* New York: International Universities Press.

Harmon, S. C., Lambert, M. J., Smart, D. M., Hawkins, E., Nielsen, S. L., Slade, K., et al. (2007). Enhancing outcome for potential treatment failures: Therapist–client feedback and clinical support tools. *Psychotherapy Research, 17,* 379–392

Hartley, D. E., & Strupp, H. H. (1983). The therapeutic alliance: Its relationship to outcome in brief psychotherapy. In J. Masling (Ed.), *Empirical studies of psychoanalytical theories* (Vol. 1, pp. 1–37). Hillsdale, NJ: Erlbaum.

Hatcher, R. L., & Barends, A. W. (1996). Patients' view of the alliance in psychotherapy: Exploratory factor analysis of three alliance measures. *Journal of Consulting and Clinical Psychology, 64,* 1326–1336.

Hatcher, R. L., & Barends, A. W. (2006). How a return to theory could help alliance research. *Psychotherapy: Theory, Research, and Practice, 43,* 292–299.

Hatcher, R. L., & Gillaspy, J. A. (2006). Development and validation of a revised short version of the Working Alliance Inventory. *Psychotherapy Research, 16,* 12–25.

Henry, W. P., & Strupp, H. H. (1994). The therapeutic alliance as interpersonal process. In A. O. Horvath & L. S. Greenberg, (Eds.), *The working alliance: Theory, research and practice* (pp. 51–84). New York: Wiley.

Horvath, A. O., & Greenberg, L. S. (1989). Development and validation of the Working Alliance Inventory. *Journal of Counseling Psychology, 36,* 223–233.

Howard, K. I., Lueger, R. J., Maling, M. S., & Martinovich, Z. (1993). A phase model of psychotherapy outcome: Causal mediation of change. *Journal of Consulting and Clinical Psychology, 61,* 678–685.

Leahy, R. L. (2001). *Overcoming resistance in cognitive therapy.* New York: Guilford Press.

Martin, D. J., Garske, J. P., & Davis, M. K. (2000). Relation of the therapeutic alliance with outcome and other variables: A meta-analytic review. *Journal of Consulting and Clinical Psychology, 68,* 438–450.

Patterson, G. R., & Forgatch, M. S. (1985). Therapist behavior as a determinant for client noncompliance: A paradox for the behavior modifier. *Journal of Consulting and Clinical Psychology, 53,* 846–851.

Rogers, C. R. (1957). The necessary and sufficient conditions of therapeutic personality change. *Journal of Consulting and Clinical Psychology, 22,* 95–103.

Rosenzweig, S. (1936). Some implicit common factors in diverse methods of psychotherapy. *American Journal of Orthopsychiatry, 6,* 412–415.

Safran, J. D., & Muran, J. C. (2000). *Negotiating the therapeutic alliance: A relational treatment guide.* New York: Guilford Press.

Safran, J. D., & Muran, J. C. (2006). Has the concept of the therapeutic alliance outlived its usefulness? *Psychotherapy: Theory, Research, Practice, Training, 43,* 286–291.

Safran, J., & Segal, Z. (1990). *Interpersonal process in cognitive therapy.* Lanham, MD: Aronson.

Shelef, K., & Diamond, G. M. (2008). Short form of the revised Vanderbilt Therapeutic Alliance Scale: Development, reliability, and validity. *Psychotherapy Research, 18,* 433–443.

Sterba, R. F. (1934) The fate of the ego in analytic therapy *International Journal of Psychoanalysis, 15,* 117–126.

Stiles, W. B., Honos-Webb, L., & Surko, M. (1998). Responsiveness in psychotherapy. *Clinical Psychology: Science and Practice, 5,* 439–458.

Summers, R. F., & Barber, J. P. (2003). Therapeutic alliance as a measurable psychotherapy skill. *Academic Psychiatry, 27,* 160–165.

Wampold, B. (2001). *The great psychotherapy debate.* Mahwah, NJ: Erlbaum.

CHAPTER 2

■ ■ ■ ■ ■

The Validity of the Alliance as a Predictor of Psychotherapy Outcome

Jacques P. Barber
Shabad-Ratan Khalsa
Brian A. Sharpless

The therapeutic alliance is considered an essential aspect of psychotherapy by many scholars (e.g., Norcross, 2002). Therefore, it is perhaps not surprising that the alliance is also one of the most commonly studied psychotherapy constructs. While other sections of this volume address the history, definition, and core components of the alliance, this chapter specifically focuses on the role of the alliance as a predictive variable for psychotherapy outcome.

It is commonly asserted in the psychotherapy literature that the alliance predicts outcome (Martin, Garske, & Davis, 2000). Indeed, a fairly recent meta-analysis of this topic (which included 79 studies) found that the average correlation between alliance and outcome is approximately .22 (Martin et al., 2000). Although it is widely assumed that a strong therapeutic alliance *predicts* subsequent improvement (and, in fact, this is how the alliance is most commonly studied), one goal of this chapter is to evaluate the adequacy of the data that underlie this assertion. Like some other previous authors (e.g., Barber, Crits-Christoph, & Luborsky, 1996; DeRubeis, Brotman, & Gibbons, 2005; DeRubeis & Feeley, 1990; Gaston, Marmar,

Gallagher, & Thompson, 1991), we are concerned that many studies do not adequately address the *temporal* relation of alliance and symptom reduction when the alliance is being studied as a predictive variable.

A second goal relates to the nature of the alliance itself. Given that the alliance arises within the context of a therapeutic encounter during which two (or more) individuals with a host of idiosyncratic life experiences, worldviews, and expectations are brought together, the alliance can be conceptualized in several ways. This "emergent" property of the alliance (Boswell et al., 2011), for lack of a better term, allows it to be viewed in several different ways familiar to psychotherapy researchers. Therefore, along with discussing the alliance as a more general predictor of outcome, we will also assess and explore the possibilities for conceptualizing the alliance in more specific terms (i.e., as a moderator and mediator of outcome, as an interaction with treatment techniques, and as an outcome variable in and of itself). We believe that an evaluation of the alliance in these several contexts is instructive and may points to ways in which alliance research may become more rigorous.

THE ALLIANCE AS A PREDICTOR OF OUTCOME

Many terms have been used in the literature to describe the predictive relation between variables of importance and therapy outcome. The term "predictors of outcome" is the most general of these terms, and in fact the alliance is most commonly referred to and assessed in this light. When the literature on prediction is reviewed, we find that some studies used outcome predictors assessed before treatment began whereas others used those assessed during treatment, primarily during the early phase (Barber, 2007). Given that many researchers would argue that the alliance is a variable that can emerge only once treatment has started, it is not generally assessed before treatment begins (see Iacoviello et al., 2007, for an exception to this rule). Thus, most of the literature on the relation between alliance and outcome is based upon the assessment of the alliance at early points in treatment (usually at Sessions 2, 5, or 10). However, as pointed out by DeRubeis et al. (2005), outcome is often assessed as a change in symptoms from pretreatment to posttreatment. Any use of the term "predictive" to describe the relation between alliance and outcome should require that the alliance actually predict the change that occurs *subsequent to its measurement only* (e.g., DeRubeis & Feeley, 1990; Kazdin, 2008a, 2008b). We therefore question the assertions of many authors who report finding that alliance predicts outcome, as they have typically not excluded changes that occurred *prior to* measurement of the alliance. We also question the nature of the conclusions one can draw from meta-analyses based upon such studies. In fact, when one considers only results from studies that have examined the temporal relation between the alliance and outcome (as will be discussed and enumerated below), we find that there are very few such studies and that their results are not necessarily what one would expect (e.g., Barber, 2009).

By failing to take the symptom change that occurs prior to the alliance's measurement into account, the possibility that the alliance could actually be a *product* of prior symptomatic change remains unaddressed. In fact, several studies have indeed demonstrated that the level of early alliance can be the product of previous symptomatic changes (e.g., Barber, Connolly, Crits-Christoph, Gladis, & Siqueland, 2000; DeRubeis & Feeley, 1990). We will now briefly review those studies that have more precisely considered the temporal sequences of symptomatic change when assessing the relation between alliance and outcome.

DeRubeis and Feeley (1990) were perhaps the first to carefully examine the temporal relation between alliance and symptom change. Data were drawn from a sample of 25 depressed patients with Beck Depression Inventory (BDI) scores greater than 20 who received cognitive therapy. They found that symptom change prior to measurement of the alliance predicted level of alliance but that alliance itself did not predict subsequent symptom change. In a replication of that study, Feeley, DeRubeis, and Gelfand (1999) also found that alliance did not predict subsequent symptom change (n = 32). However, unlike their prior findings, prior symptom change did not significantly predict alliance (although a trend in that direction was found).

In a sample of depressed older adults, Gaston and colleagues (1991) explored the association of alliance and outcome (measured as changes in BDI scores) while controlling for symptomatic change occurring prior to the measurement of the alliance. A good deal of subsequent outcome variance was explained by alliance scores measured at Sessions 5, 10, or 15 when controlling for symptomatic change in the three therapy conditions (behavioral, cognitive, and brief dynamic psychotherapy). However, only in the behavior therapy condition (with alliance measured at Session 15) was there a significant relation between alliance and subsequent change in outcome when partialling out prior symptomatic change (55% of variance explained, $p < .05$). The authors caution that they were hindered by small sample size, but this study provides limited support for the predictive value of alliance in predicting subsequent change in symptom. It is also important to note that the authors were not able to show that early treatment alliance predicted subsequent change in symptoms.

Barber et al. (1999) discerned that patients' reports of the alliance predicted decreased drug use at month 1 but not at month 6 during the pilot phase (n = 252) of the National Institute on Drug Abuse Cocaine Collaborative Treatment Study (CCTS; Crits-Christoph et al., 1999). Partialling out prior symptomatic improvement as measured by the change in drug use from

Session 1 to Session 5 (the timepoint when the alliance was assessed), Barber et al. (1999) found that the partial correlation between patients' Helping Alliance Questionnaire–II (HAq-II; Luborsky et al., 1996) and residualized outcome at month 1 was barely significant ($pr = -.23$, $p = .06$). The authors tentatively concluded that the alliance's relation to outcome at month 1 was not attributable to early symptomatic change.

Barber et al. (2001) later looked at randomized clinical trial data from the CCTS and found that symptom change (which was always measured subsequent to the alliance) was not predicted by the therapeutic alliance. In addition, alliance differentially predicted retention in different treatments within these cocaine-dependent patients.

In order to examine the potential causal role of the alliance in a more "neurotic" population, Barber et al. (2000) pooled data from four psychotherapy outcome pilot studies conducted at the University of Pennsylvania's Center for Psychotherapy Research (total patient $n = 88$). Eleven of these patients either had major depressive disorder or dysthymic disorder and major depressive disorder for 2 years; 44 had diagnoses of generalized anxiety disorder; 19 had avoidant personality disorder, and 14 had obsessive–compulsive personality disorder. It was found that early symptom change predicted alliance level at Session 5 and that alliance measured at this same time point predicted subsequent changes in depressive symptoms to the end of treatment. Furthermore, the alliance at Session 5 predicted subsequent change in depressive symptoms even after partialling out the impact of early (i.e., prior to Session 5) symptom change on the alliance. Thus, the level of early symptom reduction did in fact predict alliance levels, and the alliance remained a significant predictor (or inducer) of subsequent symptom change.

Klein et al. (2003) also found that alliance predicted subsequent change in 341 chronically depressed patients receiving cognitive-behavioral analysis system of psychotherapy. Consonant with the findings of Barber et al. (2000), Klein and colleagues (2003) found that alliance measured on a shortened version of the Working Alliance Inventory (WAI; Horvath & Greenberg, 1989) predicted subsequent change on the clinician-rated depression measure between weeks 3 and 12. Furthermore, these authors found that early alliance predicted subsequent change in depressive symptoms even after controlling for prior levels of depression, concurrent levels of depression, and a variety of important demographic and psychiatric variables (e.g., gender, personality disorder, history of abuse).

These studies represent an initial excursion into this question, but additional data are required with larger samples, alternative therapeutic modalities, and different populations in order to increase confidence that the alliance possesses a robust (and significant) causal role in psychotherapy outcome. In Table 2.1 (which has been adapted from Strunk, Brotman,

TABLE 2.1. Predicting Outcome from Alliance, Taking into Account the Temporal Sequence

Study	n	Correlation (r)	Significant?
DeRubeis & Feeley (1990)	25	.10	No
Feeley, DeRubeis, & Gelfand (1999)	25	−.27	No
Barber, Luborsky, Crits-Christoph, Thase, Weiss, et al. (1999)	252	.01[a]	No
Barber, Connolly, Crits-Christoph, Gladis, Weiss, et al. (2000)	88	.30[a]	Yes
Barber, Luborsky, Gallop, Crits-Christoph, Weiss, et al. (2001)	291	.01[a]	No
Klein, Schwartz, Santiago, Vivian, Vocisano, et al. (2003)	367	.14	Yes
Strunk, Brotman, & DeRubeis (2008)	60	.15	No

Note. From Barber (2009; adapted from Strunk, Brotman, & DeRubeis, 2008). Copyright 2009 by Taylor & Francis Group. Reprinted with permission. Available at *www.informaworld.com.*

[a]The correlation was the average of more than one correlation.

& DeRubeis, 2008, and published in Barber, 2009), we summarize all the results from the studies reviewed earlier. As can be clearly seen, only two studies (Barber et al., 2000; Klein et al., 2003) found that the alliance significantly predicted subsequent change in symptoms, and it is important to note that this correlation was relatively small. Gaston et al.'s (1991) and Barber et al.'s (1999) data are consistent with this conclusion, but their findings were not significant.

THE ALLIANCE AS A MODERATOR OF OUTCOME

Although most studies have examined the role of the alliance as a *predictor* of outcome, we decided to review the literature on whether alliance has been used as a *moderator* of outcome. Moderators of outcome are a more specific subcategory of predictors and are typically thought of as variables that specify the type of patient for whom a treatment works and/or under which particular conditions a treatment works (e.g., Baron & Kenny, 1986; Kraemer, Wilson, Fairburn, & Agras, 2002). Moderators can be either qualitative (e.g., race, sex, marital status) or quantitative (an agonistic medication dosage) and serve as third variables that affect the strength of the relation between the particular treatment and the outcome. Kraemer et al. (2002) assert that all moderating variables must precede treatment. If one accepts this definitional requirement, then in most assessments of the alliance it clearly cannot be considered a moderator. Using Baron and Kenny's (1986) somewhat less restrictive description of moderation (which only requires that the effect of treatment on outcome be affected by a third variable), one could argue that there are examples of alliance being assessed as a moderator.

For example, Caroll, Nich, and Rounsaville (1997) assessed the level of therapeutic alliance and outcome with regard to both an active (cognitive-behavioral treatment) and a control (clinical management) treatment. Although alliance scores were higher in the active condition, the therapeutic alliance was significantly associated with outcome only for the control condition. Thus, one could perhaps say that in this particular case therapeutic alliance moderated the relation between treatment condition and outcome.

One may also consider the findings from Blatt, Zuroff, Quinlan, and Pilkonis (1996, using data from the Treatment of Depression Collaborative Research Program [TDCRP]; Elkin et al., 1989) as indicating a moderating effect of the therapeutic alliance on the relation between low, medium, and high levels of perfectionism on therapy outcome. Results indicated that the alliance was not significantly related to outcome at either low or high levels of perfectionism but was significantly related to outcome in patients with medium levels of perfectionism (interestingly, as will be discussed later in this chapter, this relation between perfectionism and outcome was also shown to be mediated by alliance).

In the field of family therapy, Johnson and Ketring (2006) reported that alliance as measured very late in therapy did not moderate the relation between intake symptom severity and family therapy outcome. This last study also raises the question of what happens when alliance is not measured at intake or early during treatment.

Finally, as mentioned previously, Barber et al. (2001) reported that the therapeutic alliance predicted differential retention in supportive–expressive (SE) therapy, cognitive therapy, and individual drug counseling (IDC) for cocaine dependence. In cognitive therapy, higher alliance as measured by the HAq-II at Session 2 predicted shorter time in treatment, whereas a higher alliance in individual drug counseling was associated with greater retention. Alliance at Session 2 was not associated with retention in supportive–expressive therapy. At Session 5, alliance predicted lower retention for cognitive therapy, but greater retention in SE but did not predict retention in IDC. Using the CALPAS, this same relationship was found at Session 5. Alliance did not predict outcome differentially among treatments, but this study provides some initial evidence that alliance may have a differential impact on various treatments.

The study of alliance as a moderating variable is fairly limited. Moderators of treatment outcome are typically studied in psychotherapy research by assessing the impact of a moderator (in this case, the alliance) on one or more treatment groups and then by examining the moderator–treatment group interaction on outcome. Therefore, if researchers only examine the predictive power of a variable across groups (i.e., main effects) without examining the interaction of the predictor with treatment, general predictors of outcome are being studied instead of moderation. Considering the emergent nature of the alliance and the fact that the alliance is almost never measured at the same time as the treatment (or other predictor) variable, it is perhaps not surprising that studying the alliance as a moderator is not a simple task. Because alliance is not assessed at intake (as required by Kraemer et al., 2002) or is rarely assessed at the same time as other predictors, the study of the alliance as a moderator variable is not likely to become popular. However, if researchers follow our recommendation to study the impact of alliance on subsequent change in outcome, then there may be room for studying the moderating role of alliance. Moderation of subsequent change allows for the development of the alliance and for its assessment before outcome is evaluated.

THE ALLIANCE AS MEDIATOR OF OUTCOME

Since alliance is often considered a mechanism of change (Bordin, 1979; Frieswyk et al., 1986), it makes sense to examine whether the alliance has been studied as a potential mediator of outcome. Again, as in the case with moderation, mediation is a more specific type of prediction with a more specific relation to outcome. By definition, mediators of change are third variables through which a treatment may achieve its effect on the target of change (i.e., a dependent variable such as a symptom measure or diagnostic category). Mediators are conceptualized as causal links between particular treatments and outcome, and they further demonstrate how and why a treatment works (Baron & Kenny, 1986; Kraemer et al., 2002).

If the alliance is in fact a mediator of change, it would presumably emerge or increase through specific therapeutic interventions, and this emergence or increase would correspond to positive changes in outcome variables of interest. And, indeed, many scholars have posited that alliance is an active ingredient in therapy, meaning it is therapeutic in and of itself and accounts for at least a part of the improvement that patients experience (e.g., Castonguay, Constantino, & Grosse Holtforth, 2006).

As one example in which the alliance was examined as a potential mediator of outcome, Zuroff et al. (2000) examined the relation between perfectionism, increase in the therapeutic alliance, and outcome using the

TDCRP data set. Using guidelines established by Baron and Kenny (1986), the authors tested a mediational model (i.e., that the relationship between perfectionism and outcome was mediated by increases in patient alliance). In order to test this, it was first established that perfectionism was related to outcome and then that perfectionism was negatively correlated with an increase in alliance. When increase in alliance was entered into the model, the effect of perfectionism on outcome was weakened. In other words, perfectionism in an unmediated model predicted 9% of outcome variance, but when alliance was added to the model as a mediator, the amount of variance explained by perfectionism was reduced to 4%. This decrease in variance explained by perfectionism supports the mediational role of the alliance in this study.

Several groups of researchers have also examined alliance as a mediator of the effect of patients' expectancies on outcome. Joyce, Ogrodniczuk, Piper, and McCallum (2003) found that pretreatment expectancies were associated with outcome and that this relation was mediated by the therapeutic alliance (as rated by the patient or therapist). In this study, ratings of the alliance were obtained after each of the 20 sessions and were subsequently averaged across these 20 scores for the mediational analysis. Using data from the TDCRP, Meyer et al. (2002) also found that the effect of patient (but not therapist) expectancies for improvement on outcome was mediated by alliance (as rated by independent observers). They showed that this effect did not differ across the TDCRP treatments. Meyer and colleagues also assessed whether an overall alliance score (measured early, midway, and late in treatment) moderated expectancies' effect on outcome. The moderation hypothesis that alliance would be related to improvement in patients with positive expectancies, but not for those with negative expectancies, was not supported in this study.

In summary, these studies of the alliance as a mediator are interesting and evocative, but more research is clearly required. We would also recommend that research on the alliance as a mediator take into consideration the temporal sequence of relevant factors (e.g., the alliance, prior change in symptoms, and subsequent change in symptoms; Castonguay et al., 2006).

THE THERAPEUTIC ALLIANCE INTERACTING WITH INTERVENTIONS IN PREDICTING OUTCOME

Until this point we have reviewed how the alliance predicts or even perhaps mediates outcome. In recent years, however, some researchers have begun to investigate the role of the alliance and its relation to therapy interventions in predicting outcome. It is quite obvious that the therapeutic relationship and techniques are intertwined and indeed work together. Surprisingly, there has been relatively little empirical work in this area (for exceptions see Crits-Christoph & Connolly, 1999; Gaston, Piper, Debbane, & Garant, 1994; Gaston, Thompson, Gallagher, Cournoyer, & Gagnon, 1998).

Gaston et al. (1994) evaluated the impact of alliance and technique and their interaction on outcome and assessed whether this impact may differ in short- and long-term analytic therapy. Alliance was measured after 5, 10, and 15 weeks in short-term therapy and after 5 weeks, 12 months, and 22 months in long-term therapy. Using a sample of 17 patients receiving short-term psychotherapy and 15 patients receiving long-term psychotherapy, the investigators found that the interaction between alliance and technique differentially predicted outcome between therapies. Unfortunately, measurement of both the alliance and techniques was averaged across three phases of therapy, a decision that increased the reliability of these measurements but weakened the logic of the design. In short-term psychotherapy, 15% of the variance in outcome (measured as interpersonal problems) was explained by the interaction between alliance and exploratory techniques; however, this finding was not significant. In long-term psychotherapy, both supportive and exploratory therapist techniques interacted significantly with alliance to predict outcome. Further analyses indicated that supportive interventions were more helpful for patients with low levels of alliance, while exploratory interventions were more effective for patients with high levels. While this study is a valuable exploratory examination of the differential impact of alliance on outcome among therapies, the researchers unfortunately did not control for change that occurred prior to measurement of the therapeutic alliance. Thus, one must exercise caution in drawing any conclusions about alliance as a predictor of outcome from this study.

In another examination of the interaction of technique, alliance, and outcome, Barber et al. (2006) examined the interaction of alliance and quadratic ("U"-shaped) adherence in the individual drug counseling condition of the Treatment for Cocaine Dependence Study (Crits-Christoph et al., 1999). It was found that alliance did indeed interact with quadratic adherence to predict outcome (d = .44; Barber, 2009). Specifically, patients who had low alliance with their therapists and received moderate levels of therapist adherence had a better outcome, whereas those patients with a high alliance demonstrated a weaker relationship between adherence and outcome. In other words, for patients with low alliance, adherence to the IDC model was necessary for their improvement, while for patients with high alliance improvement was not so dependent on the counselor's adherence. While Gaston et al. (1994) had previously examined the interactions among alliance, technique, and outcome, this was the first study that did so while controlling for symptom change occurring prior to measurement of the alliance.

THE ALLIANCE AS THERAPY OUTCOME

So far we have discussed the alliance as a process variable; however, for the sake of thoroughness, it is also important to consider that alliance could be an outcome of therapy in its own right. The alliance can be viewed as an outcome in at least three ways. First, although we are not aware of many examples of this use in the literature, the achievement of a good therapeutic alliance can be a self-contained treatment goal. A strong therapeutic alliance may be an appropriate therapeutic outcome for certain types of patients (e.g., a patient with borderline personality disorder or a patient with profound levels of trauma who experiences difficulties trusting or working with others). Masterson (1978) suggested that "in psychotherapy with the borderline patient the therapeutic alliance is a goal or objective rather than a precondition" (p. 437). Although this view has not been widely implemented in the clinical literatures, establishing a good therapeutic relationship seems to be an important (and perhaps essential) goal for patients with certain psychological conditions.

Second, we could easily envision research studies where the alliance is utilized as the main variable of interest (e.g., a prediction study of factors leading to a strong therapeutic alliance). As the alliance has been repeatedly shown to be associated with outcome, an understanding of patient and therapist behaviors and characteristics leading to its development could prove useful. Studies have shown that therapist attributes like flexibility (Kivlighan, Clements, Blake, Arnzen, & Brady, 1993), experience (Hersoug, Høglend, Monsen, & Havik, 2001; Mallinckrodt & Nelson, 1991), and accurate interpretations (Crits-Christoph, Barber, & Kurcias, 1993) are associated with a stronger alliance (for a more extensive review of therapist characteristics and behaviors that contribute to the therapeutic alliance, see Ackerman and Hilsenroth [2003]). Additional knowledge about relevant patient and therapist factors could potentially yield clinically useful findings.

Third, because alliance is such an important construct, researchers such as Crits-Christoph, Connolly Gibbons, Crits-Christoph, Narducci, Schamberger, and Gallop (2006) have studied whether therapists' ability to develop better alliances with their patients can be significantly enhanced through specialized training (see Crits-Christoph, Crits-Christoph, & Connelly Gibbons, Chapter 15, this volume). This objective entails obvious clinical implications regardless of the nature of the alliance's relation to outcome, as few would argue that a strong therapeutic alliance is not beneficial to treatment. Crits-Christoph et al.'s (2006) initial excursion into alliance-fostering psychotherapy indicated that moderate to large improvements from pre- to posttraining on alliance occurred. These results, however, were not statistically significant, possibly as a result of the small sample size. Given this possibility for useful instruction, alliance training could be incorporated into the educational programs of novice psychologists and psychiatric residents (e.g., Summers & Barber, 2003). In summary, our review indicates that there are good reasons to view alliance as also an outcome variable in specialized cases.

CONCLUSION

It appears that the alliance is best investigated as a general predictor of outcome and as a potential mediator of outcome. The impact of the alliance on outcome should be studied carefully while taking the temporality of the assessed constructs into account. Specifically, when utilizing alliance as a predictor, researchers must attend to the levels of symptom change prior to and subsequent to the measurement of the strength of alliance (e.g., Kazdin, 2008b). Research that has carefully tracked measurement of the alliance and outcome temporally appears to report that the association between the two is not as robust as one might infer from the recent meta-analyses (e.g., Martin et al., 2000). In fact, there is scant evidence that the therapeutic alliance actually causes further improvement in symptoms. Whether this finding reflects the fact that some of the studies that have examined the temporal relationship between alliance and outcome, such as DeRubeis and Feeley (1990) and Feeley et al. (1999), were examining cognitive therapy rather than a more interpersonally focused therapy such as supportive–expressive is somewhat unclear. The possible implications of assessing these relationships across a variety of patient populations are also presently unclear (e.g., Castonguay et al., 2006). Possibly the lack of findings reported by Barber et al. (1999, 2001) is attributable to their having been derived only from a sample of cocaine-dependent patients—for whom the impact of the alliance may be far different than for patients with depression, for example.

On the positive side, considering that the studies from our group and Klein et al. (2003) (using a group of "neurotic" patients) were based on therapies possessing a strong interpersonal focus (e.g., supportive–expressive therapy and CBASP), one could speculate that the alliance may have more of a causal role in these types of therapies conducted with these types of patients. This line of research also merits further exploration.

If alliance is not causally related to outcome, perhaps it could be associated with good outcome in the sense that if the alliance is high, then the therapy is going well. In fact, supervisors often tell their therapist trainees that if their alliance is not going well it will be difficult to conduct effective therapy, as this likely indicates that something may be wrong with the treatment (e.g., Sharpless and Barber [2009] argue for its use as a negative clinical benchmark). If the alliance is going well, the prognosis for the outcome is not altogether clear, but a strong alliance is usually considered to be a positive indicator of the ultimate outcome.

In closing, one of the big questions for our field is whether or not the alliance is a mechanism of change. The data on this issue are seemingly equivocal. It is possible that it is a mechanism of change in supportive–expressive therapy (Barber et al., 2000) and perhaps in cognitive-behavioral analysis system of psychotherapy (Klein et al., 2003). However, the specific ways in which having a good alliance is positively associated with good outcome remain elusive. To put it another way, demonstrating that a good alliance mediates a particular psychotherapy's impact on depressive symptoms does not help us understand how the alliance made the depressed patients feel better. Hill and Knox (2009) have begun to address this question through the use of empirical data. It is possible that examining the relative role of the patient or therapist to the development of the alliance and to its association with outcome will help clarify these complex processes. Early results from Baldwin, Wampold, and Imel (2007) suggested that therapist variance was associated with outcome. However, Barber (2009) reported that most of the variance relating to the impact of the interaction between quadratic adherence and alliance on outcome was attributable to patient variance within each therapist rather than to therapist variance alone.

In summary, there are many interesting questions waiting to be answered in the research area of the therapeutic alliance, and there are even new methodologies that may prove to be quite valuable in eliciting the answers.

ACKNOWLEDGMENT

This chapter was written with support from National Institute of Mental Health Grant No. MH 070664.

REFERENCES

Ackerman, S. J., & Hilsenroth, M. J. (2003). A review of therapist characteristics and techniques positively impacting the therapeutic alliance. *Clinical Psychology Review, 23*, 1–33.

Baldwin, S. A., Wampold, B. E., & Imel, Z. E. (2007). Untangling the alliance outcome correlation: Exploring the relative importance of therapist and patient variability in the alliance. *Journal of Consulting and Clinical Psychology, 75*, 842–852.

Barber, J. P. (2007). Issues and findings in investigating predictors of psychotherapy outcome: Introduction to the special section. *Psychotherapy Research, 17*, 131–136.

Barber, J. P. (2009). Toward a working through of some core conflicts in psychotherapy research. *Psychotherapy Research, 19*(1), 1–12.

Barber, J. P., Connolly, M. B., Crits-Christoph, P., Gladis, M., & Siqueland, L. (2000). Alliance predicts patients' outcome beyond in-treatment change in symptoms. *Journal of Consulting and Clinical Psychology, 68,* 1027–1032.

Barber, J. P., Gallop, R., Crits-Christoph, P., Frank, A., Thase, M. E., Weiss, R. D., et al. (2006). The role of therapist adherence, therapist competence, and the alliance in predicting outcome of individual drug counseling: Results from the NIDA Collaborative Cocaine Treatment Study. *Psychotherapy Research, 16,* 229–240.

Barber, J. P., Luborsky, L., Crits-Christoph, P., Thase, M. E., Weiss, R., Frank, A., et al. (1999). Therapeutic alliance as a predictor of outcome in treatment of cocaine dependence. *Psychotherapy Research, 9*(1), 54–73.

Barber, J. P., Luborsky, L., Gallop, R., Crits-Christoph, P., Weiss, R. D., Thase, M. E., et al. (2001). Therapeutic alliance as a predictor of outcome and retention in the National Institute on Drug Abuse Collaborative Cocaine Treatment Study. *Journal of Consulting and Clinical Psychology, 69,* 119–124.

Baron, R. M., & Kenny, D. A. (1986). The moderator–mediator variable distinction in social psychological research: Conceptual, strategic, and statistical considerations. *Journal of Personality and Social Psychology, 51,* 1173–1182.

Blatt, S. J., Zuroff, D. C., Quinlan, D. M., & Pilkonis, P. A. (1996). Interpersonal factors in brief treatment of depression: Further analyses of the National Institute of Mental Health Treatment of Depression Collaborative Research Program. *Journal of Consulting and Clinical Psychology, 64,* 162–171.

Bordin, E. S. (1979). The generalizability of the psychoanalytic concept of the working alliance. *Psychotherapy: Theory, Research, and Practice, 16,* 252–260.

Boswell, J. F., Sharpless, B. A., Greenberg, L. G., Heatherington, L., Huppert, J. D., Barber, J. P., et al. (2011). Schools of psychotherapy and the beginnings of a scientific approach. In D. H. Barlow (Ed.), *Oxford handbook of clinical psychology.* New York: Oxford University Press.

Caroll, K. M., Nich, C., & Rounsaville, B. J. (1997). Contribution of the therapeutic alliance to outcome in active versus control psychotherapies. *Journal of Consulting and Clinical Psychology, 65,* 510–514.

Castonguay, L. G., Constantino, M. J., & Grosse Holtforth, M. (2006). The working alliance: Where are we and where should we go? *Psychotherapy: Theory, Research, Practice, and Training, 43,* 271–279.

Crits-Christoph, P., Barber, J. P., & Kurcias, J. S. (1993). The accuracy of therapists' interpretations and the development of the therapeutic alliance. *Psychotherapy Research, 3,* 25–35.

Crits-Christoph, P., & Connolly, M. B. (1999). Alliance and technique in short-term dynamic therapy. *Clinical Psychology Review, 19,* 687–704.

Crits-Christoph, P., Connolly Gibbons, M. B., Crits-Christoph, K., Narducci, J., Schamberger, M., & Gallop, R. (2006). Can therapists be trained to improve their alliances?: A preliminary study of alliance-fostering psychotherapy. *Psychotherapy Research, 16,* 268–281.

Crits-Christoph, P., Siqueland, L., Blaine, J., Frank, A., Luborsky, L., Onken, L. S., et al. (1999). Psychosocial treatments for cocaine dependence: Results of the National Institute on Drug Abuse Collaborative Cocaine Treatment Study. *Archives of General Psychiatry, 56,* 493–502.

DeRubeis, R., & Feeley, M. (1990). Determinants of change in cognitive therapy for depression. *Cognitive Therapy and Research, 14*, 469–482.

DeRubeis, R. J., Brotman, M. A., & Gibbons, C. J. (2005). A conceptual and methodological analysis of the nonspecifics argument. *Clinical Psychology: Science and Practice, 12*, 174–183.

Elkin, I., Shea, M. T., Watkins, J. T., Imber, S. D., Sotsky, S. M., Collins, J. F., et al. (1989). NIMH Treatment of Depression Collaborative Research Program: I. General Effectiveness of Treatments. *Archives of General Psychiatry, 46*, 971–982.

Feeley, M., DeRubeis, R. J., & Gelfand, L. A. (1999). The temporal relation of adherence and alliance to symptom change in cognitive therapy for depression. *Journal of Consulting and Clinical Psychology, 67*, 578–582.

Frieswyk, S. H., Allen, J. G., Colson, D. B., Coyne, L., Gabbard, G. O., Horwitz, L., et al. (1986). Therapeutic alliance: Its place as a process and outcome variable in dynamic psychotherapy research. *Journal of Consulting and Clinical Psychology, 54*, 32–38.

Gaston, L., Marmar, C. R., Gallagher, D., & Thompson, L. W. (1991). Alliance prediction of outcome beyond in-treatment symptomatic change as psychotherapy processes. *Psychotherapy Research, 1*, 104–113.

Gaston, L., Piper, W. E., Debbane, E. G., & Garant, J. (1994). Alliance and technique for predicting outcome in short- and long-term analytic psychotherapy. *Psychotherapy Research, 4*, 121–135.

Gaston, L., Thompson, L., Gallagher, D., Cournoyer, L., & Gagnon, R. (1998). Alliance, technique, and their interactions in predicting outcome of behavioral, cognitive, and brief dynamic therapy. *Psychotherapy Research, 8*, 190–209.

Hersoug, A. G., Høglend, P., Monsen, J. T., & Havik, O. E. (2001). Quality of working alliance in psychotherapy: Therapist variables and patient/therapist similarity as predictors. *Journal of Psychotherapy Practice and Research, 10*, 205–216.

Hill, C. E., & Knox, S. (2009). Processing the therapeutic relationship. *Psychotherapy Research, 19*(1), 13–29.

Horvath, A. O., & Greenberg, L. S. (1989). Development and validation of the Working Alliance Inventory. *Journal of Counseling Psychology, 36*, 223–233.

Iacoviello, B. M., McCarthy, K. S., Barrett, M. S., Rynn, M., Gallop, R., & Barber, J. P. (2007). Treatment preferences affect the therapeutic alliance: Implications for randomized controlled trials. *Journal of Consulting and Clinical Psychology, 75*, 194–198.

Johnson, L. N., & Ketring, S. A. (2006). The therapy alliance: A moderator in therapy outcome for families dealing with child abuse and neglect. *Journal of Marital and Family Therapy, 32*, 345–354.

Joyce, A. S., Ogrodniczuk, J. S., Piper, W. E., & McCallum, M. (2003). The alliance as mediator of expectancy effects in short-term individual therapy. *Journal of Consulting and Clinical Psychology, 71*, 672–679.

Kazdin, A. E. (2008a). Evidence-based treatment and practice: New opportunities to bridge clinical research and practice, enhance the knowledge base, and improve patient care. *The American Psychologist, 63*(3), 146–159.

Kazdin, A. E. (2008b). Understanding how and why psychotherapy leads to change.

Psychotherapy Research, 19(1), 418–428. Retrieved February 17, 2009, from *www.informaworld.com/10.1080/10503300802448899.*

Kivlighan, D. M., Clements, L., Blake, C., Arnzen, A., & Brady, L. (1993). Counselor sex role orientation, flexibility, and working alliance formation. *Journal of Counseling and Development, 72*, 95–100.

Klein, D. N., Schwartz, J. E., Santiago, N. J., Vivian, D., Vocisano, C., Castonguay, L. C., et al. (2003). Therapeutic alliance in depression treatment: Controlling for prior change and patient characteristics. *Journal of Consulting and Clinical Psychology, 71*, 997–1006.

Kraemer, H. C., Wilson, T., Fairburn, C. G., & Agras, S. (2002). Mediators and moderators of treatment effects in randomized clinical trials. *Archives of General Psychiatry, 59*, 877–883.

Luborsky, L., Barber, J. P., Siqueland, L., Johnson, S., Najavits, L. M., Frank, A., et al. (1996). The revised Helping Alliance Questionnaire (HAQ-II): Psychometric properties. *Journal of Psychotherapy Practice and Research, 5*, 260–271.

Mallinckrodt, B., & Nelson, M. L. (1991). Counselor training level and the formation of the psychotherapeutic working alliance. *Journal of Counseling Psychology, 38*, 135–138.

Martin, D. J., Garske, J. P., & Davis, M. K. (2000). Relation of the therapeutic alliance with outcome and other variables: A meta-analytic review. *Journal of Consulting and Clinical Psychology, 68*, 438–450.

Masterson, J. F. (1978). The borderline adult: Therapeutic alliance and transference. *American Journal of Psychiatry, 135*, 437–441.

Meyer, B., Pilkonis, P. A., Krupnick, J. L., Egan, M. K., Simmens, S. J., & Sotsky, S. M. (2002). Treatment expectancies, patient alliance, and outcome: Further analyses from the National Institute of Mental Health Treatment of Depression Collaborative Research Program. *Journal of Consulting and Clinical Psychology, 70*, 1051–1055.

Norcross, J. C. (Ed.). (2002). *Psychotherapy relationships that work: Therapist contributions and responsiveness to patients.* Oxford, UK: Oxford University Press.

Sharpless, B. A., & Barber, J. P. (2009). A conceptual and empirical review of the meaning, measurement, development, and teaching of intervention competence in clinical psychology. *Clinical Psychology Review, 29*(1), 47–56.

Strunk, D. R., Brotman, M. A., & DeRubeis, R. J. (2008). *The process of change in Cognitive Therapy for Depression: Predictors of early inter-session symptom gains and continued response to treatment.* Unpublished manuscript. Department of Psychology, Ohio State University, Columbus.

Summers, R. F., & Barber, J. P. (2003). Therapeutic alliance as a measurable psychotherapy skill. *Academic Psychiatry, 27*, 160–165.

Zuroff, D. C., Blatt, S. J., Sotsky, S. M., Krupnick, J. L., Martin, D. J., Sanislow, C. A., et al. (2000). Relation of therapeutic alliance and perfectionism to outcome in brief outpatient treatment of depression. *Journal of Consulting and Clinical Psychology, 68*, 114–124.

CHAPTER 3

■　■　■　■　■

The Alliance over Time

William B. Stiles
Jacob Z. Goldsmith

Like any human relationship, the client–therapist alliance is dynamic. To address questions about changes over time, investigators must assess the alliance at multiple points in therapy. We have organized our review of studies in which this assessment was done around three frequently addressed questions.

> First, does the alliance typically follow some predictable developmental course, such as increasing across sessions or following a U-shaped, high–low–high, pattern? Alternatively, is there some small number of distinct temporal patterns that characterizes the course of most alliances?
>
> Second, are particular developmental courses of the alliance (in particular, linear increases or U-shaped patterns) associated disproportionately with good outcomes?
>
> Third, is the strength of the alliance in a particular phase of treatment (e.g., early) or a particular session (e.g., Session 3) distinctively predictive of good outcomes?

Following an orienting discussion of the simplification involved in focusing on alliance strength, we consider some of the research on each of these three questions. We conclude with a discussion of differences between researchers' and clinical theorists' views of alliance development.

ORIENTATION: ALLIANCE STRENGTH
AS A COMMON DENOMINATOR

Most alliance research has used a drastic simplification: it has projected complex human relationships onto one evaluative dimension, called "alliance strength" or sometimes just "the alliance." Instruments developed to assess subtle and varied aspects of the alliance have tended to be collapsed into one evaluative scale. Because this simplification has shaped the empirical literature—and hence our review of it—we begin by suggesting some epistemological and methodological reasons for it.

Epistemologically, although the alliance may be understood as partly observable, it is usually considered as residing substantially within the private experience of the participants. Although some important measures have been based on ratings by observers (e.g., Luborsky, 1976; Marziali, Marmar, & Krupnick, 1981; O'Malley, Suh, & Strupp, 1983), a preponderance of research in this area has assessed the alliance with self-report instruments such as the Working Alliance Inventory (WAI; Horvath & Greenberg, 1986, 1989), the Helping Alliance Questionnaire (HAQ; Alexander & Luborsky, 1986; Luborsky et al., 1996), the California Psychotherapy Alliance Scales (CALPAS; Marmar, Weiss, & Gaston, 1989), the Agnew Relationship Inventory (ARM; Agnew, Davies, Stiles, Hardy, Barkham, & Shapiro, 1998), or the Combined Alliance Short Form (CASF; Hatcher & Barends, 1996). Self-report methods are required because the phenomenon is largely epistemologically private. As reviewed by Hatcher (Chapter 1, this volume), the instruments were developed partly from multidimensional conceptualizations of the alliance that sought to capture some of the complexity and subtlety of the relationships and partly from statistical assessments of common dimensions, as by factor analysis.

Methodologically, for alliance ratings to be comparable across respondents, all respondents must rate their alliance on the same dimensions. Factor analysis and kindred procedures seek to ensure this commonality by identifying sets of items that all or most respondents treat as parallel to one another. The internal consistency supports the assumption that different respondents are rating the same thing. In order to report results, researchers must name that thing and assume that they know what it is. But what is it?

In effect, researchers seeking to assess conceptually different dimensions by using face-valid self-report alliance instruments assume that respondents understand each item in the way it was intended by the researcher and in the same way as by one another. If this assumption is wrong, the results may be misleading. Although items may be constructed to assess conceptual subtleties, the common variance in the responses can reflect only the common elements in participants' understandings.

Evaluation is a powerful common denominator. Psychological theorists from Allport (1946) to Zajonc (1980) have agreed that assigning some degree of positive or negative valence to objects and events is automatic, universal, salient, and adaptive. Rogers (1959) described this as an *organismic valuing process*, an evaluative response to each experience that reflects its potential to enhance or damage the organism. Such theories imply that clients and therapists automatically and continually evaluate their relationship with each other and can report how they feel about it.

Researchers, clients, and therapists may each describe relationships by using detailed, complex, and subtle concepts. We suggest, however, that individual clients and therapists frequently use such concepts differently from one another and differently from the researcher who is studying their alliances. As a result, when researchers assess the *common* variance on alliance measures, the subtleties that may have gone into construction or into responding to items are lost. What all respondents understand similarly is the common evaluative component. So, when researchers aggregate across respondents, they tend to find a large evaluative dimension or a few highly intercorrelated, highly evaluative dimensions.

To put this another way, researchers who administer complex, subtly differentiated scales puzzlingly tend to obtain similar results with each scale. Items designed to make conceptual distinctions end up highly correlated. Factor analytic results tend to be unstable across studies and across instruments. Factors tend to be intercorrelated and only loosely related to a priori conceptual dimensions. We suggest these problems reflect respondents' failure to understand the conceptual distinctions in the same way as one another or as the researcher, coupled with the salience of their positive or negative feelings about the relationship. Faced with overlapping (evaluative) variance, researchers have typically abandoned the subtle distinctions. Instead, they report aggregated subscales that yield an overall score for alliance strength. Faced with a literature composed predominantly of these sorts of results, we have followed earlier reviewers in treating alliance as a single unidimensional concept.

Although alliance strength may be simple, perhaps oversimplified, it is not trivial. The qualities that make evaluation emerge reliably and coherently from factor analyses also make it meaningful and important to participants, researchers, and readers. Whether something is good or bad is often its most salient quality, as Allport (1946), Zajonc (1980), and Rogers (1959), and others have affirmed.

But the importance comes with a caveat: the behaviors and experiences that yield a strong alliance may differ dramatically across cases or even across sessions within cases, depending on participants' varying and shifting requirements (Stiles, Honos-Webb, & Surko, 1998). In this light, the notoriously low agreement across perspectives (client, therapist, observer) looks understandable, even sensible. A relationship's valence is a state of the evaluator rather than an objective characteristic. Evaluative measures are reliable (people know what they like) and valid (if what is being measured is the person's actual evaluation), so they are psychometrically sound, but different people (therapists, clients, external raters with different perspectives) may legitimately evaluate the relationships differently. The target of each different alliance measurement is a different person's evaluative experience at a point in time.

We return to this issue in our discussion. First, we summarize some of the extensive research bearing on the temporal shape of the alliance.

DEVELOPMENTAL COURSE OF THE ALLIANCE

Linear Increase

Perhaps because it is the simplest trend to test, many investigators have assessed whether the alliance tends, on the average, to increase across sessions. Some of them have reported finding evidence of such a linear pattern (Fitzpatrick, Iwakabe, & Stalikas, 2005; Golden & Robbins, 1990; Joyce & Piper, 1990; Kivlighan & Shaughnessy, 1995; Kramer, de Roten, Beretta, Michel, & Despland, 2009; Paivio & Patterson, 1999; Patton, Kivlighan, & Multon, 1997; Piper, Boroto, Joyce, McCallum, & Azim, 1995; Piper, Ogrodniczuk, Lamarche, Hilscher, & Joyce, 2005; Sauer, Lopez, & Gormley, 2003; Stiles, Agnew-Davies, Hardy, Barkham, & Shapiro, 1998). For example, Patton et al. (1997) administered the WAI to 16 clients after each session of their short-term psychoanalytic therapy and found a significant linear increase over time, using a hierarchical linear modeling (HLM) analysis. Fitzpatrick et al. (2005) gave the WAI to therapists and clients in early, middle, and late therapy and found that both clients' and therapists' ratings of alliance tended to increase across the three time points, on the average. Using a four-item alliance measure they developed, Piper et al. (2005) assessed 107 clients after each of 12 sessions of short-term interpretive and supportive group therapy for grief. HLM analysis showed a modest overall positive linear trend. Kramer et al. (2009) reported similar overall increases in somewhat longer dynamic therapies (mean = 24 sessions, range 9–40 sessions).

On the other hand, other studies have failed to find such a general pattern of improvement (Eaton, Abeles, & Gutfreund, 1988; Gaston, Piper, Debbane, Bienvenu, & Garant, 1994; Hartley & Strupp, 1982; Hilsenroth, Peters, & Ackerman, 2004; Klee, Abeles, & Muller, 1990; Marmar, Weiss, & Gaston, 1989; Morgan, Luborsky, Crits-Cristoph, Curtis, & Solomon, 1982; Sexton, Hembre, & Kvarme, 1996), suggesting that alliance strength remains more or less stable across sessions when averaged across cases. For example, Eaton et al. (1988) applied an observer-perspective measure, the Therapeutic Alliance Rating Scale (TARS; Marziali et al., 1981), to randomly chosen 15-minute segments of early, middle, and late treatment of 40 clients in outpatient therapy. They reported that that alliance was stable after early therapy, suggesting that the alliance is formed early in treatment. Sexton et al. (1996) administered the WAI to 32 clients after every session in time-limited treatments (about 10 sessions). A modest overall positive slope that was observed when all sessions were analyzed together disappeared if the first session was omitted, suggesting that that alliance was formed after the first session. Hilsenroth et al. (2004) assessed therapist and client perspectives on the alliance at three time points using, the CASF. Means of client-rated alliance were essentially stable across time points, with moderate to strong correlations between early therapy ratings and late therapy ratings.

High–Low–High (U-Shaped) Patterns

Influential theorists and reviewers have described the alliance as characteristically following a U-shaped pattern across sessions—strong in early sessions, weaker in the middle, and strong again at the end (Gelso & Carter, 1994; Horvath & Luborsky, 1993; Kivlighan & Shaughnessy, 1995, 2000; Mann, 1973; Patton et al., 1997). The more recent accounts usually cite Mann (1973), who described such a temporal pattern as it appeared clinically within a time-limited psychodynamic framework:

> In the overview, therefore, one might see the first interviews as a period in which a distinct and powerfully felt object relationship develops. During the middle phase, ambivalence is allowed to return, which then exercises pressure toward a striving for the earlier, closer, more primitive union as well as a thrust toward separation–individuation and greater autonomy. In the termination phase, mastery of separation is demanded and with that achievement goes greater sense of autonomy and a concomitant increase in self-esteem. The consequent enhancement of the ego, fortified even more by useful internalization of the therapist, serves to reduce anxiety still further. (p. 46)

Luborsky (1976) seemed to be describing something similar in saying, "The strength of the helping alliances varies from time to time, especially in relation to surges in transference which may then be diminished by the therapist's interventions" (p. 95). Likewise, Tracey and Ray (1984) proposed a high–low–high pattern of behavioral complementarity between clients and therapist.

In an important conceptual article, Gelso and Carter (1994) embraced Mann's (1973) conceptualization:

> After initial optimism, clients in time-limited interventions experience frustration and negative reactions to the limitations that are being placed upon them. This negative phase is, however, followed by a positive reaction that is also more realistic than that initially experienced. (Gelso & Carter, 1994, p. 301)

Based on this conceptualization, Gelso and Carter offered a series of summary propositions that have stimulated subsequent researchers, of which one was that alliance may well wane during the middle stage of therapy.

Articulating a version of the U-shaped pattern hypothesis, Patton et al. (1997) proposed that early therapy is marked by a period of building alliance before a middle-therapy period in which issues that emerged during the first phase of treatment are worked through. During termination, the alliance should get stronger. In addition to showing a linear increase, as noted earlier, their HLM analysis found that a quadratic term was positive and significant, reflecting a U-shaped pattern. On the other hand, Piper et al.'s (2005) HLM analysis looked for but did not find a U-shaped pattern across 12 sessions of short-term group therapy for grief. Golden and Robbins (1990) reported on two clients whose WAI scores averaged somewhat lower during the middle 4 sessions (out of 12) than during the first 4 or last 4, but their therapist's scores increased linearly across these phases. Other investigators who have looked for a consistently U-shaped course have also failed to find it (e.g., Joyce & Piper, 1990; Kramer, de Roten, Beretta, Michel, & Despland, 2008, 2009; Paivio & Patterson, 1999; Stiles et al., 2004). Thus, the evidence that alliance strength typically follows a U-shaped pattern over the course of therapy is weak.

The U-shaped pattern described by the theorists can easily be conflated with a more short-term developmental pattern, the better documented *rupture–repair pattern* (Safran & Muran, 1996; Safran, Muran, Samstag, & Stevens, 2001). Both characterizations may represent attempts to describe the same sort of clinical phenomenon. Theoretically, rupture and repair builds on a strong alliance but envisions much briefer periods of weak alliance, perhaps lasting only a few minutes or perhaps as long as a session or two. The time course might be described as V-shaped rather than U-shaped (Stiles et al., 2004; Strauss et al., 2006). Taking the U-shaped accounts literally for longer therapies would require, implausibly, that clients and therapists continue for several or many sessions with a weak, ruptured alliance. Rupture–repair sequences are addressed in this volume by other authors (Eubanks-Carter, Muran, & Safran, Chapter 5, this volume), and we defer to them for the review of relevant research.

Typologies of Temporal Patterns: Clusters

Even a superficial perusal of session-by-session plots of alliance scores shows great variation in temporal patterns (see, e.g., Stiles et al., 2004). From this perspective, the questions of whether the alliance generally has a rising or a U-shaped time course seem misleadingly broad. As an alternative to seeking general trends, some investigators have sought groups of dyads that show similar temporal patterns. For example, in a regression analysis of WAI scores across 30-session treatments with adults presenting with anxiety, depression, or interpersonal problems, Stevens, Muran, Safran, Gorman, and Winston (2007) reported that 66% of the clients showed a significantly increasing linear trend. In a study of group and individual treatments for trauma among Palestinian political ex-prisoners (*n* = 50), Kanninen, Salo, and Punamäki (2005) measured alliance at three time points (early, midway, late) in long-term (10- to 12-month) treatment and looked for temporal patterns as a function of clients' attachment style. Clients rated as having autonomous (secure) and preoccupied (anxious–avoidant) attachment styles showed a U-shaped high–low–high pattern. For clients with a dismissing (avoidant) style, alliance strength averaged about the same at the beginning and middle stages of treatment and then dropped at the end.

Kivlighan and Shaughnessy (2000) drew on Gelso and Carter's (1994) account of the U-shaped pattern to design and interpret a cluster analysis of temporal patterns. In two samples of volunteer university students (*n* = 38 and *n* = 41) who were invited to discuss their problems with a counselor for four sessions, Kivlighan and Shaughnessy (2000) distinguished three clusters whose alliance followed different temporal patterns: a stable alliance pattern (little change across sessions), a linear growth pattern (increasing strength across sessions), and the U-shaped pattern (high scores in the first and last sessions, with lower scores in the middle sessions).

In an attempted replication using data drawn from a clinical trial of 8- and 16-session versions of alternative treatments for depression (*n* = 79), Stiles et al. (2004) showed a rough replication of two of the patterns—the linear growth cluster and the stable cluster—along with two additional patterns. They did not replicate the U-shaped pattern. A striking feature in these data was the great session-to-session variability in alliance shown by some (though not all) of the clients. Of course, this variability could reflect the greater range of curve shapes possible when more than four points are considered. In their cluster analysis of four-session sequences of alliance assessed by the Helping Alliance Questionnaire (*n* = 70 outpatients), de Roten et al. (2004) also found stable alliance and linear growth patterns, consistent with Kivlighan and Shaunessy (2000) and Stiles et al. (2004), but again failed to find U-shaped patterns. Kramer et al. (2008, 2009) used cluster analysis on client and therapist HAQ scores across the first eight sessions of longer therapies and on the full therapies (mean = 24 sessions). They found clear stable alliance and linear growth patterns in client and therapist data in both analyses. More tentatively—in a relatively small number of clients—they observed a linear decreasing pattern in the early sessions, while across all sessions there was a quadratic (U-shaped) pattern.. Kalogerakos (2009) described stable linear and steep linear or quadratic patterns in patients who were seen in 16-week process–experiential and cognitive-behavioral treatments for major depression.

RELATION OF DEVELOPMENTAL COURSE TO OUTCOME

Linear Alliance Increase and Outcome

A number of studies have reported that linear increases in alliance strength were associated with positive outcomes. Klee et al. (1990), for example, found that high-outcome clients showed a significant increase from early in treatment (third session) to late in treatment (a session between 80 to 90% of the way through treatment) in their positive contributions to the alliance, as rated on the TARS. When low-outcome clients were included in the analysis, the difference was no longer significant. Studies by Eltz, Shirk, and Sarlin (1995) and Florsheim, Shotorbani, Guest-Warnick, Barratt, and Hwang (2000) found that increases in alliance were associated with positive outcome in therapy with adolescents, even though initial alliance was not. Piper et al.'s (2005) HLM analysis found that, for client ratings, the linear trend added to the power of initial alliance in predicting positive outcome (assessed as an aggregate of self-report and interview measures). Results for therapist-rated alliance were more complex, showing an interaction with initial alliance level. Kramer et al.'s (2009) HLM analyses found an association of outcome with the linear increase but not with initial level. Of course, given equivalent initial scores, clients whose alliances improve would also have had stronger average alliances across treatment. In the de Roten et al. (2004) study, patients in the linear growth cluster showed greater pre–post improvement than did patients with stable alliance.

Findings of improvement associated with linear increases haven't replicated consistently, however. Kivlighan & Shaunessy (1995) reported that clients whose alliances showed a linear increase had relatively greater residual gain on the Inventory of Interpersonal Problems (IIP; Horowitz, Rosenberg, Baer, Ureno, & Villasenor, 1988), but they failed to replicate it in a subsequent study (Kivlighan & Shaughnessy, 2000). Stiles, Agnew-Davies, Hardy, Barkham, and Shapiro (1998) replicated the Kivilghan and Shaughnessy (1995) results for therapist alliance ratings but not for client ratings. Neither Stevens et al. (2007) nor Kalogerakos (2009) found significant associations of linear increases in patient WAI ratings with outcome. Patton et al. (1997), who reported a pattern of average linear increase, found no relation of the degree of increase to outcome. In a comparative study of treatments for adolescent substance abuse, Hogue, Dauber, Stambaugh, Cecero, and Liddle (2006) found such an association in family therapy but not in individual cognitive-behavior therapy. Kramer et al. (2008) reported there were no significant outcome differences among clients whose alliance ratings showed different temporal patterns across their first eight sessions, but clients tended to improve more if their therapists showed a *stable* pattern rather than an increasing one.

U-Shaped Alliance Course and Outcome

In the relatively few studies that have looked for links of outcome with U-shaped alliance growth, the results have also been inconsistent. Using sequence analyses, Tracey and Ray (1984) showed that three successful cases conformed approximately to a three-stage model of response complementarity that suggested a U-shaped course to the alliance, whereas three unsuccessful cases did not. Patton et al. (1997) reported that outcome was significantly related to quadratic growth in their HLM analysis. However, in Kivlighan and Shaughnessy's (1995) HLM analysis, the quadratic growth effect was not significant.

Cluster analytic studies too have yielded inconsistencies. In both of their samples of university students in four-session counseling, Kivlighan and Shaughnessy (2000) found that those in the U-shaped cluster had significantly better outcomes than did those in the other two clusters. On the other hand, Stiles et al. (2004), de Roten et al. (2004), Kramer et al. (2008, 2009), and Stevens et al. (2007) did not even find U-shaped clusters; so, this effect could not be assessed. Stiles et al. (2004) did report that the minority clients who showed a sharply defined V-shaped pattern within 8- or 16-session treatments—three successive sessions in a high–low–high pattern, with the low point two standard deviations or more below the first high one—did have somewhat better outcomes than other clients, though de Roten et al. (2004), Stevens et al. (2007), and Kramer et al. (2008, 2009) failed to find an association with V-shaped patterns. Strauss et al. (2006) found a significant association of V-shaped patterns with outcomes, using a looser criterion of any one standard deviation high–low–high pattern within a series of up to eight alliance measurements that were more widely spaced (measures taken at Sessions 2, 5, 10, 20, 30, 40, 50, and 52, if clients remained in treatment).

ALLIANCE AT THE THIRD SESSION AND OUTCOME

The frequently encountered suggestion that outcome is most strongly associated with alliance at Session 3 seems traceable, through an explicitly speculative conjecture by Horvath and Luborsky (1993, p. 567), to an early study by Saltzman, Luetgert, Roth, Creaser, and Howard (1976). Although Saltzman et al. (1976) assessed the relationship by using multiple rationally constructed subscales and outcomes on several retrospectively rated dimensions of improvement, they reported correlations only with relationship assessments gathered at Session 3. That is, they did not compare predictions of outcome at different points in the treatment, though the subscales' prediction of persistence in therapy (vs. dropout) seemed marginally strongest at Session 3.

Studies that assessed alliance at only one point in time have often focused on early alliance, presumably for pragmatic reasons, and have typically found significant alliance–outcome associations (e.g., Strauss et al., 2006). Comparative studies, however, have not consistently found that early alliance is more predictive of outcome than later alliance. In a 1991 review, Horvath and Symonds (1991) reported a slightly higher effect size (ES) in associating outcomes with early alliance (assessed at Sessions 1–5, $n = 12$ studies, ES = 0.31) or late alliance (assessed at or near the end of therapy, $n = 3$ studies, ES = 0.30) than with alliance averaged across sessions ($n = 8$ presumably distinct studies, ES = 0.21). Paivio and Patterson (1999) administered the WAI at four time-points—Sessions 3, 4, 10, and at termination—to adult survivors of child abuse in emotion-focused therapy and reported alliance at Session 4 was positively correlated with some (but not all) posttreatment positive changes in different domains of functioning, whereas alliance at termination was positively correlated with all of the different outcome domains. Barber, Connolly Gibbons, Crits-Christoph, Gladis, and Siqueland (2000) reported that alliance at Sessions 2, 5, and 10 all predicted subsequent change in depression similarly, even after the effects of prior symptom improvement were partialed out. Stiles et al. (1998) assessed alliance by using the ARM at every session in 8- or 16-session therapies and found a significant tendency for correlations with outcomes to be stronger with alliance measurements made *later* in treatment. Florsheim et al. (2000) reported that in a study of adolescents in inpatient treatment high alliance at 3 weeks predicted negative outcome, whereas high alliance at 3 months predicted positive outcome. Stevens et al. (2007) reported numerically higher correlations of outcome with alliance measured in the middle phase of their 30-session treatments than for sessions in early or last phases.

OTHER STUDIES OF ALLIANCE AND TIME

Our selected questions (whether the alliance typically follows a linear or U-shaped pattern; whether these patterns are associated with positive outcomes; whether there is a critical period for alliance strength) by no means exhaust the ways researchers have investigated the alliance across time. For example, a few investigators have looked at the interdependencies of therapist and client alliance over time (e.g., Brossart, Willson, Patton, Kivlighan, & Multon, 1998; Hentschel & Bijleveld, 1995). Pos and Greenberg (2008) have explored how outcomes are related to different alliance components in the beginning, working, and ending phases of therapy. Fitzpatrick et al. (2005) reported that client and therapist alliance ratings were different and did not converge even though both alliance ratings increased over time. Iacovellio et al. (2007) reported that patients who initially preferred psychotherapy over pharmacotherapy showed increases in their alliance across sessions if they received psychotherapy but showed decreases if they received pharmacotherapy or placebo. Patients who initially preferred pharmacotherapy showed no differences in alliance development as a function of treatment type.

We have also not reviewed studies of temporal relations of alliance with other process variables, such as therapist–client behavioral connection (Sexton, Littauer, Sexton, & Tømmerås, 2005), or with outcome variables assessed on a session-by-session basis (e.g., DeRubeis, & Feeley, 1990; Feeley, DeRubeis, & Gelfand, 1999). The outcome variables have been used to help assess whether alliance strength precedes improvement—and thus may help to cause it—or whether instead alliance strength follows or is itself *a component of* improvement (see Barber, Khalsa, & Sharpless, Chapter 2, this volume).

DISCUSSION: GET REAL

To summarize the answers to our guiding questions, the literature offers some evidence of a statistical tendency for alliances to improve across therapy and for a link of such an increase with positive outcomes; however, these effects are small, variable, and inconsistent across studies. There is less evidence for a general tendency for treatments to follow a U-shaped temporal pattern or for such a pattern to be associated with positive outcomes, despite a number of theoretical articulations of why such a pattern is expectable and should be valuable. Although early alliance strength does seem to be associated with positive outcomes, it is not distinctively so, and some reports suggest that middle and late alliance are equally or more strongly associated with outcomes.

How can we account for the failure of so much research to yield clear answers to what seem like basic questions in this area? Methodological variations (e.g., samples, treatment approaches, treatment durations, rater perspectives, measures used, number of points sampled, alternative statistical procedures) might help account for the inconsistencies. However, we focus our discussion instead on a tension between psychometric precision and clinical realism in alliance research.

Researchers' versus Clinicians' Accounts of Relationship Development

We began by noting that psychometric limitations have led alliance researchers (including ourselves) to condense therapeutic relationships into a single evaluative dimension or a small number of highly intercorrelated dimensions. Other, more complex, characterizations may be accurate and more thorough, but unless respondents all use them, they do not show up as common components of ratings. Alliance measures reduce to evaluation because evaluation is a common denominator in people's diverse understanding.

Because evaluation is salient and universal—for readers as well as for researchers—alliance research has a sympathetic audience and an enthusiastic cadre of investigators, as evidenced by this volume and the reference lists at the end of each of its chapters. But condensing therapeutic relationships into a single evaluative dimension does violence to clinical conceptualizations of therapeutic relationships.

As will be evident (we hope) in the chapters in Parts II and III of this volume, clinicians use complex and sophisticated concepts when they try to describe the development of the therapeutic relationship over time. To illustrate the complexity, Gelso and Carter (1994), summarizing psychoanalytic thinking, distinguished among the real relationship, the transference, and the working alliance, suggesting that the last "may be seen as the alignment or joining of the reasonable self or ego of the client and the therapist's analyzing or 'therapizing' self or ego for the purpose of the work" (p. 297). As noted earlier, they went on to offer propositions that (among other things) described a U-shaped course for the alliance.

Kohut (1971, 1977) distinguished between *mirroring transferences* (the therapist experienced as an extension of the self) and *idealizing transferences* (the client drawing strength from being associated with the therapist's exaggerated virtues). Development, the theory suggests, involves the therapist's failing to fulfill unrealistic expectations, but rather bringing the unrealistic expectations into focus and making change possible.

Long ago, one of us (Stiles, 1979) suggested that therapeutic relationships follow a developmental course that can be described by using Erikson's (1963) Eight Ages of Man—proceeding through stages of Basic Trust versus Mistrust, Autonomy versus Shame and Doubt, Initiative versus Guilt, Industry versus Inferiority, Identity versus Role Confusion, Intimacy versus Isolation, Generativity versus Stagnation, and, as termination approaches, Ego Integrity versus Despair. The resolution of each conflict contains the seeds for the next conflict. As clients revisit this sequence of emotional issues with the therapist, they re-encounter and can address difficulties in their own ontogenetic development. For example, a shy client might have a chance to confront and overcome the sense of guilt and intrusiveness that has previously prevented him or her from taking initiative in relationships.

The alliance research we reviewed has not properly addressed such theories. For the reasons we have noted, the standard alliance measures do not distinguish among the real relationship, the transference, and the alliance; nor do they assess the proposition that the alliance involved a joining of the patient's ego with the therapist's therapizing self, track the shift from mirroring to idealizing, or make the key qualitative distinctions among shame, self-doubt, or inferiority within the therapeutic relationship.

A central problem is measurement. To say the relationship is multidimensional understates the problem. The concepts used in clinical theories (e.g., a real relationship, mirroring transference, initiative versus guilt) are not represented as dimensions but as qualitative descriptions. Treating each of the theories' qualitative descriptors as dimensions to be measured would continually entail additional dimensions, and the project would quickly become unwieldy.

Of course, participants' evaluations figure in theories, and some theoretical accounts have implications for the evaluations' developmental course; that is, a simple alliance index may inform a more realistically nuanced theory. For example, periods of negative transference may be expected to yield low alliance scores on the usual instruments. Mann's (1973) often cited description of the U-shape hypothesis was embedded in a more nuanced account of the relationship in time-limited therapy. The oversimplification comes from ignoring the further complexity of the relationship because it isn't being measured by self-report instruments.

Alliance strength can be seen as an achievement built upon many qualities and responsive actions that vary across cases and occasions (Stiles, Honos-Webb, & Surko, 1998; Stiles & Wolfe, 2006). Alliance scores might reflect different processes in different cases or at different times and with different theoretical significance. If the underlying theory isn't articulated and the context isn't examined at a level of detail commensurate with the theory, studies of global evaluations are bound to yield puzzling results.

Qualitative Case Studies

If the clinical theories are important for scientific understanding and for practice, as we, in concert with the authors of this volume's Part II and III sections, believe, then they should be subjected to research scrutiny. How can the complexity be addressed realistically? What would such research look like?

One possibility is qualitative case study research (e.g., Agnew, Harper,

Shapiro, & Barkham, 1994; Goldsmith, Mosher, Stiles, & Greenberg, 2008; McMillan & McLeod, 2006), which offers a way to assimilate the multiple and varied theoretically relevant observations that intensive case studies can yield. Whereas statistical hypothesis testing research derives just one (or a few) statements from a theory and compares it with relevant observations across many cases, case study research compares many *different* theoretical statements with observations drawn from a single case. In a metaphorical sense, both may provide equivalent degrees of freedom and hence (if observations conform to theory) may support equivalent increments of confidence in the theory as a whole (Campbell, 1979; Stiles, 2005, 2007, 2009). One illustration is McMillan and McLeod's (2006) interview study of former clients' experience of relational depth across multiple episodes of therapy. Participants described a powerful experience of connection with their therapists from the first session, a sort of leap of faith, that was common among the most facilitative episodes and rare or nonexistent in other episodes. Such an account can contribute to a theory of how early alliance may exert powerful effects on outcomes. In another illustration, Goldsmith et al. (2008) examined how therapists' empathy, manifested in empathic reflections within sessions, facilitated client assimilation of problematic experiences in person-centered therapy. They described how reflections promoted progress though a developmental sequence of stages, adding a small increment of confidence to, and simultaneously elaborating, the person-centered and assimilation theories that informed the study.

Such studies are only a beginning, of course, and they have problems of their own. Among other things, they are of interest primarily just to those who use or care about the particular theories they address. Importantly, however, the theories they strengthen and elaborate are clinically descriptive theories, not statements about central tendency or linear models of how dimensions combine. They easily accommodate variation across cases because the generalization is at the level of the theory (which explicitly encompasses variation) rather than at the level of individual statements.

In this connection, Luborsky's (1976) early and widely cited *counting signs* method of assessing alliance is of more than historical interest. By distinguishing and counting features of the therapeutic relationship, Luborsky described two types of alliance, one "based on the patient's experiencing the therapist as supportive and helpful" and one "based on a sense of working together in a joint struggle" (p. 94). Clients who improved in therapy often developed each of these in a developmental sequence. Nonimprovers developed neither type of alliance. We suggest that if the list of signs is allowed to encompass all legitimate manifestations of the alliance, then the counting signs method anticipates the degrees of freedom logic of theory-building case studies.

Alliance development is no doubt manifested in more ways than any one investigator will encounter. Contained and constrained by the theory's logical consistency and the need to respect previous results, investigators can use qualitative case studies to bring these signs within the scope of their theory (Stiles, 2009).

REFERENCES

Agnew, R. M., Harper, H., Shapiro, D. A., & Barkham, M. (1994). Resolving a challenge to the therapeutic relationship: A single-case study. *British Journal of Medical Psychology, 67*, 155–170.

Agnew-Davies, R., Stiles, W. B., Hardy, G. E., Barkham, M., & Shapiro, D. A. (1998). Alliance structure assessed by the Agnew Relationship Measure (ARM). *British Journal of Clinical Psychology, 37*, 155–172.

Alexander, L. B., & Luborsky, L. (1986). The Penn Helping Alliance Scales. In L. S. Greenberg & W. M. Pinsof (Eds.), *The psychotherapeutic process: A research handbook* (pp. 325–366). New York: Guilford Press.

Allport, G. W. (1946). Effect: A secondary principle of learning. *Psychological Review, 53*, 335–347.

Barber, J. P., Connolly Gibbons, M. B., Crits-Christoph, P., Gladis, L., & Siqueland, L. (2000). Alliance predicts patients' outcome beyond in-treatment change in symptoms. *Journal of Consulting and Clinical Psychology, 68*, 1027–1032.

Brossart, D. F., Willson, V. L., Patton, M. J., Kivlighan, D. M., & Multon, K. D. (1998). A time series model of the working alliance: A key process in short-term psychoanalytic counseling. *Psychotherapy, 35*(2), 197–205.

Campbell, D. T. (1979). "Degrees of freedom" and the case study. In T. D. Cook & C. S. Reichardt (Eds.), *Qualitative and quantitative methods in evaluation research* (pp. 49–67). Beverley Hills, CA: Sage.

de Roten, Y., Fischer, M., Drapeau, M., Beretta, V., Kramer, U., Favre, N., et al. (2004). Is one assessment enough?: Patterns of helping alliance development and outcome. *Clinical Psychology and Psychotherapy, 11*, 324–331.

DeRubeis, R. J., & Feeley, M. (1990). Determinants of change in cognitive therapy. *Cognitive Therapy and Research, 14*, 469–482.

Eaton, T. T., Abeles, N., & Gutfreund, M. J. (1988). Therapeutic alliance and outcome: Impact of treatment length and pretreatment symptomatology. *Psychotherapy, 25*, 536–542.

Eltz, M. J., Shirk, S. R., & Sarlin, N. (1995). Alliance formation and treatment outcome among maltreated adolescents. *Child Abuse and Neglect, 19*, 419–431.

Erikson, E. H. (1963). *Childhood and society.* New York: W. W. Norton.

Feeley, M., DeRubeis, R. J., & Gelfand, L. A. (1999). The temporal relation of adherence and alliance to symptom change in cognitive therapy for depression. *Journal of Consulting and Clinical Psychology, 67*, 578–582.

Fitzpatrick, M., Iwakabe, S., & Stalikas, A. (2005). Perspective divergence in the working alliance. *Psychotherapy Research, 15*, 69–79.

Florsheim, P., Shotorbani, S., Guest-Warnick, G., Barratt, T., & Hwang, W.-C. (2000).

Role of the working alliance in the treatment of delinquent boys in community-based programs. *Journal of Clinical Child Psychology, 29,* 94–107.

Gaston, L., Piper, W., Debbane, E., Bienvenu, J., & Garant, J. (1994). Alliance and technique for predicting outcome in short- and long-term analytic psychotherapy. *Psychotherapy Research, 4,* 121–135.

Gelso, C. J., & Carter, J. A. (1994). Components of the psychotherapy relationship: Their interaction and unfolding during treatment. *Journal of Counseling Psychology, 41,* 296–306.

Golden, B., & Robbins, S. (1990). The working alliance within time-limited therapy: A case analysis. *Professional Psychology: Theory, Research, and Practice, 21,* 476–481.

Goldsmith, J. Z., Mosher, J. K., Stiles, W. B., & Greenberg, L. S. (2008). Speaking with the client's voices: How a person-centered therapy used reflections to facilitate assimilation. *Person-Centered and Experiential Psychotherapies, 7,* 155–172.

Hartley, D. E., & Strupp, H. H. (1982). The therapeutic alliance: Its relationship to outcome in brief psychotherapy. In J. Masling (Ed.), *Empirical studies of psychoanalytic theories* (Vol. 1, pp. 1–37). Hillsdale, NJ: Erlbaum.

Hatcher, R. L., & Barends, A. W. (1996). Patients' view of the alliance in psychotherapy: Exploratory factor analysis of three alliance measures. *Journal of Consulting and Clinical Psychology, 64,* 1326–1336.

Hentschel, U., & Bijleveld, C. (1995). It takes two to do therapy: On differential aspects in the formation of therapeutic alliance. *Psychotherapy Research, 5,* 22–32.

Hilsenroth, M. J., Peters, E. J., & Ackerman, S. J. (2004). The development of therapeutic alliance during psychological assessment: Patient and therapist perspectives. *Journal of Personality Assessment, 83,* 332–344.

Hogue, A., Dauber, S., Stambaugh, L. F., Cecero, J. J., & Liddle, H. A. (2006). Early therapeutic alliance and treatment outcome in individual and family therapy for adolescent behavior problems. *Journal of Consulting and Clinical Psychology, 74,* 121–129.

Horowitz, L. M., Rosenberg, S. E., Baer, B. A., Ureno, G., & Villasenor, V. S. (1988). Inventory of Interpersonal Problems: Psychometric properties and clinical applications. *Journal of Consulting and Clinical Psychology, 56,* 885–892.

Horvath, A. O., & Greenberg, L. S. (1986). Development of the working alliance inventory. In L. S. Greenberg & W. M. Pinsof (Eds.), *The psychotherapeutic process: A research handbook* (pp. 529–556). New York: Guilford Press.

Horvath, A. O., & Greenberg, L. S. (1989). Development and validation of the Working Alliance Inventory. *Journal of Counseling Psychology, 36,* 223–233.

Horvath, A. O., & Luborsky, L. (1993). The role of the therapeutic alliance in psychotherapy. *Journal of Consulting and Clinical Psychology, 61,* 561–573.

Horvath, A. O., & Symonds, B. D. (1991). Relation between working alliance and outcome in psychotherapy: A meta-analysis. *Journal of Counseling Psychology, 38,* 139–149.

Iacovellio, B. M., McCarthy, K. S., Barrettt, M. S., Rynn, M., Gallop, R., & Barber, J. P. (2007). Treatment preferences affect the therapeutic alliance: Implications for randomized controlled trials. *Journal of Consulting and Clinical Psychology*, *75*, 194–198.

Joyce, A. S., & Piper, W. E. (1990). An examination of Mann's model of time-limited individual psychotherapy. *Canadian Journal of Psychiatry*, *35*, 41–49.

Kalogerakos, A. F. (2009). *An examination of therapeutic alliance patterns, client attachment, client interpersonal problems, and therapy outcome in process-experiential and cognitive-behavioral treatment for depression.* PhD dissertation, Department of Adult Education and Counseling Psychology, University of Toronto, Toronto, Canada.

Kanninen, K., Salo, J., & Punamäki, R.-L. (2000). Attachment patterns and working alliance in trauma therapy for victims of political violence. *Psychotherapy Research*, *10*, 435–449.

Kivlighan, D. M., & Shaughnessy, P. (1995). An analysis of the development of the working alliance using hierarchical linear modeling. *Journal of Counseling Psychology*, *42*, 338–349.

Kivlighan, D. M., & Shaughnessy, P. (2000). Patterns of working alliance development: A typology of working alliance ratings. *Journal of Counseling Psychology*, *47*, 362–371.

Klee, M. R., Abeles, N., & Muller, R. T. (1990). Therapeutic alliance: Early indicators, course, and outcome. *Psychotherapy*, *27*, 166–174.

Kohut, M. (1971). *The analysis of the self.* New York: International Universities Press.

Kohut, M. (1977). *The restoration of the self.* New York: International Universities Press.

Kramer, U., de Roten, Y., Beretta, V., Michel, L., & Despland, J.-N. (2008). Patient's and therapist's views of early alliance building in dynamic psychotherapy: Patterns and relation to outcome. *Journal of Counseling Psychology*, *55*, 89–95.

Kramer, U., de Roten, Y., Beretta, V., Michel, L., & Despland, J.-N. (2009). Alliance patterns over the course of short-term dynamic psychotherapy: The shape of productive relationships. *Psychotherapy Research*, *19*, 699–706.

Luborsky, L. (1976). Helping alliances in psychotherapy: The groundwork for a study of their relationship to its outcome. In J. L. Claghorn (Ed.), *Successful psychotherapy* (pp. 92–116). New York: Brunner/Mazel.

Luborsky, L., Barber, J. P., Siqueland, L., Johnson, S., Najavits, L. M., Frank, A., et al. (1996). The revised helping alliance questionnaire (HAq II). *Journal of Psychotherapy Practice and Research*, *5*, 260–271.

Mann, J. (1973). *Time-limited psychotherapy.* Cambridge, MA: Harvard University Press.

Marmar, C. R., Weiss, D. S., & Gaston, L. (1989). Toward the validation of the California Therapeutic Alliance Rating System. *Psychological Assessment*, *1*, 46–52.

Marziali, E., Marmar, C., & Krupnick, J. (1981). Therapeutic alliance scales: Development and relationship to psychotherapy outcome. *American Journal of Psychiatry*, *138*, 361–364.

McMillan, M., & McLeod, J. (2006). Letting go: The client's experience of relational depth. *Person-Centered and Experiential Psychotherapies*, *5*, 278–293.

Morgan, R., Luborsky, L., Crits-Christoph, P., Curtis, H., & Solomon, J. (1982). Predicting the outcomes of psychotherapy by the Penn Helping Alliance Rating Method. *Archives of General Psychiatry, 39*, 397–402.

O'Malley, S. S., Suh, C. S., & Strupp, H. H. (1983). The Vanderbilt Psychotherapy Process Scale: A report on the scale development and a process-outcome study. *Journal of Consulting and Clinical Psychology, 51*, 581–586.

Paivio, S. C., & Patterson, L. A. (1999). Alliance development in therapy for resolving child abuse issues. *Psychotherapy, 36*, 343–354.

Patton, M. J., Kivlighan, D. M., Jr., & Multon, K. D. (1997). The Missouri psychoanalytic counseling research project: Relation of changes in counseling process to client outcome. *Journal of Counseling Psychology, 44*, 189–208.

Piper, W. E., Boroto, D. R., Joyce, A. S., McCallum, M., & Azim, H. F. A. (1995). Pattern of alliance and outcome in short-term individual psychotherapy. *Psychotherapy: Theory, Research, Practice, Training, 4*, 639–647.

Piper, W. E., Ogrodniczuk, J. S., Lamarche, C., Hilscher, T., & Joyce, A. S. (2005). Levels of alliance, pattern of alliance, and outcome in short-term group therapy. *International Journal of Group Psychotherapy, 55*, 527–550.

Pos, A., & Greenberg, L. (2008, September). The changing role of the alliance across therapy phases during experiential treatment for depression. In L. Angus (Moderator), *Addressing the complexity of client change in psychotherapy: Understanding the contributions of alliance, emotion and meaning-making processes to treatment outcomes in the York I & II Depression Studies*. Panel presented at the North American Society for Psychotherapy Research meeting, New Haven, CT.

Rogers, C. R. (1959). A theory of therapy, personality, and interpersonal relationships as developed by the client-centered framework. In S. Koch (Ed.), *Psychology: A study of a science: Vol. III. Formulations of a person and the social context* (pp. 184–256). New York: McGraw-Hill.

Safran, J. D., & Muran, J. C. (1996). The resolution of ruptures in the therapeutic alliance. *Journal of Consulting and Clinical Psychology, 64*, 447–458.

Safran, J. D., Muran, J. C., Samstag, L. W., & Stevens, C. (2001). Repairing alliance ruptures. *Psychotherapy, 38*, 406–412.

Saltzman, C., Luetgert, M. J., Roth, C. H., Creaser, J., & Howard, L. (1976). Formation of a therapeutic relationship: Experiences during the initial phase of psychotherapy as predictors of treatment duration and outcome. *Journal of Consulting and Clinical Psychology, 44*, 546–555.

Sauer, E. M., Lopez, F. G., & Gormley, B. (2003). Respective contributions of therapist and client adult attachment orientations to the development of the early working alliance: A preliminary growth modeling study. *Psychotherapy Research, 13*, 371–382.

Sexton, H., Littauer, H., Sexton, A., & Tømmerås, E. (2005). Building an alliance: Early therapy process and the client–therapist connection. *Psychotherapy Research, 15*, 103–116

Sexton, H. C., Hembre, K., & Kvarme, G. (1996). The interaction of the alliance and therapy microprocess: A sequential analysis. *Journal of Consulting and Clinical Psychology, 64*(3), 471–480.

Stevens, C. L., Muran, J. C., Safran, J. D., Gorman, B. S., & Winston, A. (2007).

Levels and patterns of the therapeutic alliance in brief psychotherapy. *American Journal of Psychotherapy*, *61*, 109–129.

Stiles, W. B. (1979). Psychotherapy recapitulates ontogeny: The epigenesis of intensive interpersonal relationships. *Psychotherapy: Theory, Research, and Practice*, *16*, 391–404.

Stiles, W. B. (2005). Case studies. In J. C. Norcross, L. E. Beutler, & R. F. Levant (Eds.), *Evidence-based practices in mental health: Debate and dialogue on the fundamental questions* (pp. 57–64). Washington, DC: American Psychological Association.

Stiles, W. B. (2007). Theory-building case studies of counselling and psychotherapy. *Counselling and Psychotherapy Research*, *7*, 122–127.

Stiles, W. B. (2009). Logical operations in theory-building case studies. *Pragmatic Case Studies in Psychotherapy*, *5*(3), 9–22. Available at *http://jrul.libraries.rutgers.edu/index.php/pcsp/article/view/973/2384*.

Stiles, W. B., Agnew-Davies, R., Hardy, G. E., Barkham, M., & Shapiro, D. A. (1998). Relations of the alliance with psychotherapy outcome: Findings in the Second Sheffield Psychotherapy Project. *Journal of Consulting and Clinical Psychology*, *66*, 791–802.

Stiles, W. B., Glick, M. J., Osatuke, K., Hardy, G. E., Shapiro, D. A., Agnew-Davies, R., et al. (2004). Patterns of alliance development and the rupture–repair hypothesis: Are productive relationships U-shaped or V-shaped? *Journal of Counseling Psychology*, *51*, 81–92.

Stiles, W. B., Honos-Webb, L., & Surko, M. (1998). Responsiveness in psychotherapy. *Clinical Psychology: Science and Practice*, *5*, 439–458.

Stiles, W. B., & Wolfe, B. E. (2006). Relationship factors in treating anxiety disorders. In L. G. Castonguay & L. E. Beutler (Eds.), *Principles of therapeutic change that work* (pp. 155–165). New York: Oxford University Press.

Strauss, J. L., Hayes, A. M., Johnson, S. L., Newman, C. R., Brown, G. K., Barber, J. P., et al. (2006). Early alliance, alliance ruptures, and symptom change in a non-randomized trial of cognitive therapy for avoidant and obsessive–compulsive personality disorders. *Journal of Consulting and Clinical Psychology*, *74*, 337–345.

Tracey, T. J., & Ray, P. B. (1984). Stages of successful time-limited counseling: An interactional examination. *Journal of Counseling Psychology*, *31*, 13–27.

Zajonc, R. B. (1980). Feeling and thinking: Preferences need no inferences. *American Psychologist*, *35*, 151–175.

CHAPTER 4

■   ■   ■   ■   ■

Qualitative Studies of Negative Experiences in Psychotherapy

Clara E. Hill

Therapist techniques, client involvement, and the therapeutic relationship seem to be inextricably intertwined (Hill, 2005). In talking about the processes involved in building and repairing problems in the alliance, then, we can take a look at what happens for therapists and clients during negative events in sessions. The purpose of this chapter is therefore to describe the results of several qualitative studies from our research program about what works in terms of improving the alliance when clients and therapists experience negative reactions in therapy. In this chapter, I present evidence that negative experiences do in fact occur in therapy; then I provide a justification for using qualitative methods for investigating negative experiences; and finally I present the results from three qualitative studies examining the process of working with these negative experiences.

EVIDENCE FOR THE OCCURRENCE OF NEGATIVE EXPERIENCES

There is evidence that about 5–10% of clients deteriorate in therapy (see review in Cooper, 2008), which would suggest that some clients have negative experiences. In addition, more direct evidence exists for negative experiences. One set of studies found that clients had and hid negative feelings about their therapies (Hill, Thompson, Cogar, & Denman, 1993; Regan & Hill, 1992; Rennie, 1994). In another set of studies, when therapists were aware of clients' negative experiences, the outcome was actually worse, suggesting that therapists did not manage the process related to these problematic experiences well (Hill, Thompson, & Corbett, 1992; Martin, Martin, Meyer, & Slemon, 1985; Martin, Martin, & Slemon, 1987; Regan & Hill, 1992; Thompson & Hill, 1991).

Furthermore, in a sample of 132 clients who had trauma, 72% reported that they had been angry at their therapists at least once during therapy, and 64% reported that their therapists had been unjustly angry with them at least once during therapy (Dahlenberg, 2004). Similarly, Castonguay, Goldfried, Wiser, Raue, and Hayes (1996) found evidence of strains in the alliance (e.g., clients were negative, unresponsive, avoidant) in some cases of cognitive therapy. Therapists addressed these problems by adhering more closely to the cognitive therapy protocol and emphasizing the impact of the client's distorted thoughts, which then led to power struggles between the therapist and client. Likewise, in interpretive individual psychotherapy, Piper et al. (1999) found that during the session immediately preceding premature termination, clients talked about dropping out. They also expressed frustration about unmet expectations and the therapists' repeated focus on painful feelings. Therapists responded by focusing on the therapeutic relationship and transference, which the clients resisted, resulting in power struggles. Because of these dramatic findings regarding negative experiences in therapy, it seems important to investigate further the process of working with such events in the hope of distilling some wisdom about what therapists might do to repair problems in therapeutic relationships.

RATIONALE FOR USING A QUALITATIVE APPROACH

When we talk about negative experiences, by definition we are talking about perceptions of events. Hence, to investigate these events, we need a methodology that allows us to capture inner experiences in a rich way and enables participants to tell their stories without being constrained by preexisting ideas. Qualitative methods are ideal for this type of investigation because they involve open-ended questioning of participants and coding of data based on a bottom-up approach (i.e., learning from the data) rather than a top-down approach (i.e., testing hypotheses) that only allows for finding what the researcher has set out to find.

In particular, in this chapter, I review studies that investigated negative experiences using consensual qualitative research (CQR; Hill et al., 2005; Hill, Thompson, & Williams, 1997). In this approach, researchers first interview participants by using semistructured interviews (which involve asking a limited number of predetermined open-ended questions about a delimited topic and also probing for in-depth information about the individual participant based on the participant's responses). A primary team of at least three judges then (1) constructs domains (i.e., topics) from the data, (2) develops core ideas (i.e., summaries, abstracts) for all the raw data within each domain for each participant, and (3) conducts a cross-analysis (i.e., develops categories reflecting themes) within domains across participants. One or two auditors check the data at each step to ensure that the primary team stays as close to the data as possible. A final feature is that judges continually return to the raw data to ensure that all findings are justified based on the data.

QUALITATIVE STUDIES
FROM OUR RESEARCH PROGRAM

I focus here on three studies that we have conducted on negative experiences. All three studies used CQR, as described above.

Misunderstandings

Rhodes, Hill, Thompson, and Elliott (1994) did a qualitative study of instances in which therapists or therapists-in-training felt misunderstood by their therapists. Of the 19 cases, 11 were resolved and 8 were unresolved, so we could look at differences between these two sets of cases to suggest factors associated with resolution.

In the resolved cases, before the misunderstanding event, clients typically said that they had a good relationship (e.g., felt safe, felt supported, could communicate negative feelings) with the therapist. In contrast, clients in the unresolved cases either mentioned a poor relationship (e.g., a rocky relationship, no empathic connection) or made no mention at all of the relationship.

The precipitant of the misunderstanding events in both the resolved and unresolved cases was that the therapist either did something that the client did not like (e.g., was critical of something the client did) or did not do something that the client wanted or expected (e.g., did not remember important facts). Thus, misunderstanding events were characterized by these clients as therapists being out of tune with or not responsive to the clients' needs.

Following the event, most clients in the resolved cases immediately asserted their dissatisfaction (e.g., told their therapists they felt criticized), although a few initially "went underground" (i.e., hid their negative reaction) and then later asserted their feelings. In response to the clients' assertions, therapists in the resolved cases sometimes accommodated clients by apologizing, accepting appropriate responsibility for the problem, or changing the offensive behavior (e.g., lateness). Likewise, clients sometimes accommodated the therapist by accepting the therapist's perspective or by deciding that the behavior was not all that egregious or relevant to therapy. After the immediate resolution of the event, most clients reported that they continued to work with their therapist to understand the misunderstanding event, and thus were able to grow from the experience. Clients also indicated that the therapeutic relationship was enhanced as a result of working through the misunderstanding event. Thus, it seemed that there was a mutual repair process, such that the therapist and client negotiated their relationship with some give and take on both parts.

An example of a resolved event is the following situation. A therapist who thought the client was intellectualizing interrupted the client and challenged her, asking what she was really feeling. The client immediately told the therapist that the interruption and challenge made her feel that "she had not been given a chance" and that she experienced the therapist as "abrupt, disrespectful, and admonishing." The therapist acknowledged that she had been too abrupt and indicated that something was going on for her personally that caused her to approach the client in such an abrupt and challenging manner. The therapist and client kept talking about this event over the next several months, trying to understand it. The client said that the event was important because "it addressed the issue of how I defend myself against my feelings in therapy, and it had an impact on our relationship, that is, I was able to express my negative feelings toward my therapist, and we were able to process these feelings in a helpful way." Importantly, this event occurred in the context of a generally good therapeutic relationship; the work was process-oriented, so the client was aware of the importance of processing the relationship and was used to dealing openly with problems in the relationship as they arose.

In contrast, in the unresolved cases, a few clients immediately asserted their dissatisfaction. Unfortunately, their therapists were not responsive but rather maintained their original stance without considering the client's viewpoint. In other cases, the clients "went underground" and never said anything to the therapists about their dissatisfaction. Not surprisingly, their therapists never knew about the clients' dissatisfaction and were unresponsive; these clients soon terminated the therapy.

From the results of the Rhodes et al. (1994) study, then, it appeared that it was important for the therapy dyad to have the foundation of a good relationship and then to negotiate and repair the relationship after the misunderstanding event. The client needed to assert his or her dissatisfaction and let the therapist know that there was a problem. The therapist had to listen, respect, and be responsive to the client's assertion and make accommodations. In particular, therapists apologized, took appropriate responsibility, and changed problematic behaviors.

Impasses

As a follow-up to the Rhodes et al. (1994) study, Hill, Nutt-Williams, Heaton, Thompson, and Rhodes (1996) interviewed each of 11 therapists about their experiences with a case where there was a therapeutic impasse (defined as a deadlock or stalemate) that resulted in the termination of therapy. The therapists reported that the impasse clients had considerable pathology (both Axis I and personality disorders), a history of problems with their families-of-origin, troubled current intimate relationships, and general interpersonal problems (dependency, guilt, anger, unassertiveness). For most of the cases, the therapists reported that the initial therapeutic relationship was limited and superficial (e.g., one therapist reported an underlying competitiveness even though the client was friendly on the surface) or poor (e.g., one client was angry and withholding, and there was a bad connection between the therapist and the client).

The impasse generally involved a lack of agreement about the goals and tasks of therapy (e.g., one client demanded but rejected the therapist's suggestions; another client was angry about the strategy that her therapist and daughter had developed to deal with her crisis). Rather than being a single event, these impasses thus involved general disagreement and power struggles related to the way that therapy should be conducted. According to the therapists, the clients were angry, impatient, contemptuous, upset, confused, and uncomfortable with the therapists. In addition, clients seemed to feel blamed, abandoned, and criticized by the therapists, as well as disappointed, hopeless, and discouraged about the lack of progress of the therapy. For their part, therapists reported feeling frustrated, confused, disappointed, angry, hurt, and incompetent. The therapists often spent a lot of time thinking about the impasses, trying to figure out what went wrong. Thus, these impasses involved a lot of negative emotions for both therapists and clients.

All but one therapist tried to discuss problems in the relationship with the clients, reengage them in therapy, and help them gain insight about the problems (e.g., one therapist tried to explore with the client what had happened, help the client understand the impasse in light of past and present relationships, and help the client reconceptualize the problem). A few therapists also became more active and directive and advised clients about what to do. Unfortunately, these strategies did not seem to work, and the therapeutic relationships continued to deteriorate and clients unilaterally terminated. Therapists were often caught off guard because they had not been aware of the extent of the clients' dissatisfaction.

All therapists indicated that one possible reason for the impasses was a therapist mistake of not providing the client with what he or she needed or wanted. They mentioned being too pushy or unsupportive (e.g., one therapist was disapproving, active, pushy, and expected too much of the client); too cautious or nondirective (e.g., one therapist thought that she should have helped the client explore her feelings more); unclear, changing strategies too much, or losing neutrality (e.g., one therapist thought that he might have confused the client when he shifted from an active to a neutral stance); or misdiagnosing the client (e.g., one therapist overestimated the client's strengths and did not recognize the depth of the client's pain). Other reasons for impasses were triangulation (i.e., the intrusion of other people into the therapeutic relationship such that the client had to choose between the therapist and the other person), transference issues (i.e., the client reacted strongly and negatively to the therapist, as she or he had to parents), and countertransference (i.e., personal issues of the therapist).

A comparison of the findings of the Hill et al. (1996) study with the Rhodes et al. (1994) study is striking. There is no mention in the Hill et al. study of the clients asserting their dissatisfaction or their feelings. And although the Hill et al. therapists did try to discuss and explore problems in the therapeutic relationship with clients, they did not seem to be aware of their possible mistakes until much later. In addition, these therapists did not apologize, accept responsibility, or change offending behaviors. They also used insight-oriented techniques that might have come across as distancing and intellectualizing, given that the relationship rupture had not been resolved (note that Cashdan [1988] suggested that insight only be approached much later after ruptures have been resolved).

Dealing with Angry Clients

Hill et al. (2003) interviewed 13 experienced therapists about their experiences in working with client anger. We suspected that experiences would be very different if clients hostilely expressed their anger directly to the therapist versus withholding their anger; so, we interviewed therapists about one case of each type.

Not surprisingly, therapists indicated that they had more difficulty working with clients who expressed hostile anger than with those who did not assert their anger. In addition, relationships were not as good with hostile as compared with unassertive cases. The precipitant of the event was most often a challenging therapist intervention in the hostile than unassertive cases, such that therapists tended to respond to client hostility with mutual hostility. Therapists also reported having more negative feelings (e.g., anxiety, incompetence, annoyance, frustration) in the hostile rather than unassertive cases. And therapists less often encouraged their clients to express and work through their feelings in the hostile rather than unassertive cases.

In addition, the resolution process proceeded somewhat differently in the hostile versus unasserted anger cases. Hostile cases were more often resolved when the client was not presenting problematic behaviors (e.g., acting out or pushing boundaries); therapists tended to feel anxious and angry in such situations and would challenge the clients, which resulted in negative interactions. In addition, resolution was more likely when therapists turned negative feelings outward (e.g., felt annoyed or frustrated at the client) instead of inward (e.g., felt anxious or incompetent); when therapists had a goal of connecting with the client, made a major effort to talk about the anger with the client, and provided an explanation for their own behaviors; and when therapists attributed the event to problems in the therapeutic relationship rather than to personality problems within the client.

An example of a resolved hostile event was a situation in which the therapist was 20 minutes late for a session and the client had to sit in the waiting room with another client, an obese woman eating a sausage in a manner that the client perceived to be rude and disgusting. When the session began, the client was furious and accused the therapist of using the obese woman as a confederate to test the client's ability to deal with anger. The therapist apologized for being late, explaining that she had had a crisis with the preceding client. The client accepted her apology, and they were able to talk about other situations in which the client became angry with others outside of therapy. The therapist also made a point of changing her behavior so that she was not late for sessions with this client again. It seemed important that this event occurred in the context of a good therapeutic relationship so the client could tolerate the processing of the event.

In terms of unasserted anger events, resolution was more likely when there was a good therapeutic relationship and when therapists raised the topic of anger and tried to help the client explore the anger and gain insight, particularly in relating the current anger to other situations. An example here of a resolved case is a situation in which there was a good therapeutic relationship and the client was particularly open, trusting, and motivated for therapy. When the client suddenly became very quiet and broke eye contact, the therapist commented about the quietness and asked the client what was going on. The client stated that she did not like the therapist's calling her mother "Mother" as if it were her name (e.g., "Mother did such, and so …") because it seemed too familiar. The client acknowledged that she easily became upset when talking about her mother. After exploring the situation, the client apologized for getting angry and expressed fear that the therapist would not see her any more if she expressed negative feelings toward her. The therapist reassured the client and encouraged her to talk about her feelings, which relieved the client and drew them closer together.

Thus, therapists were able to empathize with and encourage unassertive clients but became upset at hostile clients. It makes sense that therapists would feel more kindly toward unassertive clients who clearly need their help and that they might have difficulty being empathic with clients who lash out at them. Similarly, in the interpersonal circle (see Benjamin, 1974; Kiesler, 1996) friendliness begets friendliness and hostility begets hostility.

SUMMARY OF FINDINGS

Extracting insights from these studies, it appears that therapists have a great deal of difficulty working with negative events in therapy. Even therapists who are quite good at working with clients during productive times experience anxiety, self-doubt, and feelings of incompetence when faced with clients who are angry at them for some perceived mistake.

These findings also suggest that it is important for therapists to be aware of their inner emotions and then to actively acknowledge and work with clients to help them resolve the negative emotions. If therapists can actively work with clients on these relationship problems, the relationship is enhanced; so, it is important for therapists to learn what to do in these situations. Based on the findings of our qualitative studies, the following interventions seemed to be helpful for therapists for working with negative events:

- If therapists make a mistake, they can apologize, accept responsibility for the mistake, and change the offending behavior.
- If therapists are working with clients who express hostility, they can try to empathize and connect with these clients, help the clients talk about their anger, provide an explanation for their behavior to help clients understand it better, and attribute problems to relationship issues rather than to personality problems on the part of the clients.
- If clients do not overtly express anger but therapists suspect that the clients are angry, therapists can help clients explore the possible anger and relate the anger to other situations.

In contrast, it appears that it would be best for therapists to avoid

- being too pushy,
- being unsupportive,
- being too cautious,
- changing strategies too often,
- misdiagnosing clients,

- not being alert to the influence of other people on the therapeutic relationship, and
- not being alert to problems that arise in the transference and countertransference.

The results reported here for qualitative studies on negative experiences should be considered in conjunction with task analysis studies on rupture repair (see Eubanks-Carter, Muran, & Safran, Chapter 5, this volume; Safran, Muran, Samstag, & Stevens, 2002). In addition, readers are referred to the broader domain of studies involved in processing the therapeutic relationship (see review in Hill & Knox, 2009). In combination, these studies suggest that it is beneficial to directly address negative experiences that arise in the therapeutic relationship, although there is not yet agreement about best practices in this area.

FUTURE DIRECTIONS

Reflecting Bordin's (1979, 1994) ideas, I would assert that negative experiences are bound to occur in psychotherapy, which involves a human relationship between two people. What is important is to use these experiences for positive growth in therapy. Similarly, our goal as researchers is not only to document that negative experiences occur in therapy (with an emphasis on learning more about what types of negative experiences are most likely to occur in specific situations with different types of clients seen by different types of therapists) but also to learn more about what interventions help clients to grow and benefit once these negative experiences are uncovered. Our current work looking at corrective relational experiences in therapy (Berman et al., in press; Knox, Hill, Hess, Crook-Lyon, & Burkard, in press) may shed some light on these questions.

Relatedly, we need to train therapists in how to cope effectively when they have negative reactions in therapy and when they perceive that clients are having negative experiences in therapy. In a preliminary study, Hess, Knox, and Hill (2006) investigated three approaches to training (supervisor-facilitated learning, self-training, and biblio-training) for helping graduate trainees manage client anger directed at them. In a current study, we (Spangler et al., in preparation) are examining the effects of instruction, modeling, practice, and feedback (these components were used based on the review by Hill and Lent [2007] of the literature on training students in helping skills) in training undergraduate trainees in how to use immediacy (i.e., talking about the therapeutic relationship in the here-and-now). More studies are needed that assess the effects of training programs not only on progress in terms of trainees applying the skills—but also in terms of client change once the skills are applied (see also Hill & Lent, 2007).

REFERENCES

Benjamin, L. S. (1974). Structural analysis of social behavior. *Psychological Review*, *81*, 392–425.

Berman, M., Hill, C. E., Liu, J., Jackson, J., Sim, W., & Spangler, P. (in press). Corrective relational events in the treatment of three cases of anorexia nervosa. In L. G. Castonguay & C. E. Hill (Eds.), *Transformation in psychotherapy: Corrective experience across cognitive-behavioral, humanistic, and psychodynamic approaches*. Washington, DC: American Psychological Association.

Bordin, E. S. (1979). The generalizability of the psychoanalytic concept of the working alliance. *Psychotherapy: Theory, Research, and Practice*, *16*, 252–260.

Bordin, E. S. (1994). Theory and research on the therapeutic working alliance: New directions. In A. O. Horvath & L. S. Greenberg (Eds.), *The working alliance: Theory, research, and practice* (pp. 13–37). New York: Wiley.

Cashdan, S. (1988). *Object relations therapy: Using the relationship*. New York: Norton.

Castonguay, L. G., Goldfried, M. R., Wiser, S., Raue, P. J., & Hayes, A. M. (1996). Predicting the effect of cognitive therapy for depression: A study of unique and common factors. *Journal of Consulting and Clinical Psychology*, *64*, 497–504.

Dahlenberg, C. J. (2004). Maintaining the safe and effective therapeutic relationship in the context of distrust and anger: Countertransference and complex trauma. *Psychotherapy: Theory, Research, Practice, Training*, *41*, 438–447.

Hess, S., Knox, S., & Hill, C. E. (2006). Teaching graduate students how to manage client anger: A comparison of three types of training. *Psychotherapy Research*, *16*, 282–292.

Hill, C. E. (2005). Therapist techniques, client involvement, and the therapeutic relationship: Inextricably intertwined in the therapy process. *Psychotherapy: Theory, Research, Practice, Training*, *42*, 431–442.

Hill, C. E., Kellems, I. S., Kolchakian, M. R., Wonnell, T. L., Davis, T. L., & Nakayama, E. Y. (2003). The therapist experience of being the target of hostile versus suspected-unasserted client anger: Factors associated with resolution. *Psychotherapy Research*, *13*, 475–491.

Hill, C. E., & Knox, S. (2009). Processing the therapeutic relationship. *Psychotherapy Research*, *19*, 13–29.

Hill, C. E., Knox, S., Thompson, B. J., Williams, E. N., Hess, S., & Ladany, N. (2005). Consensual qualitative research: An update. *Journal of Counseling Psychology*, *52*, 196–205.

Hill, C. E., & Lent, R. W. (2006). A narrative and meta-analytic review of helping skills training: Time to revive a dormant area of inquiry. *Psychotherapy: Theory, Research, Practice, Training*, *43*, 154–172.

Hill, C. E., Nutt-Williams, E., Heaton, K. J., Thompson, B. J., & Rhodes, R.

H. (1996). Therapist retrospective recall of impasses in long-term psychotherapy: A qualitative analysis. *Journal of Counseling Psychology, 43,* 207–217.

Hill, C. E., Thompson, B. J., Cogar, M. M., & Denman, D. W., III. (1993). Beneath the surface of long-term therapy: Client and therapist report of their own and each other's covert processes. *Journal of Counseling Psychology, 40,* 278–288.

Hill, C. E., Thompson, B. J., & Corbett, M. M. (1992). The impact of therapist ability to perceive displayed and hidden client reactions on immediate outcome in first sessions of brief therapy. *Psychotherapy Research, 2,* 143–155.

Hill, C. E., Thompson, B. J., & Williams, E. N. (1997). A guide to conducting consensual qualitative research. *The Counseling Psychologist, 25,* 517–572.

Kiesler, D. J. (1996). *Contemporary interpersonal theory and research: Personality, psychopathology, and psychotherapy.* New York: Wiley.

Knox, S., Hill, C. E., Hess, S., Crook-Lyon, R. E., & Burkhard, A. W. (in press). Corrective relational experiences of therapists or therapists-in-training. In L. G. Castonguay & C. E. Hill (Eds.), *Transformation in psychotherapy: Corrective experience across cognitive-behavioral, humanistic, and psychodynamic approaches.* Washington, DC: American Psychological Association.

Martin, J., Martin, W., Meyer, M., & Slemon, A. (1986). Empirical investigation of the cognitive mediational paradigm for research on counseling. *Journal of Counseling Psychology, 33,* 115–123.

Martin, J., Martin, W., & Slemon, A. (1987). Cognitive mediation in person-centered and rational–emotive therapy. *Journal of Counseling Psychology, 34,* 251–260.

Piper, W. E., Ogrudniczuk, J. S., Joyce, A. S., McCallum, M., Rosie, J. S., O'Kelly, J. H., et al. (1999). Prediction of dropping out in time-limited, interpretive individual psychotherapy. *Psychotherapy: Theory, Research, Practice, Training, 36,* 114–122.

Regan, A. M., & Hill, C. E. (1992). An investigation of what clients and counselors do not say in brief therapy. *Journal of Counseling Psychology, 39,* 168–174.

Rennie, D. L. (1994). Clients' deference in psychotherapy. *Journal of Counseling Psychology, 41,* 427–437.

Rhodes, R., Hill, C. E., Thompson, B. J., & Elliott, R. (1994). Client retrospective recall of resolved and unresolved misunderstanding events. *Journal of Counseling Psychology, 41,* 473–483.

Safran, J. D., Muran, J. C., Samstag, L. W., & Stevens, C. (2002). Repairing alliance ruptures. In J. C. Norcross (Ed.), *Psychotherapy relationships that work: Therapist contributions and responsiveness to patients* (pp. 235–255). New York: Oxford University Press.

Spangler, P., Dunn, M., Hummel, A., Salahuddin, N., Walden, T., Liu, J., et al. (in preparation). Training undergraduate students in learning the skill of immediacy.

Thompson, B., & Hill, C. E. (1991). Therapist perceptions of client reactions. *Journal of Counseling and Development, 69,* 261–265.

CHAPTER 5

■　■　■　■　■

Alliance Ruptures and Resolution

Catherine Eubanks-Carter
J. Christopher Muran
Jeremy D. Safran

A number of studies have demonstrated that a strong alliance is a robust predictor of good outcome and that, conversely, weakened alliances are correlated with unilateral termination by the patient (Horvath & Bedi, 2002; Martin, Garske, & Davis, 2000; Samstag, Batchelder, Muran, Safran, & Winston, 1998; Samstag et al., 2008; Tryon & Kane, 1990, 1993, 1995; however, note that several studies of substance abuse patients have not demonstrated a clear and consistent relationship between alliance and outcome, e.g., Barber et al., 1999, 2001; Horvath & Bedi, 2002). Over the past two decades, a body of research has developed that explores what happens when there is a weakening in the quality of the alliance. Several terms have been used to describe this phenomenon: challenges (e.g., Harper, 1989a, 1989b), misunderstanding events (e.g., Rhodes, Hill, Thompson, & Elliott, 1994); impasses (e.g., Hill, Nutt-Williams, Heaton, Thompson, & Rhodes, 1996); alliance threats (e.g., Bennett, Parry, & Ryle, 2006); and markers of enactments (e.g., Safran, 2002). These moments are most commonly referred to as alliance "ruptures" (see Safran, Crocker, McMain, & Murray, 1990; Safran & Muran, 1996, 2000; Safran, Muran, & Samstag, 1994).

Research on alliance ruptures has been strongly influenced by Bordin's

(1979) conceptualization of the alliance as being composed of interdependent factors: the agreement between patient and therapist on the tasks and goals of treatment and the affective bond between patient and therapist. A rupture is a deterioration in the alliance, manifested by a lack of collaboration between patient and therapist on tasks or goals, or by a strain in the emotional bond. Although the word "rupture" connotes a major breakdown in the relationship, the term is also used to describe minor tensions of which one or both of the participants may be only vaguely aware (Safran et al., 1990). Ruptures can be obstacles to treatment and can contribute to patient dropout. However, successful resolution of a rupture can serve as a corrective emotional experience (Alexander & French, 1946), providing a powerful opportunity for therapeutic change. In this chapter, we review the existing body of research on alliance ruptures and rupture resolution. We highlight the different methodologies that have been employed in rupture research, and we suggest directions for future work in this growing area of study.

METHODS OF RESEARCHING ALLIANCE RUPTURES

Alliance ruptures and the processes by which they are resolved can be subtle and complex events that are not always transparent even to the patient and therapist who are involved. Accordingly, several different research methods have been employed in an effort to elucidate these phenomena. Qualitative methods have been employed to examine patients' and therapists' recountings of rupture events, most notably by Clara Hill, as described in Chapter 4 of this volume. Hill and colleagues' work points to the difficulties that therapists often have in identifying when a rupture is taking place. For example, they have found that therapists are often not aware of patient dissatisfaction with treatment and that therapists' failure to address patient dissatisfaction adequately can lead to patient termination (Hill et al., 1996; Rhodes et al., 1994).

In addition to qualitative analyses of reports of ruptures, rupture research has predominantly followed one of three methodological paradigms: (1) the task analytic paradigm, which has been used to develop and refine models of rupture resolution; (2) the randomized controlled trial (RCT) paradigm, used to test the effectiveness of particular rupture resolution interventions and treatments; and (3) the naturalistic observation paradigm, used to track the natural occurrence of rupture and resolution processes in therapy and to examine their relationships to outcome. In this chapter we review the research associated with each of these methodologies in turn and then discuss their strengths and weaknesses and summarize what they have contributed to our understanding of ruptures and rupture resolution.

TASK ANALYSIS OF RUPTURES AND THEIR RESOLUTION

The task analytic paradigm analyzes the processes involved in producing change (Greenberg, 1986; Rice & Greenberg, 1984; Safran, Greenberg, & Rice, 1988). Task analysis begins with a preliminary rational model based largely on clinical theory. This model is progressively refined and revised, based on the analysis of empirical data, ultimately yielding a rational–empirical model of the components of the performance of a particular task. Several researchers have employed this method to study the task of rupture resolution.

Although they did not identify their method as task analysis, one of the earliest studies of ruptures and resolution, conducted by Foreman and Marmar (1985), employed an approach that is consistent with the task analytic paradigm. Foreman and Marmar began by developing a list of therapeutic interventions that could be used to address a poor alliance. They then selected six cases of short-term dynamic therapy in which the early alliance was rated as poor by observers; in half of these cases the alliance remained weak and the outcome was poor, while in the other half the alliance improved and a good outcome was achieved. Coders rated the extent to which the identified interventions were employed in the two groups of cases and found that addressing and drawing links among the patient's defenses, guilt and expectation of punishment, and problematic feelings in relation to the therapist most strongly differentiated between good and poor outcome cases. The exploration of problematic feelings in the patient's other relationships did not differentiate between the two groups.

Safran, Muran, and colleagues built upon Foreman and Marmar's study by undertaking a more rigorous and intensive examination of the process of rupture resolution in a series of studies following the task analytic paradigm. In the first study (Safran et al., 1990), a pool of 29 patients being treated for depression or anxiety disorders with a 20-session protocol of integrative cognitive–interpersonal therapy (Safran, 1990a, 1990b; Safran & Segal, 1990) was identified. A subset of patients was selected from this pool, based on fluctuations in scores on six items from the Working Alliance Inventory (WAI; Horvath & Greenberg, 1989) that were administered to both patients and therapists after each session. Patients and therapists were asked to make alliance ratings for each third of the session; sessions in which the alliance scores for both patient and therapist dropped at least 20% from the first to the middle third of the session and then increased again at least 20% from the second to the final third, were selected as representing ruptures that were successfully resolved. Fifteen resolved rupture sessions from 10 cases were identified. After listening to audiotapes of these sessions, the researchers developed a preliminary stage process model of rupture resolution. The model was tested on another subset of cases drawn from the original pool and was subsequently revised (Safran et al., 1994). Safran and Muran (1996) tested the revised model by conducting confirmatory lag 1 sequential analyses, which found that all predicted sequences within model stages and between model stages emerged as statistically significant. Safran and Muran then conducted a replication study by using a new set of cases that were selected based on patient and therapist self-reports of ruptures. In support of the model, confirmatory lag 1 sequential analyses demonstrated a difference between resolution and nonresolution sessions. In addition, analyses confirmed the hypothesized sequence of events within stages of resolution sessions—but not the predicted sequences between stages. Based on close examination of the cases in the replication study, Safran and Muran made further revisions to the resolution model.

The current rupture resolution model (Safran & Muran, 2000) consists of four stages. In Stage 1, the therapist recognizes a rupture and tries to disengage from it by inviting the patient to explore the event. In Stage 2, the therapist and patient explore the nuances of their perceptions of the rupture. Exploration can lead the patient to become concerned that the therapist will reject him or her; this concern often leads the patient to try to avoid further exploration of the rupture event. In Stage 3, the therapist and patient explore avoidance maneuvers and their function. In Stage 4, the therapist and patient move toward clarifying the wish or need that underlies the patient's problematic interpersonal behaviors. For example, a patient who desires intimacy but fears rejection may distance him- or herself from the therapist in an effort at self-protection. Clarification of the underlying wish for closeness enables the patient to recognize and understand how he or she is relating to others and to identify more effective ways to achieve his or her interpersonal goals.

The nature of the clarification in Stage 4 usually differs, based on the type of rupture. Safran and Muran (1996) categorized rupture markers into two overarching subtypes of withdrawal and confrontation, using Harper's coding system (1989a, 1989b). These two subtypes can be differentiated by drawing on Horney's (1950) neurotic trends. In withdrawal ruptures, the patient either moves *away* from the therapist (e.g., by avoiding the therapist's questions) or else *toward* the therapist, but in a way that denies an aspect of the patient's experience (e.g., by being overly deferential and appeasing). In confrontation ruptures, the patient moves *against* the therapist, either by expressing anger or dissatisfaction in a non-collaborative manner (e.g., hostile complaints about the therapist or the treatment) or by trying to pressure or control the therapist (e.g., making demands of the therapist). In the resolution of a withdrawal rupture, clarifying the underlying wish or need involves helping the patient move from qualified to clearer expressions of self-assertion (e.g., the patient learns to tell the therapist what he or she needs from him or her). Confrontation ruptures, by contrast, often begin with the patient asserting a complaint; clarifying the underlying wish or need involves helping the patient to gain access to more vulnerable feelings, such as a fear that one cannot be helped. Throughout, the therapist maintains an open, nondefensive posture and demonstrates a willingness to acknowledge and explore how he or she also contributes to ruptures in the alliance.

Building on the work of Safran and Muran and colleagues, three additional teams of researchers have developed similar rupture resolution procedures that use the task analytic paradigm. Agnew, Harper, Shapiro, and Barkham (1994) tested a psychodynamic–interpersonal model of resolution of confrontation ruptures by using one good outcome case of eight-session psychodynamic–interpersonal therapy from the Sheffield study of treatment for depression. One rupture and one resolution session were selected, based on changes in alliance scores, and confrontation rupture markers in those sessions were identified by using Harper's coding system (Harper, 1989a). Similar to Safran and Muran's model, Agnew et al.'s model begins the resolution process with acknowledgment of the rupture, followed by collaborative exploration of the rupture in order to reach a shared understanding with the patient. However, while Safran and Muran's model depicts resolution as a progression toward clarification of the patient's underlying wish or need, Agnew et al. place greater focus on linking the alliance rupture to situations outside of therapy and discussing new ways to handle those situations.

Bennett et al. (2006) used task analysis to examine rupture resolution in six cases of cognitive-analytic therapy (CAT; Ryle, 1997) for borderline personality disorder. Rupture sessions were selected based on deviations in scores on the Therapy Experience Questionnaire (TEQ; Ryle, 1995). Judges, who were experienced CAT therapists, listened to audiotapes of the sessions and identified ruptures and resolutions; these were then used to refine a rational model of rupture resolution. Consistent with Safran and Muran's research, Bennett et al. found that in good outcome cases therapists recognized and focused attention on the majority of ruptures while in poor outcome cases they usually failed to notice or draw attention to the alliance threat. Bennett et al. also stressed a collaborative, nondefensive stance on the part of the therapist. However, in contrast to Safran and Muran's focus on the immediate process and progressive clarification of the patient's underlying needs, Bennett et al. placed greater emphasis on linking the rupture to a preestablished case formulation and to the patient's other relationships.

Aspland, Llewelyn, Hardy, Barkham, and Stiles (2008) used task analysis to refine a preliminary model of rupture resolution in cognitive-behavioral therapy (CBT). They examined ruptures and resolution in two positive-outcome cases of CBT for depression from the Second Sheffield Psychotherapy Project (Shapiro et al., 1994). Cases were identified based on changes in alliance scores, following the naturalistic observation method employed by Stiles et al. (2004), which will be discussed later in this chapter. For each of the two cases, a rupture session (when the alliance score dropped) and a resolution session (when the alliance score improved) were selected. Using transcripts, experienced clinicians identified confrontation and withdrawal markers, following Harper's (1994) and Safran and Muran's (2000) descriptions of these types of ruptures, as well as resolution markers. After close examination of rupture and resolution markers, the preliminary rupture resolution model was revised. Aspland et al. (2008) observed that most ruptures appeared to arise from unvoiced disagreements about the tasks and goals of therapy, which led to negative complementary interactions in which the therapist focused on the task and the patient withdrew. Resolution occurred when therapists shifted their focus from the therapy task to issues that were salient for the patient. Consistent with Safran and Muran, Aspland et al. emphasized the therapist's collaborative stance. However, in contrast to Safran and Muran, as well as Agnew et al. (1994) and Bennett et al. (2006), Aspland et al.'s final resolution model did not include any overt recognition or discussion of the rupture itself, because none of the therapists in their sample employed this strategy. The Aspland et al. model is an example of an *indirect* approach to rupture resolution, in contrast to the *direct* strategies described in the other models (Safran & Muran, 2000).

RCTs OF RUPTURE RESOLUTION INTERVENTIONS

Recognizing the negative impact that unresolved ruptures can have on treatment outcome, several researchers have followed the randomized controlled trials paradigm to investigate whether integrating rupture resolution techniques can improve the efficacy of a particular treatment. With the RCT approach, an integrative rupture resolution treatment is compared to another treatment, such as treatment as usual or treatment by the therapist prior to receiving rupture resolution training. If the rupture resolution treatment is determined to be more effective, then this finding provides indirect support for the resolution techniques and rupture resolution model that undergird the treatment.

An early example of the RCT approach is the set of Vanderbilt studies conducted by Strupp, Henry, and colleagues. In the Vanderbilt I study, Henry, Schacht, and Strupp (1986) found that therapists responded to patients' negative feelings by expressing their own negative feelings in a defensive fashion. Concerned by this evidence of therapists' difficulties with managing alliance ruptures, in the Vanderbilt II study the researchers developed and tested a manualized time-limited dynamic therapy that aimed to reduce expression of therapist hostility toward difficult patients by focusing on the management of interpersonal patterns in the therapeutic relationship (Henry, Schacht, Strupp, Butler, & Binder, 1993; Henry, Strupp, Butler, Schact, & Binder, 1993; Strupp, 1993). However, the results were contrary to expectations in that therapists trained in this modality manifested an increase in hostile messages toward clients as well as complex communications that could be interpreted as either helpful or critical, or both. They also tended to be less warm and friendly and to express more negative attitudes.

The findings of the Vanderbilt studies demonstrated how difficult it can be to train therapists to resolve alliance ruptures. The authors observed that therapists seemed to adhere to manuals in a rigid fashion that interfered with their normally supportive style (Henry, Strupp, et al., 1993). Similarly, Castonguay, Goldfried, Wiser, Raue, and Hayes's (1996) study of cognitive therapy for depression and Piper and colleagues' (Piper, Azim, Joyce, & McCallum, 1991; Piper et al., 1999) and Schut et al.'s (2005) studies of psychodynamic therapy have found evidence that some therapists attempt to resolve ruptures by increasing their adherence to a theoretical model (e.g., challenging distorted cognitions in cognitive therapy or making transference interpretations in dynamic therapy). These studies found that high adherence in the context of a rupture was linked to poor outcome and premature termination.

However, there is also evidence that training therapists in manualized approaches that emphasize the formation and maintenance of a strong alliance may improve some therapists' abilities to manage alliance ruptures successfully. Hilsenroth and colleagues (Hilsenroth, Ackerman, Clemence, Strassle, & Handler, 2002) examined the effect of providing structured training in short-term dynamic psychotherapy to graduate student clinicians. The training included a focus on a therapeutic model of assessment that sought to incorporate collaborative goal setting and the development of a therapeutic bond into the assessment phase of treatment. Analysis of alliance ratings made after the third or fourth session of therapy found that the structured training was associated with higher alliance scores (as rated by both patients and therapists) than a standard supervision condition.

In a study by Bambling and colleagues (2006), the impact of therapeutic alliance-focused supervision was evaluated on the performance of 127 therapists conducting an eight-session problem solving treatment with 127 depressed patients. The therapists were randomly assigned to either a no supervision control group or one of two supervision conditions: (1) skill-focused supervision (which focused on providing therapists with concrete advice about how to enhance the alliance, and (2) process-focused supervision (which focused on helping therapists develop greater awareness of interpersonal processes impacting on the alliance during the session). The results indicated differences in treatment outcome for patients treated by therapists in the two different alliance-focused supervision groups. Patients treated by unsupervised therapists, however, had significantly poorer outcomes than those treated by therapists in either of the two supervision conditions.

In a pilot study, Crits-Christoph and colleagues (2006) found support for training therapists in alliance-fostering therapy, a 16-session treatment for depression that combines psychodynamic–interpersonal interventions with alliance-focused techniques such as responding to ruptures directly by encouraging patients to express their underlying feelings and the interpersonal issues connected to them (see Crits-Christoph, Crits-Christoph, & Connolly Gibbons, Chapter 15, this volume, for more details). Crits-Christoph et al. found that the training resulted in increases in alliance scores that were moderate to large in size but not statistically significant, as well as small improvements in depressive symptoms and larger improvements in quality of life. However, there was variability among the therapists in the study, with one therapist showing decreased alliance scores after the training.

Beginning in the early 1990s, Safran and Muran developed a short-term alliance-focused psychotherapy treatment informed by their findings from task analytic work and brief relational therapy, and tested its effectiveness (BRT; Muran & Safran, 2002; Safran & Muran, 2000; Safran, 2002). By closely attending to ruptures, therapists and patients in BRT work collaboratively to identify and understand the patient's problematic interpersonal patterns and to experiment in the session with new ways of interacting. The emphasis in BRT is on helping the patient to develop a generalizable skill of awareness, or mindfulness, often through the use of metacommunication, in which the therapist explicitly draws the patient's attention to the interpersonal patterns that are emerging in the patient–therapist interaction.

Muran, Safran, and colleagues conducted an RCT comparing BRT, CBT, and a short-term dynamic therapy in a sample of 128 patients with Cluster C personality disorders and personality disorder not otherwise specified (Muran, Safran, Samstag, & Winston, 2005; see also Muran, 2002). This study found that BRT was as effective as CBT and short-term dynamic therapy on standard statistical analyses of change and was more successful than the other two treatments with respect to retention. With another sample of patients with personality disorders, Safran, Muran, Samstag, and Winston (2005) reported additional evidence that BRT successfully keeps challenging patients engaged in therapy. In the first phase of the Safran et al. study, 60 patients were randomly assigned to short-term dynamic therapy or CBT, and their progress was monitored. Eighteen treatment failures were identified on the basis of a number of empirically defined criteria. In the second phase of the study, these identified patients were offered the opportunity to change treatments. The 10 patients who agreed to the change were randomly assigned either to BRT or to a control condition (the other standard treatment, CBT or dynamic therapy). Results showed that all 5 patients reassigned to CBT or dynamic therapy and 7 of the 8 patients who declined reassignment terminated treatment prematurely. By contrast, only

1 of the 5 patients reassigned to BRT dropped out of treatment. One BRT patient ended treatment early in order to accept a job offer in another country; this patient appeared to be progressing toward a good outcome. The three patients who completed BRT all achieved good outcomes.

While Safran, Muran, and colleagues continue to investigate the effectiveness of BRT, they are also exploring ways to integrate relational alliance-focused principles into standard cognitive therapy. Currently, a study funded by the National Institute of Mental Health (Muran, Safran, Gorman, Eubanks-Carter, & Banthin, 2008) is under way to see if integrating rupture resolution training into CBT training improves therapy process and outcome. Similar efforts to integrate rupture resolution into CBT have been conducted by Castonguay, Constantino, Newman, and colleagues In an effort to improve cognitive therapists' ability to respond to alliance ruptures, Castonguay developed integrative cognitive therapy for depression (ICT; Castonguay, 1996), which integrates Safran and Muran's rupture resolution strategies (Safran & Muran, 2000; Safran & Segal, 1990) as well as strategies developed by Burns (1989) into traditional cognitive therapy. When ruptures are identified, the therapist breaks from the cognitive therapy protocol and addresses the rupture by inviting the patient to explore the rupture, empathizing with the patient's emotional reaction, and reducing the patient's anger or dissatisfaction by validating negative feelings or criticisms and taking at least partial responsibility for the rupture. In a pilot study, Castonguay et al. (2004) found that patient symptom improvement was greater in ICT than in a wait-list condition and compared favorably to previous findings for CT. In a randomized trial comparing ICT to CT, Constantino et al. (2008) found that ICT patients had greater improvement on depression and global symptoms and more clinically significant change than CT patients. ICT also yielded better patient-rated alliance quality and therapist empathy, and there was a trend toward better patient retention in ICT than in CT.

A similar effort to integrate rupture resolution strategies into CBT for generalized anxiety disorder (GAD) was undertaken by Newman, Castonguay, Borkovec, Fisher, and Nordberg (2008). The researchers tested the efficacy of an integrative treatment package consisting of CBT and an interpersonal/emotional processing module that included rupture resolution methods drawn from Safran and Muran's work (Safran & Muran, 2000) and emotion-focused interventions influenced by the work of Greenberg and Safran (1987) and Greenberg, Rice, and Elliot (1993). The study found that the integrative treatment significantly decreased GAD symptoms, yielding a higher effect size than the average effect size of CBT for GAD in the treatment literature. Participants also showed clinically significant improvements in GAD symptoms and interpersonal problems, with continued gains at 1-year follow-up.

NATURALISTIC OBSERVATION
OF RUPTURES AND RESOLUTION

The third main method of researching alliance ruptures is naturalistic observation. With this method, researchers observe the natural occurrence of ruptures and rupture resolution in psychotherapy and examine the link between these phenomena and outcome. Although task analytic and RCT studies may use naturalistic observation methods to identify rupture and resolution markers, their aims are different. Task analytic studies aim to refine and confirm a rational model of the resolution process, and RCT studies aim to demonstrate the superiority of a particular treatment or form of training; naturalistic observation studies, by contrast, focus on simply observing a process and clarifying its relationship to outcome. Naturalistic observation includes three methods for identifying ruptures and resolutions: direct patient and therapist self-reports of ruptures and resolutions, observer-based measures to identify ruptures and resolutions, and indirect self-reports based on measures of the overall alliance.

Direct Self-Report Methods

Muran et al. (2009) applied the naturalistic observation approach to data from their RCT comparing BRT, CBT, and short-term dynamic therapy (Muran et al., 2005). After each session, patients and therapists completed postsession questionnaires (PSQ; Muran, Safran, Samstag, & Winston, 1992) that included self-report measures of the alliance as well as self-report indices measuring the occurrence of ruptures, rupture intensity, and the extent to which ruptures were resolved. They found that ruptures occurred frequently across the three therapy treatments: during the first six sessions of treatment, ruptures were reported by 37% of patients and 56% of therapists. Ruptures were also found to be significantly related to outcome. Higher rupture intensity, as reported jointly by patients and therapists, was associated with poor outcome on measures of interpersonal functioning. Failure to resolve these ruptures was predictive of dropout.

Eames and Roth (2000) also administered the PSQ to 11 therapists and 30 of their patients receiving treatment as usual at outpatient clinics in the United Kingdom. Similar to Muran et al. (2009), they found that therapists reported ruptures more often, reporting them in 43% of sessions, while patients reported them in 19%. They also examined the relationship between report of ruptures and patient attachment style and found a significant positive correlation between preoccupied attachment style and therapist report of ruptures and a negative correlation between dismissing attachment dimension and therapist report of ruptures.

Observer-Based Methods

The differences between patient and therapist self-reports of ruptures noted above and also presented in Table 5.1 are consistent with findings that patients usually give higher alliance ratings than therapists (e.g., Barber et al., 1999; Fitzpatrick, Iwakabe, & Stalikas, 2005; Hatcher, Barends, Hansell, & Gutfreund, 1995; Kivlighan & Shaughnessy, 1995; Mallinckrodt & Nelson, 1991). This discrepancy may be due to the "theoretical lens"

TABLE 5.1. Prevalence of Alliance Ruptures and Rupture–Repair Sequences

Study	n	Method of detecting ruptures	Frequency of ruptures
Colli & Lingiardi (2009)	16 patients, 32 sessions	Observer-based	Indirect ruptures: 100% of sessions Direct ruptures: 43% of sessions Therapist negative interventions: 31% of sessions
Eames & Roth (2000)	30 patients, Sessions 2–5	Direct self-report, patient Direct self-report, therapist	19% of sessions 43% of sessions
Eubanks-Carter, Mitchell, Muran, & Safran (2010)	20 patients, 48 sessions	Direct self-report, patient Observer-based	35% of sessions Withdrawal ruptures: 100% of sessions Confrontation ruptures: 75% of sessions
Muran, Safran, Gorman, Samstag, Eubanks-Carter, et al. (2009)	128 patients, Sessions 1–6	Direct self-report, patient Direct self-report, therapist	37% of cases 56% of cases
Sommerfeld, Orlach, Zim, & Mikulincer (2008)	5 patients, 151 sessions	Direct self-report, patient Observer-based	42% of sessions 77% of sessions
Stevens, Muran, Safran, Gorman, & Winston (2007)	44 patients	Indirect self-report	Rupture–repair sequences: 50% of cases
Stiles, Glick, Osatuke, Hardy, Shapiro, et al. (2004)	79 patients	Indirect self-report	Rupture–repair sequences: 21.5% of cases
Strauss, Hayes, Johnson, Newman, Brown, et al. (2006)	25 patients	Indirect self-report	Rupture–repair sequences: 56% of cases

through which therapists view the relationship (Horvath, 2000; see also Muran et al., 2009). However, the difference between patient and therapist perspectives of the alliance also raises the concern that patients may underreport ruptures due to a lack of awareness of them or discomfort with acknowledging them. One way to address this problem is to use observer-based methods to detect ruptures and resolution processes.

An early example of the use of an observer-based method is Lansford's (1986) exploratory study of "weakenings" in the therapeutic alliance in six cases of time-limited dynamic therapy. Using audiotapes of the sessions, raters identified ruptures and repairs and then examined the relationship between the occurrence of ruptures and treatment outcome. The study found that the most successful outcomes were associated with patients and therapists who actively dealt with alliance ruptures.

Sommerfeld, Orbach, Zim, and Mikulincer (2008) directly examined the difference between patient self-report of ruptures and observer-based report. In a study of 151 sessions from five patients in psychodynamic therapy, patients completed a brief version of the PSQ that included items from the Session Evaluation Questionnaire (SEQ; Stiles, 1980) that assessed the depth of the session. Patients reported ruptures in 42% of the sessions. Using transcripts of these same sessions, judges identified confrontation and withdrawal ruptures by using Harper's coding system (1989a, 1989b); rupture markers were identified by observers in 77% of sessions. There was no significant association between the observer and client perspectives. Sommerfeld et al. also found that sessions where both patient and observer saw a rupture were rated as having greater depth by the patient. As ruptures that are identified by both self-report and observer report are likely ones that are explicitly discussed in the session, this finding suggests that patients find therapy more helpful when therapists are sensitive to subtle indications of ruptures and encourage patients to explore them. Sommerfeld et al. (2008) also found a significant association between the occurrence of ruptures and the appearance of dysfunctional interpersonal schemas involving the therapist, identified by using the CCRT method (Luborsky & Crits-Christoph, 1998). This finding suggests that when ruptures occur dysfunctional interpersonal schemas are likely to be active; thus, ruptures provide critical opportunities to identify, explore, and change patients' self-defeating patterns of thought and behavior.

Colli and Lingiardi (2009) have developed a transcript-based method of assessing alliance ruptures and resolutions, the Collaborative Interaction Scale (CIS). A strength of the CIS is that it assesses both patients' and therapists' positive and negative contributions to the therapeutic process. The CIS has also demonstrated good interrater reliability with graduate student raters (Colli & Lingiardi, 2009). The patient rupture markers and therapist intervention items were largely derived from the work of Safran, Muran, and colleagues, in particular the Rupture Resolution Scale developed by

Samstag, Safran, and Muran (2000) and the therapist resolution strategies described by Safran and Muran (2000). A study of 32 session transcripts from 16 patients receiving either cognitive or psychodynamic psychotherapy revealed significant correlations between negative therapist interventions (e.g., showing hostility) and patient rupture markers. Positive therapist interventions (e.g., focusing on the here-and-now of the relationship) were correlated with both collaborative patient processes (e.g., talking about feelings or thoughts) and with indirect rupture markers, in which the patient indirectly expresses a form of emotional disengagement from the process, similar to a withdrawal rupture.

Given that most observer-based methods for coding ruptures and resolutions rely on the use of transcripts (e.g., Colli & Lingiardi, 2009; Sommerfeld et al., 2008) or the use of highly experienced clinicians as judges (e.g., Aspland et al., 2008; Bennett et al., 2006), Eubanks-Carter, Muran, and Safran (2009) developed a coding system that does not require transcription of sessions and can be used by beginning graduate student raters. The Rupture Resolution Rating System (3RS) draws on Harper's (1989a, 1989b) manuals for coding confrontation and withdrawal ruptures as well as the Rupture Resolution Scale developed by Samstag et al. (2004). Preliminary findings from the 3RS are consistent with Sommerfeld et al.'s (2008) evidence of a discrepancy between lower patient self-report of ruptures and higher observer report. In a pilot study of 48 sessions from early treatment of 20 CBT cases (Eubanks-Carter, Mitchell, Muran, & Safran, 2010), while patients reported ruptures in only 35% of sessions, observers detected withdrawal rupture markers in every session and confrontation rupture markers in 75% of sessions. Studies examining the relationship between ruptures detected by the 3RS and treatment outcome are currently under way.

Indirect Self-Report

In addition to observer-based measures, another way to detect ruptures without relying on patients' and therapists' ability and willingness to directly self-report alliance problems is to use indirect self-report methods. These methods involve having participants complete measures of the overall alliance and then identifying ruptures and resolutions based on fluctuations in alliance scores. As noted above, early task analytic studies (e.g., Agnew et al., 1994; Safran et al., 1990, 1994) used fluctuations in alliance scores to identify rupture and resolution sessions. Over the past decade, more sophisticated methods, described below, have been developed. These methods grew out of work on patterns of alliance development and their association with outcome (e.g., Golden & Robbins, 1990; Kivlighan & Shaughnessy, 1995, 2000; Kramer, de Roten, Beretta, Michel, & Despland, 2008; Kramer, de Roten, Beretta, Michel, & Despland, 2009; Patton, Kivlighan, & Multon, 1997).

Stiles and colleagues (2004) were not able to replicate Kivlighan and

Shaughnessy's (2000) findings that a U-shaped (high–low–high) alliance pattern over time was predictive of good outcome. Thus, they shifted their focus from the global alliance pattern to the examination of discrete high–low–high or V-shaped rupture–repair episodes. Stiles et al. (2004) identified rupture–repair sequences using criteria based on shape-of-change parameters calculated for each patient's profile of patient-reported alliance scores on the Agnew Relationship Measure (ARM; Agnew-Davies, Stiles, Hardy, Barkham, & Shapiro, 1998). In a sample of 79 clients receiving either CBT or psychodynamic–interpersonal therapy for depression, Stiles et al. identified rupture–repair episodes in 17 (21.5%) of the cases. The authors examined the relationship between this rupture–repair profile and outcome and found that this group of patients averaged larger gains than the rest of the sample, suggesting that the process of resolving ruptures contributes to good outcome.

Following Stiles et al., Strauss et al. (2006) sought to identify rupture–repair episodes in a sample of 30 patients with avoidant and obsessive–compulsive personality disorders who received up to a year of CT. Strauss et al. developed different criteria for rupture and resolution sessions, looking for fluctuations in scores on the California Psychotherapy Alliance Scale (CALPAS; Marmar, Weiss, & Gaston, 1989) that were at least as large as the mean standard deviation of alliance scores across the sample. Of the 25 patients with at least three alliance assessments, Strauss et al. identified rupture–repair sequences in 14 cases (56%), and, similar to Stiles, they found that these patients reported greater symptom reduction than patients who did not experience rupture–repair episodes.

Stevens, Muran, Safran, Gorman, and Winston (2007) also developed criteria for identifying rupture–repair sequences from fluctuations in WAI scores: ruptures were defined as decreases of at least 1.00 on the WAI, and were deemed to be resolved if the alliance score rose to within 0.25 points of the prerupture score in three to five sessions. Using a sample of 44 patients drawn from the personality disorder cases examined in Muran et al. (2005) and Muran et al. (2009), Stevens et al. (2007) found that rupture–repair sequences were very common, appearing in 50% of the cases. However, in contrast to Stiles et al. (2004) and Strauss et al. (2006), the presence of rupture–repair episodes was not significantly related to treatment outcome.

In addition to the foregoing criterion-based approaches to identifying ruptures and resolution from alliance scores, Eubanks-Carter, Gorman, & Muran (2009) have identified methods from fields as diverse as economics, epidemiology, climatology, and manufacturing and have demonstrated how they can be employed to detect changes in the alliance. Through the use of sophisticated software programs, these methods permit researchers to analyze change across large samples and examine the extent to which the field's current understanding of how ruptures develop and how they are resolved generalizes across different patient and therapist populations.

SUMMARY AND FUTURE DIRECTIONS

Research on alliance ruptures and resolution has demonstrated that these are common clinical phenomena that can pose significant challenges to therapists (see Table 5.1) but can also provide opportunities for therapeutic change. The body of rupture research is small, and the use of small samples, different clinical populations and treatments, and varying methods of identifying rupture and resolution markers place limits on the generalizability of the findings. However, there are several points of consensus across the studies. First, the findings from most of the task analytic studies (Agnew et al., 1994; Bennett et al., 2006; Safran & Muran, 1996) and the RCT studies support the value of therapists openly acknowledging and exploring ruptures rather than avoiding or ignoring them. Consistent with this conclusion, the naturalistic observation findings linking rupture resolution to good outcome provide further support for the view of ruptures as opportunities for positive change when managed appropriately.

A second point of consensus across a number of studies is the importance of therapists maintaining an open and nondefensive stance in the context of ruptures. The task analytic models emphasize the need for therapists to be willing to accept responsibility for their contributions to ruptures. The findings from the Vanderbilt studies and other related research demonstrating the negative impact of therapist rigidity in the context of ruptures offer more support for therapist awareness of the role they play in creating and maintaining ruptures.

An area where there is lack of consensus among approaches to rupture resolution is the question of whether therapists should try to link alliance ruptures to parallel situations in the patient's other relationships (e.g., Agnew et al., 1994; Bennett et al., 2006) or they should maintain a focus on the patient–therapist interaction (e.g., Foreman & Marmar, 1985; Safran et al., 1994). Future research could examine these two approaches to see whether one is consistently more effective or whether the appropriate choice depends on the clinical situation. Patient variables such as diagnosis or attachment style (e.g., Eames & Roth, 2000) and therapist variables such as personality characteristics or theoretical orientation (see Aspland et al., 2008) may influence what kinds of ruptures occur and which resolution processes are most effective. The coding systems developed by Harper (1989a, 1989b) have made a significant contribution to the field's ability to identify patient behaviors that mark ruptures. However, as the Vanderbilt studies and other research have demonstrated, therapists can play an important role in the emergence of alliance strains. The use of measures such as the CIS, which includes therapist rupture markers, to examine the relationships between therapist behaviors and the development of alliance ruptures would be a valuable next step.

Although most research on alliance ruptures supports the explicit exploration of ruptures, as noted above, Aspland et al.'s (2008) findings of the value of indirect means to achieve resolution are worthy of further examination. Task analytic studies have examined resolution processes through the lens of the authors' preliminary models; this approach may have led researchers to prefer direct resolution therapeutic techniques over indirect methods as well as resolution strategies initiated by patients. Naturalistic observation studies that identify where resolution has occurred without reliance on a particular resolution model, and then trace the events that preceded resolution, may offer new insights into previously unexamined therapist *and* patient behaviors that contribute to rupture resolution.

The small but growing body of research on alliance ruptures and resolution has benefited from close and careful attention to process, particularly as exemplified by the task analytic studies. As the field pursues methods to study the occurrence and resolution of ruptures in larger samples through clinical trials of rupture–resolution treatments and large-scale natural observation studies, it is our hope that the ethos of the task analytic model will continue to wield influence: research as an iterative process, with theory sharpening the focus of empirical investigation and empirical results refining and grounding the theory—partners in constant dialogue and negotiation.

REFERENCES

Agnew, R. M., Harper, H., Shapiro, D. A., & Barkham, M. (1994). Resolving a challenge to the therapeutic relationship: A single-case study. *British Journal of Medical Psychology*, 67, 155–170.

Agnew-Davies, R., Stiles, W. B., Hardy, G. E., Barkham, M., & Shapiro, D. A. (1998). Alliance structure assessed by the Agnew Relationship Measure (ARM). *British Journal of Clinical Psychology*, 37, 155–172.

Alexander, F., & French, T. M. (1946). *Psychoanalytic therapy*. New York: Ronald Press.

Aspland, H., Llewelyn, S., Hardy, G. E., Barkham, M., & Stiles, W. (2008). Alliance ruptures and rupture resolution in cognitive-behavior therapy: A preliminary task analysis. *Psychotherapy Research*, 18, 699–710.

Bambling, M., King, R., Raue, P., Schweittzer, R., & Lambert, W. (2006). Clinical supervision: Its influence on client-rated working alliance and client symptom reduction in the brief treatment of major depression. *Psychotherapy Research*, 16, 317–331.

Barber, J. P., Luborsky, L., Crits-Christoph, P., Thase, M. E., Weiss, R., Frank, A., et al. (1999). Therapeutic alliance as a predictor of outcome in treatment of cocaine dependence. *Psychotherapy Research*, 9, 54–73.

Barber, J. P., Luborsky, L., Gallop, R., Crits-Christoph, P., Frank, A., Weiss, R. D., et al. (2001). Therapeutic alliance as a predictor of outcome and retention in the National Institute on Drug Abuse Collaborative Cocaine Treatment Study. *Journal of Consulting and Clinical Psychology*, 69, 119–124.

Bennett, D., Parry, G., & Ryle, A. (2006). Resolving threats to the therapeutic alliance in cognitive analytic therapy of borderline personality disorder: A task analysis. *Psychology and Psychotherapy: Theory, Research, and Practice, 79,* 395–418.

Book, H. (1988). *How to practice brief psychodynamic psychotherapy: The core conflictual relationship theme method.* Washington, DC: American Psychological Association.

Bordin, E. (1979). The generalizability of the psychoanalytic concept of the working alliance. *Psychotherapy: Theory, Research, and Practice, 16,* 252–260.

Burns, D. D. (1989). *The feeling good handbook.* New York: William Morrow.

Castonguay, L. G. (1996). *Integrative cognitive therapy for depression treatment manual.* Unpublished manuscript, The Pennsylvania State University, University Park, PA.

Castonguay, L. G., Goldfried, M. R., Wiser, S., Raue, P., & Hayes, A. M. (1996). Predicting outcome in cognitive therapy for depression: A comparison of unique and common factors. *Journal of Consulting and Clinical Psychology, 64,* 497–504.

Castonguay, L. G., Schut, A. J., Aikins, D., Constantino, M. J., Lawrenceau, J. P., Bologh, L., et al. (2004). Repairing alliance ruptures in cognitive therapy: A preliminary investigation of an integrative therapy for depression. *Journal of Psychotherapy Integration, 14,* 4–20.

Colli, A., & Lingiardi, V. (2009). The Collaborative Interactions Scale: A new transcript-based method for the assessment of therapeutic alliance ruptures and resolutions in psychotherapy. *Psychotherapy Research, 19,* 718–734.

Constantino, M. J., Marnell, M. E., Haile, A. J., Kanther-Sista, S. N., Wolman, K., Zappert, L., et al. (2008). Integrative cognitive therapy for depression: A randomized pilot comparison. *Psychotherapy: Theory, Research, Practice, Training, 45,* 122–134.

Crits-Christoph, P., Gibbons, M. B., Crits-Christoph, K., Narducci, J., Schamberger, M., & Gallop, R. (2006). Can therapists be trained to improve their alliances?: A preliminary study of alliance-fostering psychotherapy. *Psychotherapy Research, 16,* 268–281.

Eames, V., & Roth, A. (2000). Patient attachment orientation and the early working alliance—a study of patient and therapist reports of alliance quality and ruptures. *Psychotherapy Research, 10,* 421–434.

Eubanks-Carter, C., & Gorman, B. S. (2009). *New methods for detecting change in the alliance.* Manuscript in preparation.

Eubanks-Carter, C., Gorman, B. S., & Muran, J. C. (2010). *Quantitative naturalistic methods for detecting change points in psychotherapy research.* Manuscript submitted for publication.

Eubanks-Carter, C., Mitchell, A., Muran, J. C., & Safran, J. D. (2010). *Development of a new observer-based system for rating confrontation and withdrawal rupture markers and rupture resolution strategies.* Manuscript in preparation.

Eubanks-Carter, C., Muran, J. C., & Safran, J. D. (2009). *Rupture Resolution Rating System (3RS): Manual.* Unpublished manuscript, Beth Israel Medical Center, New York.

Fitzpatrick, M. R., Iwakabe, S., & Stalikas, A. (2005). Perspective divergence in the working alliance. *Psychotherapy Research, 15,* 69–79.

Foreman, S. A., & Marmar, C. R. (1985). Therapist actions that address initially poor therapeutic alliances in psychotherapy. *American Journal of Psychiatry*, *142*, 922–926.

Golden, B. R., & Robbins, S. B. (1990). The working alliance within time-limited therapy. *Professional Psychology: Research and Practice, 21*, 476–481.

Greenberg, L. S. (1986). Change process research. *Journal of Consulting and Clinical Psychology, 54*, 4–11.

Greenberg, L. S., Rice, L. N., & Elliott, R. (1993). *Facilitating emotional change: The moment-by-moment process.* New York: Guilford Press.

Greenberg, L. S., & Safran, J. D. (1987). *Emotion in psychotherapy.* New York: Guilford Press.

Harper, H. (1989a). *Coding Guide I: Identification of confrontation challenges in exploratory therapy.* Sheffield, UK: University of Sheffield.

Harper, H. (1989b). *Coding Guide II: Identification of withdrawal challenges in exploratory therapy.* Sheffield, UK: University of Sheffield.

Harper, H. (1994). *The resolution of client confrontation challenges in exploratory psychotherapy: Developing the new paradigm in psychotherapy research.* Unpublished doctoral dissertation, University of Sheffield, Sheffield, UK.

Hatcher, R. L., Barends, A., Hansell, J., & Gutfreund, M. J. (1995). Patients' and therapists' shared and unique views of the therapeutic alliance: An investigation using confirmatory factor analysis in a nested design. *Journal of Consulting and Clinical Psychology, 63*, 636–643.

Henry, W. P., Schacht, T. E., & Strupp, H. H. (1986). Structural analysis of social behavior: Application to a study of interpersonal process in differential psychotherapeutic outcome. *Journal of Consulting and Clinical Psychology, 54*, 27–31.

Henry, W. P., Schacht, T. E., Strupp, H. H., Butler, S. F., & Binder, J. L. (1993). Effects of training in time-limited dynamic psychotherapy: Mediators of therapists' responses to training. *Journal of Consulting and Clinical Psychology, 61*, 441–447.

Henry, W. P., Strupp, H. H., Butler, S. F., Schacht, T. E., & Binder, J. L. (1993). Effects of training in time-limited dynamic psychotherapy: Changes in therapist behavior. *Journal of Consulting and Clinical Psychology, 61*, 434–440.

Hill, C. E., Nutt-Williams, E., Heaton, K. J., Thompson, B. J., & Rhodes, R. H. (1996). Therapist retrospective recall of impasses in long-term psychotherapy: A qualitative analysis. *Journal of Counseling Psychology, 43*, 207–217.

Hilsenroth, M. J., Ackerman, S. J., Clemence, A. J., Strassle, C. G., & Handler, L. (2002). Effects of structured clinician training on patient and therapist perspectives of alliance early in psychotherapy. *Psychotherapy: Theory, Research, Practice, Training, 39*, 309–323.

Horney, K. (1950). *Neurosis and human growth.* New York: Norton.

Horvath, A. O. (2000). The therapeutic relationship: From transference to alliance. *Journal of Clinical Psychology, 56*, 163–173.

Horvath, A. O., & Bedi, R. P. (2002). The alliance. In J. C. Norcross (Ed.), *Psychotherapy relationships that work* (pp. 37–70). New York: Oxford University Press.

Horvath, A. O., & Greenberg, L. S. (1989). Development and validation of the Working Alliance Inventory. *Journal of Counseling Psychology, 36*, 223–233.

Kivlighan, D. M., & Shaughnessy, P. (1995). Analysis of the development of the working alliance using hierarchical linear modeling. *Journal of Counseling Psychology, 42,* 338–349.

Kivlighan, D. M., & Shaughnessy, P. (2000). Patterns of working alliance development: A typology of client's working alliance ratings. *Journal of Counseling Psychology, 47,* 362–371.

Kramer, U., de Roten, Y., Beretta, V., Michel, L., & Despland, J.-N. (2008). Patient's and therapist's views of early alliance building in dynamic psychotherapy: Patterns and relation to outcome. *Journal of Counseling Psychology, 55,* 89–95.

Kramer, U., de Roten, Y., Beretta, V., Michel, L., & Despland, J.-N. (2009). Alliance patterns over the course of short-term dynamic psychotherapy: The shape of productive relationships. *Psychotherapy Research, 19,* 699–706.

Lansford, E. (1986). Weakenings and repairs of the working alliance in short-term psychotherapy. *Professional Psychology: Research and Practice, 17,* 364–366.

Luborsky, L. (1984). *Principles of psychoanalytic psychotherapy: A manual for supportive/expressive treatment.* New York: Basic Books.

Luborsky, L., & Crits-Christoph, P. (1998). *Understanding transference: The Core Conflictual Relationship Theme Method* (2nd ed.). Washington, DC: American Psychological Association.

Mallinckrodt, B., & Nelson, M. L. (1991). Counselor training level and the formation of the psychotherapeutic working alliance. *Journal of Counseling Psychology, 38,* 133–138.

Marmar, C. R., Weiss, D. S., & Gaston, L. (1989). Toward the validation of the California Therapeutic Alliance Rating System. *Psychological Assessment, 1,* 46–52.

Martin, D. J., Garske, J. P., & Davis, M. K. (2000). Relation of the therapeutic alliance with outcome and other variables: A meta-analytic review. *Journal of Consulting and Clinical Psychology, 68,* 438–450.

Muran, J. C. (2002). A relational approach to understanding change: Plurality and contextualism in a psychotherapy research program. *Psychotherapy Research, 12,* 113–138.

Muran, J. C., & Safran, J. D. (2002). A relational approach to psychotherapy. In F. W. Kaslow (Ed.), *Comprehensive handbook of psychotherapy* (pp. 253–281). New York: John Wiley.

Muran, J. C., Safran, J. D., Gorman, B. S., Samstag, L. W., Eubanks-Carter, C., & Winston, A. (2009). The relationship of early alliance ruptures and their resolution to process and outcome in three time-limited psychotherapies for personality disorders. *Psychotherapy: Theory, Research, Practice, Training, 46,* 233–248.

Muran, J. C., Safran, J. D., Gorman, B. S., Eubanks-Carter, C., & Banthin, D. (2008, June). *Identifying ruptures and their resolution from postsession self-report measures.* In J. C. Muran (Chair), *Recent developments in rupture resolution research.* Panel conducted at the annual meeting of the Society for Psychotherapy Research, Barcelona, Spain.

Muran, J. C., Safran, J. D., Samstag, L. W., & Winston, A. (1992). *Patient and therapist postsession questionnaires, Version 1992.* Beth Israel Medical Center, New York.

Muran, J. C., Safran, J. D., Samstag, L. W., & Winston, A. (2005). Evaluating an alliance-focused treatment for personality disorders. *Psychotherapy: Theory, Research, Practice, Training, 42,* 532–545.

Newman, M. G., Castonguay, L. G., Borkovec, T. D., Fisher, A. J., & Nordberg, S. S. (2008). An open trial of integrative therapy for generalized anxiety disorder. *Psychotherapy: Theory, Research, Practice, Training, 45*, 135–147.

Patton, M. J., Kivlighan, D. M., & Multon, K. D. (1997). The Missouri Psychoanalytic Counseling Research Project: Relation of changes in counseling process to client outcomes. *Journal of Counseling Psychology, 44*, 189–208.

Piper, W. E., Azim, H., Joyce, A. S., & McCallum, M. (1991). Transference interpretations, therapeutic alliance, and outcome in short term individual psychotherapy. *Archives of General Psychiatry, 48*, 946–953.

Piper, W. E., Ogrodniczuk, J. S., Joyce, A. S., McCallum, M., Rosie, J. S., O'Kelly, J. G., et al. (1999). Prediction of dropping out in time-limited, interpretive individual psychotherapy. *Psychotherapy, 36*, 114–122.

Rhodes, R., Hill, C., Thompson, B., & Elliott, R. (1994). Client retrospective recall of resolved and unresolved misunderstanding events. *Counseling Psychology, 41*, 473–483.

Rice, L. N., & Greenberg, L. S. (1984). *Patterns of change: Intensive analysis of psychotherapy process.* New York: Guilford Press.

Ryle, A. (1995). Transference and counter-transference variations in the course of cognitive-analytic therapy of two borderline patients: The relation to the diagrammatic reformulation of self-states. *British Journal of Medical Psychology, 68*, 109–124.

Ryle, A. (1997). *Cognitive analytic therapy and borderline personality disorder: The model and the method.* Chichester, UK: Wiley.

Safran, J. D. (1990a). Towards a refinement of cognitive therapy in light of interpersonal theory: I. Theory. *Clinical Psychology Review, 10*, 87–105.

Safran, J. D. (1990b). Towards a refinement of cognitive therapy in light of interpersonal theory: II. Practice. *Clinical Psychology Review, 10*, 107–121.

Safran, J. D. (2002). Brief relational psychoanalytic treatment. *Psychoanalytic Dialogues, 12*, 171–195.

Safran, J. D., Crocker, P., McMain, S., & Murray, P. (1990). Therapeutic alliance rupture as a therapy event for empirical investigation. *Psychotherapy: Theory, Research, and Practice, 27*, 154–165.

Safran, J. D., Greenberg, L. S., & Rice, L. N. (1988). Integrating psychotherapy research and practice: Modeling the change process. *Psychotherapy, 25*, 1–17.

Safran, J. D., & Muran, J. C. (1996). The resolution of ruptures in the therapeutic alliance. *Journal of Consulting and Clinical Psychology, 64*, 447–458.

Safran, J. D., & Muran, J. C. (2000). *Negotiating the therapeutic alliance: A relational treatment guide.* New York: Guilford Press.

Safran, J. D., Muran, J. C., & Samstag, L. W. (1994). Resolving therapeutic alliance ruptures: A task analytic investigation. In A. O. Horvath & L. S. Greenberg (Eds.), *The working alliance: Theory, research, and practice* (pp. 225–255). New York: Wiley.

Safran, J. D., Muran, J. C., Samstag, L. W., & Winston, A. (2005). Evaluating alliance-focused intervention for potential treatment failures: A feasibility study and descriptive analysis. *Psychotherapy: Theory, Research, Practice, Training, 42*, 512–531.

Safran, J. D., & Segal, Z. V. (1990). *Interpersonal process in cognitive therapy.* New York: Basic Books.

Samstag, L. W., Batchelder, S. T., Muran, J. C., Safran, J. D., & Winston, A. (1998). Early identification of treatment failures in short-term psychotherapy: An assessment of therapeutic alliance and interpersonal behavior. *Journal of Psychotherapy Practice and Research, 7*, 126–143.

Samstag, L. W., Muran, J. C., Wachtel, P. L., Slade, A., Safran, J. D., & Winston, A. (2008). Evaluating negative process: A comparison of working alliance, interpersonal behavior, and narrative coherency among three psychotherapy outcome conditions. *American Journal of Psychotherapy, 62*, 165–194.

Samstag, L. W., Safran, J. D., & Muran, J. C. (2000). *Rupture Resolution Scale and Coding Manual.* Unpublished manuscript, Beth Israel Medical Center, New York.

Schut, A. J., Castonguay, L. G., Flanagan, K. M., Yamasaki, A. S., Barber, J. P., Bedics, J. D., et al. (2005). Therapist interpretation, patient–therapist interpersonal process, and outcome in psychodynamic psychotherapy for avoidant personality disorder. *Psychotherapy: Theory, Research, Practice, Training, 42*, 494–511.

Shapiro, D. A., Barkham, M., Rees, A., Hardy, G. E., Reynolds, S., & Startup, M. (1994). Effects of treatment duration and severity of depression on the effectiveness of cognitive-behavioral and psychodynamic interpersonal psychotherapy. *Journal of Consulting and Clinical Psychology, 62*, 522–534.

Sommerfeld, E., Orbach, I., Zim, S., & Mikulincer, M. (2008). An in-session exploration of ruptures in working alliance and their associations with clients' core conflictual relationship themes, alliance-related discourse, and clients' postsession evaluation. *Psychotherapy Research, 18*, 377–388.

Stevens, C. L., Muran, J. C., Safran, J. D., Gorman, B. S., & Winston, A. (2007). Levels and patterns of the therapeutic alliance in brief psychotherapy. *American Journal of Psychotherapy, 61*, 109–129.

Stiles, W. B. (1980). Measurement of the impact of psychotherapy sessions. *Journal of Consulting and Clinical Psychology, 48*, 176–185.

Stiles, W. B., Glick, M. J., Osatuke, K., Hardy, G. E., Shapiro, D. A., Agnew-Davies, R., et al. (2004). Patterns of alliance development and the rupture–repair hypothesis: Are productive relationships U-shaped or V-shaped? *Journal of Counseling Psychology, 51*, 81–92.

Strauss, J. L., Hayes, A. M., Johnson, S. L., Newman, C. F., Brown, G. K., Barber, J. P., et al. (2006). Early alliance, alliance ruptures, and symptom change in a nonrandomized trial of cognitive therapy for avoidant and obsessive–compulsive personality disorders. *Journal of Consulting and Clinical Psychology, 74*, 337–345.

Strupp, H. H. (1993). The Vanderbilt Psychotherapy Studies: Synopsis. *Journal of Consulting and Clinical Psychology, 61*, 33–36.

Tryon, G. S., & Kane, A. S. (1990). The helping alliance and premature termination. *Counselling Psychology Quarterly, 3*, 233–238.

Tryon, G. S., & Kane, A. S. (1993). Relationship of working alliance to mutual and unilateral termination. *Journal of Counseling Psychology, 40*, 33–36.

Tryon, G. S., & Kane, A. S. (1995). Client involvement, working alliance, and type of therapy termination. *Psychotherapy Research, 5*, 189–198.

PART II

. . . . .

PRACTICE AND THE THERAPEUTIC ALLIANCE

CHAPTER 6

■ ■ ■ ■ ■

A Psychodynamic Perspective on the Therapeutic Alliance

Theory, Research, and Practice

Stanley B. Messer
David L. Wolitzky

Our aim in this chapter is to present the history, current theoretical status, empirical standing, and practice implications of the concept of the therapeutic alliance in psychodynamic psychotherapy. We start with a historical overview highlighting the controversies surrounding the therapeutic alliance and discuss it in relation to the nature of the therapeutic action of psychoanalytic treatment. We then review the empirical literature to indicate its implications for empirically based psychodynamic therapy with adults.

CONCEPTUAL FACTORS

Historical Introduction

From early on, Freud (1913) understood that the uncovering work he considered essential to successful psychoanalytic treatment required an attitude of collaboration and cooperation between patient and therapist. Locating this attitude within the "unobjectionable positive transference" (Freud, 1912a, p. 105), "rapport" was the term Freud used to refer to this important aspect of the patient–therapist relationship. He called it the "vehicle for success" in treatment, which need not, and probably should not, be analyzed.

To foster the rapport necessary for a patient to be receptive to his or her interpretations and other interventions, the therapist had to (1) show a serious interest in the patient, (2) clear away the resistances, (3) count on the patient associating the therapist with at least one affectionate, benign figure from his past, (4) maintain an attitude of sympathetic understanding, (5) avoid a moralistic stance, and (6) not advocate for some contending third party. We now know that, even with these factors in place, patients will vary in the degree to which they *feel* the rapport, how long it will take for it to develop, and how closely the therapist has to adhere to the conditions listed above for an effective alliance to take hold. In any case, these six factors contribute to what has come to be called the "therapeutic alliance."

Perhaps the major theoretical change since Freud concerning the role of the therapeutic alliance is the current emphasis on its curative aspects per se, compared to the earlier view of the alliance as a precondition for the main curative factor, namely, interpretations leading to insight. In this regard, there has been significant empirical research that supports the idea that the skill with which the therapist fosters the alliance and handles its inevitable ruptures makes an essential contribution to the success of the treatment (e.g., Safran & Muran, 2000).

The early elaboration of the therapeutic alliance construct saw it as occurring between the analyst's analyzing function and the patient's capacity and willingness to identify with this function by engaging in the self-reflection that the analyst encouraged. Both patient and therapist were expected to oscillate flexibly between experiencing and reflecting on their experience. Sterba (1934) described this as a split in the ego between an "experiencing ego" and a "self-reflective ego." On the therapist's side, he or she should be able to immerse him- or herself empathically in the patient's psychic reality but also be able to step back from that stance and reflect on the possible meanings of the patient's experiences. The patient, likewise, needs to verbalize his or her experiences and periodically, either spontaneously and/or in response to the therapist's interventions, take him- or herself as an object and reflect on the meanings of his or her experiences. Viewed in this manner, this aspect of the analytic work, in the context of mutual agreement on tasks and goals (Bordin, 1979), contributes to a good alliance, which in turn facilitates the patient's receptivity to the analyst's insight-promoting interpretations.

Various Terms for the Therapeutic Alliance

Terms for the therapeutic alliance have varied, and each has been based on similar, but differently nuanced, conceptualizations. The different terms used include the "therapeutic alliance" (Zetzel, 1956, 1966), the "working alliance" (Greenson, 1965), the "treatment alliance" (Sandler, Dare, & Holder, 1992), and the "helping alliance" (Luborsky, 1976, 1984). In a pantheoretical conceptualization, Bordin (1979) differentiated three components of the therapeutic alliance—agreement on goals, assignment of tasks, and development of a bond. Relatively speaking, Greenson's concept is closer to the goals and tasks components identified by Bordin (1979), whereas Zetzel's (1956, 1966) formulation is more focused on the development of a therapeutic bond and the role of "ego identification" and trust in that development. Greenson's concept of "working alliance" would seem to imply that agreement on goals and taking on the responsibilities of being a patient presupposes a degree of trust in the therapist's good intentions and a sense of common purpose. Luborksy (1984, p. 79) has used the term "helping alliance" to refer to "the degree to which the patient experiences the relationship with the therapist as helpful or potentially helpful in achieving the patient's goals in psychotherapy." As is well known, he has provided empirical evidence that a positive helping alliance, measured early in treatment, correlates with a favorable therapy outcome (Luborsky, 1994).

Although there are conceptual distinctions to be made among these various terms used to refer to the therapeutic alliance, for ease of exposition, we will use these terms interchangeably or simply refer to the "therapeutic alliance" or "the alliance." We should note that the alliance concept, as has been the case with many constructs that originated in psychodynamic therapy, has found its way into a variety of therapies, including cognitive-behavioral therapy (Gilbert & Leahy, 2007).

Alliance, Transference, and the Real Relationship

Many authors have attempted to demarcate three overlapping components of the analytic relationship—the transference, the alliance, and the real relationship (Meissner, 2007). The traditional concept of "transference" refers to the patient's distortions of the analyst based on his or her own neurotic issues (Greenson, 1967), although Gill (1994) takes issue with the view of transference as a "distortion".) The "alliance" refers to the mutual collaboration of patient and therapist in the therapeutic tasks. The "real relationship" refers to transactions and attitudes based on veridical perceptions of the analyst. Greenson and Wexler (1969) believed it was important to recognize and to acknowledge the transference-free aspects of the therapy relationship. They note that dealing with nontransference reactions might involve "non-interpretive or non-analytic interventions" but maintain that such interventions are not "anti-analytic" (Greenson & Wexler, 1969, p. 28). An interesting implication of these statements is that an exclusive reliance on transference interpretation and a consequent failure to accord due recognition to the realistic aspects of the relationship could actually "stifle" the transference and interfere with the "maturation" of the patient's non-distorted perceptions of the analyst. We see here an implicit concern with iatrogenic (i.e., therapy-induced) transference reactions that cannot readily be analyzed and the suggestion that there be greater mutuality in the therapy relationship.

The idea of greater mutuality in the context of the inevitably and irreducibly asymmetrical nature of the therapy relationship has been a major emphasis of the American relational movement (Aron, 1996). The therapist wants to be experienced as a "good enough" new object so that the patient can have a "corrective emotional experience" (Alexander & French, 1946). Freudian analysts influenced by Strachey (1934) also realize that their transference interpretations are more effective if the patient regards the analyst as a new object as well as an old one but do not seem to think they need to make special efforts to achieve this aim.

The object relations view regards the therapeutic alliance as more of an inherently curative factor in a good therapeutic relationship. In this approach, the quality of the dyadic interaction is always at the forefront of analytic attention. Here we concur with Wallerstein (2003, p. 395), who noted with regard to the therapeutic alliance that

> within other theoretical perspectives in psychoanalysis (Kleinian, British object relational, etc.), the concept has never seemed useful at all, probably because two-person approaches to the therapeutic situation have no need of an alliance concept which emerged within ego psychology specifically to take account of the "real" interaction between the patient and the second person, the analyst.

Gill (1994) suggested that many traditional analysts have been wary of the alliance concept, or more specifically its technical implications, because it entails a "somewhat grudging concession" (p. 40) that the analytic situation involves a "two-person relationship" in which the analyst is as much a participant as an observer. In a similar vein, Gill (1994) further noted his belief that "the rise to explicit prominence of the alliance concept was an attempt to correct what had come to be considered the overly rigid, withdrawn, silent stance of the analyst" (p. 41). Gill (1994) claims the analyst cannot, and should not try to, remain a detached observer who somehow takes a position outside the interaction. This claim is especially true if the analyst is attempting to actively foster an alliance and not just waiting silently for the unfolding of the transference. For example, whether one explains to the patient the rationale for not answering questions or just chooses to remain silent, one is engaging in an interaction with the patient. In other words, silence is as much a form of interaction as speaking, a point

Gill (1994) made repeatedly. Insofar as traditional analysts tried to limit their interactions to interpretations, active facilitation of the therapeutic alliance was done reluctantly, partly out of a desire (misguided, we believe) not to contaminate the field of observation.

Greenson's Conception of the "Working Alliance"

Formulated during the 1960s, Greenson's views are presented here not only for historical reasons but because the issues he raised more than four decades ago have continued to be actively discussed and debated. The contemporary relevance of Greenson's views is evidenced by the fact that in 2008 the *Psychoanalytic Quarterly* reprinted his original article with commentaries by Cooper (2008) and Goldberger (2008).

Given the limited success of some psychoanalytic treatments, Greenson (1965, 1967), influenced by Zetzel's (1956) concept of the "therapeutic alliance" and Stone's (1961) critique of the excessively austere atmosphere of the psychoanalytic situation, emphasized the importance of what he called the "working alliance." Greenson (1967, p. 102) defines the working alliance as "the relatively nonneurotic, rational rapport which the patient has with his analyst. It is this reasonable and purposeful part of the feelings the patient has for the analyst which makes for the *working alliance*."

According to Greenson (1967, p. 102), the bases for the working alliance are (1) the "patient's motivation to overcome his illness," (2) "his sense of helplessness," (3) "his conscious and rational willingness to cooperate," and (4) "his ability to follow the instructions and insights of the analyst." A history of good-quality object relationships facilitates the establishment and maintenance of a decent working alliance. Here, Zetzel's notion of "therapeutic alliance" is relevant in that she stresses the desirability of the analyst, like a good mother, to show "intuitive adaptive responses" (Zetzel, 1966, p. 92) to patients' anxieties and deficiencies in basic trust stemming from a poor history of early relationships. She suggests that the initial phase of the treatment is preliminary to the analysis proper, "an essential prerequisite to the analytic process itself" (Zetzel, 1966, p. 99). For Zetzel, the alliance is *both* a precondition for fostering the analytic process and is therapeutic in its own right insofar as the patient develops a special object relationship to the therapist with whom he or she comes to identify.

Following Sterba (1934), Greenson (1967, p. 102) saw the alliance as one between the "reasonable ego" of the patient and the "analyst's analyzing ego." The patient's ability to maintain a working alliance depends on his or her ability to effect a split between the "experiencing ego" and the "observing ego." For example, even in the midst of an intense transference reaction, the patient needs to be able to step back from that reaction and reflect on its motives and meanings.

Greenson (1967, p. 103) made a point that has sparked controversy concerning the usefulness of distinguishing between the working alliance and the transference. He states that the "differentiation between transference reactions and working alliance is not an absolute one since the working alliance may contain elements of the infantile neurosis which will eventually require analysis." For example, insofar as the patient's cooperative attitude is based on a desire to win the analyst's love and/or an overidealization of the analyst, it likely will become an issue that needs to be analyzed. There are, however, differences of opinion in how long, or to what degree, an idealizing transference should be analyzed.

One has to appreciate that by the late 1950s classical psychoanalytic treatment was regarded by many as being carried out in an unnecessarily depriving atmosphere, with the analyst taking an excessively remote, aloof stance in relation to the patient, based on the (misguided) assumption that this would prevent transference gratification and thereby make the transference more analyzable. Thus, Stone (1961) and Greenson (1967) felt the need to speak out in favor of the "humanness" of the analyst as being as important as his or her analyzing function. They argued that an unwavering pursuit of insight oblivious to the analytic atmosphere would be counterproductive with any patient, but especially with more disturbed patients. Greenson (1967, p. 243) wrote:

> Essentially the humanness of the analyst is expressed in his compassion, his concern, and his therapeutic intent toward his patient. It matters to him how the patient fares, he is neither just an observer nor a research worker. ... The humanness is also expressed in the attitude that the patient has rights and is to be respected as an individual. He is to be treated with ordinary courtesy; rudeness has no place in psychoanalytic therapy. If we want the patient to work with us as a co-worker on the regressive material he produces, we must take care that the mature aspects of the patient are consistently nurtured in the course of our analytic work.

The technical implication of this view, which it was apparently necessary to articulate in 1967, is that we recognize the inherent asymmetry of the analytic relationship and not do anything to exacerbate it further.

It follows from this view that the analyst should express empathy for the pain imposed by the analytic situation, that he or she explain the procedures of the analysis and their rationale (e.g., the reasons for asking for "free associations," for not offering reassurance, and for preferring the patient be on the couch). Although Greenson was not worried that such an approach would provide undue gratification for the patient, he did suggest that "there must be a predominance of deprivation" (Greenson, 1967, p. 216) in order to foster a regressive transference neurosis.

As Richards and Lynch (2008) note, among traditional analysts, the issue of the relative importance of insight versus the therapeutic benefits of the relationship per se, not just as a precondition for insight, has been an ongoing dialectic since the 1930s. Is attachment preliminary to understanding, or is a good object relationship that is implied by a strong alliance a therapeutic element in its own right? Sterba, Strachey, Gitelson, and others dealt with this issue at the Marienbad symposium of 1936 (Glover, 1937; Strachey, 1937) and the Edinburgh symposium of 1961 (Gitelson, 1962). Strachey's (1934) now classic article on the therapeutic action of psychoanalysis stressed the relational factor of the analyst's benign, accepting attitude as essential in reducing the harshness of the patient's superego.

Meissner (2007) asserts that the therapeutic alliance is often poorly understood or ignored in conceptions of psychotherapy, maintaining that it is "indispensable in all forms of therapy" (Meissner, 2007, p. 231) as well as in all healing contexts (e.g., medical treatment, forensic psychiatry, child treatment, supervision). In the context of psychoanalytic therapy, Meissner cites Strachey's (1934, p. 502) classic paper that suggests that "the introjected, reasonable analyst, reconstituted within the superego, becomes the beneficent agent of cure." Meissner regards this change as definitely attributable to a good alliance.

Meissner's (2007) account of the therapeutic alliance includes multiple factors—the therapeutic contract (e.g., time, frequency of sessions, fee, and boundaries), authority (i.e., the analyst as the facilitator of the therapy process), empathy (which he regards as the *"sine qua non* of analytic work" (p. 234), trust, autonomy and initiative, freedom (the patient's voluntary participation in the process), neutrality, abstinence, and ethical considerations (e.g., confidentiality). This conceptualization of the therapeutic alliance is much broader than those that focus on the collaborative aspects of the relationship in developing specific goals and in pursuing the general goal of exploration. Although the elements cited by Meissner are relevant to the therapeutic alliance, to define it so broadly makes it harder to differentiate it from the real relationship. Furthermore, it is not clear to what extent these factors need to be present at the outset in order for the alliance to form versus the extent to which they are outcomes of a good therapeutic alliance. For example, it makes sense to think that some modicum of trust facilitates the development of a good alliance. However, it is less clear that abstinence (i.e., reticence) on the part of the therapist should be regarded as one of the "inherent qualities of the alliance" (Meissner, 2007, p. 235) or as contributing to a positive alliance. In fact, for some patients the therapist's emotional restraint could induce a negative alliance.

THE ALLIANCE CONCEPT: CONTROVERSY AND CRITIQUE

The idea of an alliance between patient and therapist has had both a long and, at times, controversial history in psychoanalysis. Several writers, most notably Brenner (1979), disagree with the concept and implications of the working or therapeutic alliance, seeing it as an avoidance of and substitute for analytic work. They claim that an emphasis on the alliance leads to unanalyzed transference gratification and inhibition in the expression of negative attitudes toward the analyst. For example, Brenner (1979) takes issue with a case report by Zetzel (1956) regarding an anxious woman who felt disappointed in the fee she was charged, expecting it to be lower. Zetzel (1956) approvingly noted that when the analyst became less silent and recognized the patient's anxiety she felt better. Instead of accepting this as evidence for the analyst's less rigid, more "human attitude" (Zetzel, 1966, p. 99), Brenner chided Zetzel for not relying on interpretation of the patient's feelings about the fee (e.g., feeling deprived or victimized), which he believed would have been more productive. In other words, Brenner questions whether it is desirable to distinguish the therapeutic alliance from transference, let alone take measures to foster the therapeutic alliance before, or instead of, interpreting the transference.

Brenner offers a similar critique in his review of some of Greenson's (1965) cases. He argues that case material offered by Greenson in which the latter shows how disruptions or deficiencies in the working alliance present obstacles to understanding and insight are best regarded not as failures in fostering the alliance but as failures in alertness to interpreting conflicts responsible for impairments in the alliance. He concludes, "I am convinced by all the available evidence that the concepts of therapeutic alliance and working alliance ... are neither valid nor useful" (Brenner, 1979, p. 149). An often cited example he presents concerns the question of reacting to a patient's loss of a loved one. In everyday life, the ordinary human inclination and response to learning of the death of a significant person in the patient's life is to express sympathy for the patient's loss. Brenner (1979) advises restraint in this regard. He writes: "For an analyst to express sympathy for a patient who has just lost a close relative may make it more difficult than it would otherwise be for the patient to express pleasure or spite or exhibitionistic satisfaction over the loss" (p. 152). In other words, "In analysis, it is best for the patient if one approaches *everything* analytically" (emphasis in original) (p. 150).

Several other critics of the therapeutic alliance concept have raised the same concerns (e.g., Adler & Bachant, 1998; Curtis, 1979; Kanzer, 1975; Stein, 1981), namely, that *an emphasis on fostering and safeguarding the alliance runs the risk of failing to recognize and to analyze subtle transference reactions and gratifications*. As Adler and Bachant (1998, p. 208) stated it, "The alliance cannot be exempt from examination or isolated from the analytic process." And, "There is an *inherent risk* that in deepening the therapeutic alliance, the emotional enticement of gratifying union will draw the analytic couple away from the rigors of further interpretive work" (Adler & Bachant, 1998, p. 208, emphasis added). They suggest that "the place of love in the analytic relationship is ubiquitous," and that there is a "pull to live out, rather than analyze, relational dynamics" that is "ever compelling"; therefore, an emphasis on understanding is necessary as "an essential safeguard of the patient's autonomy" (p. 208).

What does this view imply? It suggests that these authors fear that the analyst–patient dyad will not want to interrupt the pleasures of collaborative dialogue to explore the possible neurotic elements in it. For example, suppose the phone rings during a session. An irate patient who storms out would be seen as overreacting, based perhaps on experiencing the disruption as the intrusion of an unwelcome rivalrous sibling. An underreaction in which the patient continues talking as though not disturbed in any way by the intrusion might be harder to detect because the continuation of the collaborative dialogue is also desired by the analyst. In a similar vein, Stein (1981) warns that the supposedly "unobjectionable positive transference" might not be so unobjectionable. For example, the "good" patient who is following the rules of the analysis might be partly doing so out of motives to compete with other, unseen patients (siblings) and become the analyst's favorite patient, to use but one of many examples to illustrate this point. After all, as Freud (1916–1917, p. 455) pointed out in trying to account for the patient's motivation to cooperate in the analysis, "What turns the scale in his struggle is not intellectual insight—which is neither strong enough nor free enough for such achievement—but simply and solely his relationship to the doctor." The degree to which one should analyze this motivational base for the patient's cooperation, versus capitalizing on it by allowing it to remain silent until it becomes a resistance, is an open empirical question.

In a similar vein, whether it will be harder to explore dynamic issues when the patient has experienced some degree of transference gratification is an empirical question. Non-Freudian contemporary analysts (e.g., relational analysts) are not very concerned about this possibility. In fact, many would say that the greater danger is excessive frustration of transference wishes, as such deprivation could lead to iatrogenic regression, especially with patients whose early needs for nurturance have remained largely unmet.

The Therapeutic or Working Alliance in the Context of a Theory of Therapeutic Action

The argument for exclusive reliance on interpretation is rooted in the belief that insight is the key or only curative factor in psychodynamic treatment, particularly for patients in the neurotic range. Relationship factors, however, have taken their place alongside insight—and in many accounts have eclipsed it—in theories of the therapeutic action of psychoanalytic treatment, especially with more disturbed patients. This situation is particularly the case in the variety of object relational approaches to treatment and in self-psychology. In relational theories, experiencing the therapist as a new, benign object is considered essential. In Kohut's (1984) self psychology, the value of interpretation is based primarily on its capacity to generate in the patient a feeling of being understood. Insight has been dethroned as the primary curative agent.

Although most analytic writers today do not dismiss the value of insight, they put the benefits to be derived from a relationship with a "good enough" therapist at least on a par with insight. The usual formulation is that the analyst has to be perceived as a "bad" object (i.e., as having negative qualities) in order for the transference to develop, but it also is vital that the therapist be experienced as a "good" object (i.e., in some respects more benign and understanding than one's parents). There are at least two reasons why it is essential and beneficial for the therapist to be experienced as a "good" object for the transference to be resolved or, at least, attenuated: (1) it will promote and maintain a "good enough" therapeutic alliance for the patient to be receptive to recognizing and gaining insight into the transferential aspects of his behavior, and (2) experiencing a good, benign, new object relationship is considered therapeutic in its own right.

The controversial issues regarding the therapeutic alliance raised by Brenner and others (e.g., Stein, 1981) do not seem problematic from a relational perspective. From this perspective the rule of abstinence is generally more relaxed because the issue of transference gratification is of less concern, self-disclosure appears to be more common, and major emphasis is placed on the mutual reciprocal interaction of two subjectivities. In self-psychological approaches (Kohut, 1984), there also are aspects of the relationship that are considered curative, for example, feeling "mirrored" by the analyst and using the analyst as an idealized selfobject. In addition, Kohut (1984) states that the healing aspect of the analyst's interpretation is that the patient feels understood.

An ultimate theory of the therapeutic action of analytic therapy will have to consider the extent to which the importance of the therapeutic alliance lies in its making interpretive work possible versus the extent to which it is a curative factor in its own right, at least with some and perhaps with all patients. Of course, one need not choose between these alternatives. Consider, for example, the work on rupture and repair of the therapeutic alliance by Safran and Muran (2000). Transference–countertransference enactments are inevitable during the course of treatment and often give rise to periodic ruptures in the alliance. The uniqueness of the therapy relationship as a microcosm of other interpersonal relationships lies in the collaborative examination of the dynamics of the interaction of the two participants. Thus, when the analyst and/or patient realize that they have slipped into and are engaged in a transference–countertransference enactment that disrupts the alliance, they have the opportunity to examine it and learn about their respective contributions to it. If these ruptures do not occur too frequently, do not go too deep, and are reparable, they can actually strengthen the therapeutic relationship and be a good model for negotiating difficulties in other interpersonal relationships. Here is where emotional experience and cognitive understanding can come together.

The literature discussed to this point has been almost entirely clinical and theoretical. As such, it raises interesting issues but without an adequate means of confirming or disconfirming different views. Fortunately, the alliance is an area in psychodynamic psychotherapy that lends itself to systematic empirical study. In what follows, we review research that bears on the role of the alliance in psychodynamic therapy.

PRACTICE GUIDELINES BASED ON PSYCHODYNAMICALLY ORIENTED RESEARCH ON THE THERAPEUTIC ALLIANCE

The empirical research on the therapeutic alliance is copious, complex, and often inconsistent. Among the most salient reasons for the complexity and inconsistency are different conceptualizations of the alliance and what makes up its components (e.g., therapist empathy, bonds, tasks, goals); the use of different assessment tools (there are many of these) and who does the rating (patient, therapist, or researcher); different results, depending on the phase of therapy studied (early, middle, late); the variety of therapy outcome measures to which the alliance is correlated (e.g., symptom reduction, interpersonal changes, target complaints); the varied length of therapy; and variations reflecting the clinical group studied (various or combined diagnostic categories). (See Stiles, Agnew-Davies, Hardy, Barkham, and Shapiro [1998] for empirical examples of variations in results attributable to differences in some of these dimensions.) Despite such challenges, our effort in this section is to glean from the psychodynamically oriented research on the therapeutic alliance, findings that can guide the practicing clinician.

Before proceeding, we should note that some challenge this area of research on conceptual grounds. Wallerstein (2003), for example, questions the notion of the therapeutic alliance as a "bounded measurable entity" (p. 397). He objects to the therapeutic alliance's being treated as a thing "that can be better or worse, stronger or weaker, and that, therefore some metric can be established to assess this entity in its fluctuations over time. I conceive the alliance rather as a subtle and complex (and at times much contested) process, not easily reducible to some linear metric" (p. 397). Although he does not say so, if what Wallerstein means by "subtle and complex" is that aspects of it are unconscious and not readily tapped by pencil-and-paper measures, he would have a point. In fact, this circumstance might be one reason that the alliance accounts for less variance in treatment outcome (about 5%) than one would expect from the emphasis it receives in the clinical literature. On the other hand, Wallerstein's (2003) view, as stated, could be applied to virtually any psychodynamic concept or phenomenon (e.g., transference, resistance) and is one we reject, as it constitutes an empirical dead end.

Therapist Factors

Therapist Personal Attributes

In a review of therapist personal attributes associated with a good alliance in therapies that were mostly psychodynamic, Ackerman and Hilsenroth (2003) found the following: being flexible, experienced, honest, respectful, trustworthy, confident, interested, alert, friendly, warm, and open. Interestingly, there was very little variation according to the therapist's theoretical orientation, reinforcing the notion of the therapeutic alliance as a pantheoretical construct. The implication of these findings is that therapists who have these attributes to begin with or who can acquire or refine them will do better at establishing a collaborative relationship with their patients. These findings are also in keeping with the emphasis on the relationship as a key factor leading to successful outcomes apart from, or in concert with, therapist techniques. The authors caution that many of the studies measured the alliance in only one or two sessions, thus limiting the generalizability of the results. Since perceptions of the therapeutic alliance are quite likely to change over time, more data points are required for a fuller picture of alliance development.

Similarly, Ackerman and Hilsenroth (2001) reviewed the literature and reported on therapist attributes associated with a poorer alliance: showing disregard for patients, being distracted, self-focused, and less involved in the treatment process; and being uncertain of one's ability to help one's patients. Other therapist negative attributes included being tense, tired, and bored; distant and aloof; critical, defensive, and blaming; and unable to provide a supportive therapeutic environment. As with the positive attributes, there was little variation among different theoretical orientations in the negative attributes that affect the alliance. These findings provide a cautionary note as to how therapists should *not* relate to their patients if they wish to establish a good working relationship with them.

Therapist Techniques

Despland, de Roten, Despars, Stigler, and Perry (2001) studied a small sample of patients in a four-session assessment for psychodynamic therapy known as brief psychodynamic investigation. It focuses on the reasons for the consultation and the early interaction between therapist and patient. Whereas neither patient defensive functioning nor supportive or exploratory interventions alone differentiated early alliance development, the degree of adjustment of therapists' interventions to patients' level of defensive functioning discriminated a low therapeutic alliance from either an improving or high alliance. They present examples of two patients with relatively high-level defenses (and one with less mature defenses) to illustrate their findings. In an initial session with a 25-year-old student, the therapist tried to help her express her feelings in an overly supportive way, not interpreting the conflict between her wish to be able to control her emotions independently and her antithetical wish to be helped passively without having to ask for it. "Not addressing her wish to remain in control and instead relying on a highly supportive approach actually triggered a counter dependent reaction. The alliance remained at a low level" (Despland et al., 2001, p. 159).

By contrast, in a second case of a 20-year-old student, the therapist often confronted the patient, interpreting to her how she tried to maintain her independence in order to avoid her fear of being rejected whenever she adopted a more a passive style. "The moderately high degree of questioning, clarification, and interpretation of her conflicts was well adjusted to her level of defensive functioning. The patient's alliance continuously improved over the four sessions, and there was a large decrease in distress" (Despland et al., 2001, p. 160). These findings suggest that therapists should strive to adjust their level of interventions to the maturity of the patients' defenses to help establish a good alliance.

In a study of a subsample of patients with personality disorder early on in long-term psychodynamic therapy, Bond, Banon, and Grenier (1998) examined "turning points" indicated by either a change in the alliance, in emotional elaboration, or in the level of patient defensiveness. They found that the impact of transference interpretations was influenced by the state of the alliance. Transference interpretations were tolerated well in the context of a strong positive alliance but not in the absence of such an alliance. They concluded that, when the alliance is tenuous, transference interpretations are damaging to it, especially in personality-disordered patients (e.g., borderline ones). Such interpretations can prematurely disrupt the development of a fantasized merger with the therapist or an idealizing transference that may be necessary during the initial stages of building an alliance, particularly with more fragile patients.

Bender (2005) reviewed the literature on the role of the therapeutic alliance in the treatment of personality disorders and came to a similar conclusion, namely, that transference interpretations should be used sparingly with the more disturbed personality disorders (e. g., those with borderline and narcissistic features) during the early phase of treatment, a cautionary outlook recommended previously by Kohut (1984). These recommendations are supported by the findings of Piper, Azim, Joyce, and McCallum (1991) for a mixed diagnostic group, namely, that a higher proportion of transference interpretations are associated with a poorer alliance and that, for patients with a poor quality of object relations, close correspondence of transference interpretations to the dynamic formulation is predictive of a poor therapeutic alliance.

Bender recommends that supportive, empathic interventions are more likely to build the alliance, although those with milder personality disorders (e.g., obsessive–compulsive, avoidant, dependent) can tolerate interpretations of repressed conflicts earlier in treatment. She describes the kinds of alliance challenges posed by the different personality disorders or trait clusters and ways to engage these patients in treatment. (For a more extensive review of empirically supported psychodynamic interventions with personality disordered patients, see Messer and Abbass, 2010.)

Returning to the articles by Ackerman and Hilsenroth (2001, 2003), in addition to reviewing the association between therapist attributes and alliance, they surveyed studies on the relationship of therapist *techniques* to both a positive (2003) and a negative (2001) alliance. The following techniques were found to be associated with a positive therapeutic alliance: exploration of interpersonal themes, being reflective and supportive, acting collaboratively to develop specific goals, noting past therapy success, making accurate interpretations, facilitating expression of affect, being active, and affirming, understanding, and attending to the patient's experience. A later report by Ackerman, Hilsenroth, and Knowles (2005) supports and extends these findings. It demonstrated that early use of psychodynamic–interpersonal interventions, such as expressive and affect-oriented techniques, an emphasis on past experiences, and identifying patterns and the therapeutic relationship, were predictive of later alliance.

Techniques that contributed negatively to the alliance were overstructuring or failing to provide a frame for the therapy, inappropriate use of self-disclosure or silence, making superficial interventions, belittling the patient, and overuse of transference interpretations, as noted above. They found that these factors apply to nonpsychodynamic forms of therapy as well. The authors point out that these techniques are similar to the ones that lead to strains and ruptures in the alliance and derive from a lack of attentiveness to the ongoing therapeutic relationship. They underscore that therapists should not avoid bringing negative sentiments into the room and/or discourage the patient to from doing so and should acknowledge their own part in the rupture and explore its elements. In this vein, Safran and Muran (2000) developed a psychodynamic therapy, brief relational therapy, that focuses on alliance ruptures and their repair, which has garnered empirical support even with personality disordered patients (Muran, Safran, Samstag, & Winston, 2005).

In brief, to enhance development of the therapeutic alliance, psychodynamic therapists should adjust their interventions to patients' defenses, explore interpersonal themes, develop specific goals, facilitate affect, and attend to patterns and past experiences. In the case of the more severely personality disordered patients, they should use transference interpretations only infrequently, at least during the initial phases of therapy. Therapists should not be too self-disclosing or silent, should encourage expression of patients' negative feelings, and in this connection should explore their own role in any rupture of the alliance.

Patient Factors

There have been four main patient factors studied in relation to therapeutic alliance: interpersonal functioning, defensive functioning, pretreatment symptom level, and expectations for improvement.

Interpersonal Functioning

Two early studies showed a positive relationship between patients' ability to engage in positive interpersonal relationships and the therapeutic alliance (Marmar, Weiss, & Gaston, 1989; Marziali, 1984). Similarly, Gibbons et al. (2003) found that patients with less interpersonal distress formed better alliances (while controlling for prior symptomatic change and pretreatment expectations of improvement). The obverse was also true: those with a hostile/dominant interpersonal style had poorer alliances.

In a sample of elderly depressed patients, however, pretreatment quality of interpersonal functioning was found not to be related to the therapeutic alliance (Gaston, Marmar, Thompson, & Gallagher, 1988). The authors point out that interpersonal relationships were self-reported in this study and that the patients were not seeking help with interpersonal relations but with depression. Piper, Boroto, Joyce, McCallum, and Azim (1995) compared patterns of change in the therapeutic alliance in two samples of psychiatric patients (with low or high quality of object relations) in a 20-session time-limited psychodynamic therapy. In patients with low-quality object relations, they found a direct relationship between increasing alliance and favorable outcome. In those with high-quality object relations, there was no association between patterns of change in the alliance and outcome, but there was considerable evidence of a direct relationship between average alliance level and favorable outcome. Both these authors and Gibbons et al. (2003) concluded that strengthening the alliance during the course of therapy may be particularly important for patients with long-term relationship difficulties, especially those who are hostile/dominant.

More recently, Beretta et al. (2005) studied the alliance, Core Conflictual Relationship Themes (CCRT), and interpersonal relations (through the Inventory of Interpersonal Problems) in a sample of patients with mood and anxiety disorders, half of whom also had Cluster C personality disorders (dependent and avoidant). This study focused on a four-session brief psychodynamic intervention (or investigation; see above). The perception by the patient that there existed a helping alliance was dependent on the type of patient object representations; that is, those who saw others as helpful, cooperative, and trustworthy had better therapeutic alliances. Contrariwise, those who saw others as hurtful and untrustworthy had lower-quality alliances. Furthermore, those with low affiliation had more difficulty in establishing an early alliance (although they did wish to be connected to others). Those who had lower dominance needs were more likely to show progress in the development of the alliance, perhaps because they were less likely to engage in power struggles and more likely to relinquish control in order to engage more deeply in a productive alliance.

Defensive Functioning

Whereas *defensive interpersonal style* was associated with relatively poorer alliance in one study (Gaston et al., 1988), no such relationship was found in two others (Hersoug, Sexton, & Høglend, 2002; Siefert, Hilsenroth, Weinberger, Blagys, & Ackerman, 2006). Siefert et al. (2006) surmise that this discrepancy was attributable either to different measurement sources (patient vs. clinician ratings) or that the use of specific defenses such as idealization or devaluation may impact the alliance, whereas overall level of defensive functioning may not. Another explanation comes from a study discussed earlier by Despland et al. (2001), who found that defensive functioning per se was not related to the quality of the alliance but that how the therapist intervened (exploration vs. support) in response to patients' level of defenses *was* related.

Pretreatment Symptom Level

Reviewing several studies of *pretreatment symptom levels* and therapeutic alliance, Crits-Christoph and Gibbons (2003) found higher levels to be associated with alliance in one study, lower levels in another, and no relation in two others. In a study by Gibbons et al. (2003), pretreatment symptoms were not found to predict TA for patients in manualized supportive–expressive therapy. In a recent study by Puschner, Wolf, and Kraft (2008), initial symptom status and early symptom change did not affect early status of the therapeutic alliance. The weight of the evidence seems to be that pretreatment symptom level is not a good predictor of alliance.

Expectations for Improvement

Expectations have been found to be correlated positively with the therapeutic alliance (Joyce & Piper, 1998). Supporting this finding, Gibbons et al. (2003) reported that those with greater pretreatment expectations of improvement formed better alliances both early and later on in therapy over and above early symptomatic improvement. Positive expectations also predicted growth in the alliance over time. Joyce, Ogrodniczuk, Piper, and McCallum (2003) studied the relationships among expectations of improvement, alliance, and outcome in a combination of patients who received either an interpretive form of brief therapy or a more supportive variety. Expectations for outcome were directly associated with the alliance as rated by patient or therapist and with treatment outcome. The therapist alliance served to mediate the effect of patient outcome expectations on therapy benefits, whether the outcome was assessed by the patient or the therapist. It seems clinically desirable for therapists early on in treatment to evaluate and explore patient expectations regarding therapy.

Other Patient Factors

Those factors associated *positively* with the therapist alliance include the stability of self concept and better differentiation of self and other (Marmar, Horowitz, Weiss, & Marziali, 1986); motivation for psychotherapy (Marmar et al., 1986; Marmar, Weiss, & Gaston, 1989); and gender, with women forming stronger alliances (Gibbons et al., 2003). Patient factors associated *negatively* with the alliance include avoidance and depressive thoughts (Constantino, Castonguay, & Schut, 2002).

In general, and not surprisingly, those with good interpersonal relations and positive object representations form better alliances—and the obverse. Particularly with patients who are hostile or dominant, the therapist needs to pay special attention to the alliance. Therapists also need to attend to the nature of patient defenses, matching the mode of intervention (e.g., support or exploration) to them. The more positive patient expectations and motivation for therapy are, the better the alliance, suggesting the desirability of the therapist's being aware of these patient attitudes.

The Therapeutic Alliance as a Predictor of Therapy Process and Outcome

The correlation between the therapeutic alliance and outcome is one of the most consistent empirical findings in the field of psychotherapy, although it is typically modest in size (Castonguay, Constantino, & Holtforth, 2006). The results of meta-analyses and comprehensive reviews of scores of studies, which run the theoretical gamut, are that the average correlation of the therapeutic alliance and outcome across studies ranges from .17 to .26, which accounts for roughly 5% of the outcome variance (e.g., Beutler et al., 2004; Horvath & Bedi, 2002; Martin, Garske, & Davis, 2000). Nevertheless, the literature is rife with contradictory findings, and the range of correlations between alliance and outcome in individual studies is very wide. To illustrate with one recent negative example, a study (Puschner et al., 2008) involving a large group of patients ($n = 259$), most of whom were seen in psychodynamic or psychoanalytic therapy (and some in CBT) and who rated the therapeutic alliance several times over a 2-year period, found that the alliance did not predict outcome as assessed by symptom reduction. Neither change in the alliance nor change in symptom distress at a given point in treatment affected subsequent change in the other variable. Although this is just one study, and one that relied on patient ratings only, it does possess the virtue of having assessed the alliance and symptoms at various intervals over a considerable period of time with a large sample of patients, a majority of whom were treated psychodynamically.

On the other hand, Nuetzel, Randy, Larsen, and Prizmic (2007) came to a much more positive conclusion about the predictive ability of the therapeutic alliance. Carried out and conceptualized within a more purely psychoanalytic conceptual framework, the study assessed 13 patients' views of the therapeutic relationship *on a weekly basis* for 6–33 months (perhaps the only study to do so this frequently for this long a time period). Factor analysis of the (new) relationship scale employed revealed four factors that were labeled Therapeutic Alliance, Resistance, Transference Love and Negative Transference, with Therapeutic Alliance explaining by far the largest percentage of variance. Supporting the validity of the scale and theoretical predictions, this factor was negatively correlated with the factors of Resistance and Negative Transference, as reported by the patients, and positively correlated with the factor of Transference Love.

In contrast to the situation in the previous study, the weekly form filled out by patients went far beyond symptom change. It also contained questions and rating scales covering important life domains, such as patients' emotional states, physical symptoms, self-esteem, social connectedness, major life events, optimism, life satisfaction, work productivity, and perceptions of pleasant and unpleasant life events. It was found that these variables—other than pleasantness and unpleasantness of weekly best and worst events—made up a single factor, referred to as General Adjustment. Increases in Therapeutic Alliance emerged as a significant, and by far the best, predictor of simultaneous improvements in General Adjustment and of increases in Pleasantness of Good Events. The study also found that, despite the Therapeutic Alliance factor's starting out high, it continued to climb in a linear fashion for 1 1/2 years in the full sample and longer in those five patients whose therapies went to at least 2 years, with occasional dips along the way attributable to increased resistance.

Nuetzel et al. (2007) point out that the Therapeutic Alliance factor appears to be consistent with the friendly rapport that Freud (1912a) described as helping treatment progress. Key components include positive feelings about the therapist and the experience (called "bonds" by Bordin) and a sense of productivity (akin to Bordin's tasks and goals). In sum, when patients' perceptions of the alliance are stronger, the patients also perceive their lives to be better in a variety of spheres. Other data in this study suggest that the alliance contains elements of both transference and reality (see Greenson, 1967, as discussed above) and that the alliance helps the patient to continue the work in the face of powerful resistances. While one cannot draw causal attributions from the findings, they do reinforce the idea of a close connection between the therapeutic alliance and General Adjustment variables as gauged on a week-to-week basis in psychoanalytic therapy. That the results are so different from those of Puschner et al. (2008) may be due to the different method, design, and statistics used in these studies.

In another study of open-ended psychodynamic therapy, Saunders (2000) drew upon the data set reported by Howard, Kopta, Krause, and Orlinsky (1986) to examine the relationship among three alliance variables related to the bond between patient and therapist, session quality, and therapy outcome. Clients assessed both the quality and helpfulness of the sessions and filled out the alliance rating forms based on three variables: role investment, empathic resonance, and mutual affirmation. Results indicated that different aspects of the bond predicted session quality and treatment outcome. Clients who felt motivated and invested in therapy and who reported a friendly and affirmative therapeutic environment were likely to rate the session as helpful and productive. Those who had a relatively high sense of understanding and of being understood (an aspect of alliance), experienced a greater sense of subjective well-being and symptom improvement, thus affirming the link between alliance and therapeutic progress and outcome.

In a more recent study, Ambresin, de Roten, Drapeau, and Despland (2007) examined the early change in maladaptive defense style and its relationship to alliance in a brief (four-session) psychodynamic intervention, as described above. Those patients whose alliance improved over the four sessions were found to decrease their use of maladaptive defenses significantly. In a study of brief (about 20-session) psychodynamic therapy (Marcolino & Iacoponi, 2003), patients who perceived their therapists as understanding them and being involved in their issues had the best results in lowering depressive symptoms. In addition, patients with a greater capacity to form a working alliance had the best overall outcomes. In other studies, the aspect of alliance that refers to the level of confidence and commitment a patient feels toward the therapy and the degree to which therapy is experienced as worthwhile (Confident Collaboration) was related to perceived improvement in therapy, as rated by both patient and therapist (Clemence, Hilsenroth, Ackerman, Strassle, & Handler, 2005; Hatcher & Barends, 1996), further supporting the alliance–outcome link.

There have also been studies of the therapeutic alliance and outcome in specific patient populations. Barber et al. (2001) examined the relationship between the therapeutic alliance, retention, and outcome in 308 cocaine-dependent outpatients. Alliance was not a significant predictor of outcome but did predict patient retention, depending on when the alliance was measured. Zuroff and Blatt (2006) examined data from the National Institute of Mental Health Treatment for Depression Collaborative Research program to ascertain the impact of the alliance in depressed patients on treatment outcome. A positive therapeutic alliance early in treatment predicted a more rapid decline in maladjustment subsequent to the assessment. It occurred in interpersonal therapy (the therapy in this study closest to a psychodynamic approach) as well as the other conditions. Therapeutic alliance also predicted better adjustment throughout the 18-month follow-up as well as development of greater enhanced adaptive capacities (that is, it went beyond symptom change only). Importantly, controlling for a wide range of patient characteristics and for symptom change prior to the measurement of alliance did not eliminate the effect of the alliance on rate of improvement. The authors concluded that the quality of the therapeutic alliance and other measures of the therapeutic relationship is "a real and substantial factor that plays a significant role in determining therapeutic outcome" (Zuroff & Blatt, 2006, p. 137). Because the results were the same in each of the conditions, which included CBT as well as clinical management without any specific techniques, "The results also argue against the view that the relationship is simply a facilitator of or enhancer of the effects of specific treatment techniques" (p. 138). The authors speculate that the subjective experience of a positive therapeutic relationship may transform patients' mental representations (cognitive–emotional schemas) of themselves and others.

Nevertheless, there has been controversy over whether the therapeutic alliance is an artifact of prior symptom improvement or a sturdy predictor or cause of outcome in and of itself. While Zuroff and Blatt (2006) and Barber, Connolly, Crits-Christoph, Gladis, and Siqueland (2000) posited that alliance itself predicted symptom change, with other factors such as previous symptom improvement factored out, Barber (2009), upon review of all relevant studies, concluded that there is little support for the notion that alliance causes subsequent symptom improvement. According to Barber, it is more likely that the therapeutic alliance is simply a thermometer indicating that therapy is going well or poorly.

CONCLUSION

Recall that at the outset we cited Freud's (1913, pp. 139–140) view that the analyst needed to "show a serious interest in the patient," "maintain an attitude of sympathetic understanding," and "avoid a moralistic stance" in order to promote rapport. Clinical experience and empirical studies of at least the first two factors indicate that these attitudes foster an alliance. However, whereas Freud and many of his followers believed that such attitudes were preconditions for the operation of the main therapeutic ingredient of interpretation leading to insight, there has been a growing tendency to regard the alliance as having a therapeutic benefit in its own right, particularly with more disturbed patients. Zuroff and Blatt's (2006) hypotheses, based on their analysis of the data from the NIMH Collaborative Depression Study, that a positive therapeutic relationship may transform patients' mental representations (cognitive–emotional schemas) of themselves and others accords with the research findings of Wallerstein (1986) and implies that attaining insight should not necessarily be considered the sole or even prime factor in the therapeutic action of dynamic psychotherapy.

Not surprisingly, psychodynamic therapists, particularly those with an object relations orientation, have focused increasingly on how to promote and sustain a positive relationship with their patients. This focus includes a greater inclination to offer even mildly disturbed patients explicit support, to offer the patient more in the way of personal self-disclosure (e.g., to acknowledge one's role in being drawn into a maladaptive interaction with the patient), to be more empathically attuned to patients' needs to be understood, and to accept some responsibility for the therapist's contribution to inevitable ruptures in the therapeutic alliance. These trends are consistent with the transition from a "one-person" psychology to a "two-person" psychology (Aron, 1996) and with the corresponding dominance of object relational approaches to treatment.

As noted above, a positive therapeutic alliance is correlated not only with the therapist's being supportive and attending to the patient's experience but also with being reflective, exploring interpersonal themes, and making accurate interpretations. This pattern of findings is consistent with the conclusion drawn by Eagle and Wolitzky (1981) that interpretations take place in the context of a relationship, making it impossible, other than heuristically, to separate the effects of insight from the effects of a good alliance, which includes feeling understood. Thus, it becomes unclear to what extent the therapeutic impact of an interpretation derives from its content per se versus its contribution to the patient's feeling understood, as advocated by Kohut (1984)—which we underline to place the alliance in the larger context of a theory of action of psychodynamic psychotherapy.

REFERENCES

Ackerman, S. J., & Hilsenroth, M. J. (2001). A review of therapist characteristics and techniques negatively impacting the therapeutic alliance. *Psychotherapy: Theory, Research, Practice, Training, 38,* 171–185.

Ackerman, S. J., & Hilsenroth, M. J. (2003). A review of therapist characteristics and techniques positively impacting the therapeutic alliance. *Clinical Psychology Review, 23,* 1–33.

Ackerman, S. J., Hilsenroth, M. J., & Knowles, E. S. (2005). Ratings of therapist dynamic activities and alliance early and late in psychotherapy. *Psychotherapy: Theory, Research, Practice, Training, 42,* 225–231.

Adler, E., & Bachant, J. L. (1998). *Working in depth: A clinician's guide to framework and flexibility in the analytic relationship.* Northvale, NJ, and London: Jason Aronson.

Alexander, F., & French, T. M. (1946). *Psychoanalytic therapy: Principles and applications.* New York: Ronald Press.

Ambresin, G., de Roten, Y., Drapeau, M., & Despland, J. (2007). Early change in maladaptive defence style and development of the therapeutic alliance. *Clinical Psychology and Psychotherapy, 14,* 89–95.

Aron, L. (1996). *A meeting of minds: Mutuality in psychoanalysis.* Hillsdale, NJ: Analytic Press.

Barber, J. P. (2009). Toward a working through of some core conflicts in psychotherapy research. *Psychotherapy Research, 19,* 1–12.

Barber, J. P., Connolly, M. B., Crits-Christoph, P., Gladis, L., & Siqueland, L. (2000). Alliance predicts patients' outcome beyond in-treatment change in symptoms. *Journal of Consulting and Clinical Psychology, 68,* 1027–1032.

Barber, J. P., Luborsky, L., Gallop, R., Crits-Christoph, P., Frank, A., Weiss, R. D., et al. (2001). Therapeutic alliance as a predictor of outcome and retention in the National Institute on Drug Abuse Collaborative Cocaine Treatment Study. *Journal of Consulting and Clinical Psychology, 69,* 119–124.

Bender, D. S. (2005). The therapeutic alliance in the treatment of personality disorders. *Journal of Psychiatric Practice, 11,* 73–87.

Beretta, V., de Roten, Y., Stigler, M., Drapeau, M., Fischer, M., & Despland, J. (2005). The influence of patient's interpersonal schemas on early alliance building. *Swiss Journal of Psychology, 64,* 13–20.

Beutler, L., Matik, M., Alimohamed, S., Harwood, T. M., Talebi, H., Noble, S., et al. (2004). Therapist variables. In M. Lambert (Ed.), *Bergin & Garfield's handbook of psychotherapy and behavior change* (pp. 227–306). New York: Wiley.

Bond, M., Banon, E., & Grenier, M. (1998). Differential effects of interventions on the therapeutic alliance with patients with personality disorders. *The Journal of Psychotherapy Practice and Research, 7,* 301–318.

Bordin, E. (1979). The generalizability of the psychoanalytic concept of the working alliance. *Psychotherapy: Theory, Research, and Practice, 16,* 252–260.

Brenner, C. (1979). Working alliance, therapeutic alliance, and transference. *Journal of the American Psychoanalytic Association, 27*(Suppl.), 137–157.

Castonguay, L. G., Constantino, M. J., & Holtforth, M. G. (2006). The working alliance: Where are we and where should we go? *Psychotherapy: Theory, Research, Practice, Training, 43,* 271–279.

Clemence, A. J., Hilsenroth, M. J., Ackerman, S. J., Strassle, C. G., & Handler, L. (2005). Facets of the therapeutic alliance and perceived progress in psychotherapy: Relationship between patient and therapist perspectives. *Clinical Psychology and Psychotherapy, 12,* 443–454.

Constantino, M. J., Castonguay, L. G., & Schut, A. J. (2002). The working alliance: A flagship for the "scientist-practitioner" model in psychotherapy. In G. S. Tryon (Ed.), *Counseling based on process research: Applying what we know* (pp. 81–131). Boston: Allyn & Bacon.

Cooper, A. (2008). Commentary on Greenson's "The Working Alliance and the Transference Neurosis." *Psychoanalytic Quarterly, 77,* 103–119.

Crits-Christoph, P., & Gibbons, M. B. C. (2003). Research developments on the therapeutic alliance in psychodynamic psychotherapy. *Psychoanalytic Inquiry, 23,* 332–349.

Curtis, H. C. (1979). The concept of the therapeutic alliance: Implications for the "widening scope." *Journal of the American Psychoanalytic Association, 27*(Suppl.), 159–192.

Despland, J., de Roten, Y., Despars, J., Stigler, M., & Perry, J. C. (2001). Contribution of patient defense mechanisms and therapist interventions to the development of early therapeutic alliance in a brief psychodynamic investigation. *Journal of Psychotherapy Practice and Research, 10,* 155–164.

Eagle, M., & Wolitzky, D. L. (1981). Therapeutic influences in dynamic psychotherapy: Overview and synthesis. In S. Slipp (Ed.), *Curative factors in dynamic psychotherapy* (pp. 349–378). New York: McGraw-Hill.

Freud, S. (1912a). The dynamics of transference. *Standard Edition, 12,* 97–108.

Freud, S. (1912b). Recommendations of physicians practicing psycho-analysis. *Standard Edition, 12,* 109–120.

Freud, S. (1913). On beginning the treatment (Further recommendations on the technique of psycho-analysis I). *Standard Edition, 12,* 121–144.

Freud, S. (1916–1917). Introductory lectures on psycho-analysis. *Standard Edition, 15,* 1–239.

Gaston, L., Marmar, C. R., Thompson, L. W., & Gallagher, D. (1988). Relation of patient pretreatment characteristics to the therapeutic alliance in diverse psychotherapies. *Journal of Consulting and Clinical Psychology, 56,* 483–489.

Gibbons, M. B. C., Crits-Christoph, P., de la Cruz, C., Barber, J. P., Siqueland, L., & Gladis, M. (2003). Pretreatment expectations, interpersonal functioning, and symptoms in the prediction of the therapeutic alliance across supportive–expressive psychotherapy and cognitive therapy. *Psychotherapy Research*, *13*, 59–76.

Gilbert, P., & Leahy, R. L. (Eds.). (2007). *The therapeutic relationship in the cognitive behavioral therapies*. New York: Routledge.

Gill, M. M. (1994). *Psychoanalysis in transition: A personal view*. Hillsdale, NJ, and London: Analytic Press.

Gitelson, M. (1962). The curative factors in psycho-analysis: I: The first phase of psycho-analysis. *International Journal of Psychoanalysis*, *43*, 194–205.

Glover, E. (1937). Symposium on the theory of the therapeutic results of psycho-analysis. *International Journal of Psychoanalysis*, *18*, 125–132.

Goldberger, M. (2008). Discussion of "The working alliance and the transference neurosis" by Ralph R. Greenson. *Psychoanalytic Quarterly*, *77*, 121–138.

Greenson, R. R. (1965). The working alliance and the transference neurosis. *Psychoanalytic Quarterly*, *34*, 155–181.

Greenson, R. R. (1967). *The technique and practice of psychoanalysis* (Vol. 1). New York: International Universities Press.

Greenson, R. R., & Wexler, M. (1969). The non-transference relationship in the psychoanalytic situation. *International Journal of Psychoanalysis*, *50*, 27–39.

Hatcher, R. L., & Barends, A. (1996). Patients' view of the alliance in psychotherapy: Exploratory factor analysis of three alliance measures. *Journal of Consulting and Clinical Psychology*, *64*, 1326–1336.

Hersoug, A. G., Sexton, H. C., & Høglend, P. (2002). Contribution of defensive functioning to the quality of working alliance and psychotherapy outcome. *American Journal of Psychotherapy*, *56*, 539–554.

Horvath, A. O., & Bedi, R. P. (2002). The alliance. In J. C. Norcross (Ed.), *Psychotherapy relationships that work* (pp. 37–70). New York: Oxford University Press.

Howard, K. I., Kopta, S. M., Krause, M. S., & Orlinsky, D. E. (1986). The dose–effect relationship in psychotherapy. *American Psychologist*, *41*, 159–164.

Joyce, A. S., Ogrodniczuk, J. S., Piper, W. E., & McCallum, M. (2003). The alliance as mediator of expectancy effects in short-term individual therapy. *Journal of Consulting and Clinical Psychology*, *71*, 672–679.

Joyce, A. S., & Piper, W. E. (1998). Expectancy, the therapeutic alliance, and treatment outcome in short-term individual psychotherapy. *Journal of Psychotherapy Practice and Research*, *7*, 236–248.

Kanzer, M. (1975). The therapeutic and working alliances. *International Journal of Psychoanalytic Psychotherapy*, *4*, 48–68.

Kohut, H. (1984). *How does analysis cure?* Chicago and London: University of Chicago Press.

Luborsky, L. (1976). Helping alliances of psychotherapy. In J. P. Claghorn (Ed.), *Successful psychotherapy* (pp. 92–116). New York: Brunner/Mazel.

Luborsky, L. (1984). *Principles of psychoanalytic psychotherapy: A manual for supportive–expressive treatment*. New York: Basic Books.

Luborsky, L. (1994). Therapeutic alliances as predictors of psychotherapy outcome: Factors explaining the predictive success. In A. O. Horvath & L. S. Greenberg (Eds.), *The working alliance: Theory, research, and practice* (pp. 38–50). Oxford, UK: Wiley.

Marcolino, J. A. M., & Iacoponi, E. (2003). The early impact of therapeutic alliance in brief psychodynamic psychotherapy. *Revista Brasileira de Psiquiatria, 25,* 78–86.

Marmar, C. R., Horowitz, M. J., Weiss, D. S., & Marziali, E. (1986). The development of the therapeutic alliance rating system. In L. S. Greenberg & W. M. Pinsof (Eds.), *The psychotherapeutic process: A research handbook* (pp. 367–390). New York: Guilford Press.

Marmar, C. R., Weiss, D. S., & Gaston, L. (1989). Toward the validation of the California Therapeutic Alliance Rating System. *Psychological Assessment, 1,* 46–52.

Martin, D. J., Garske, J. P., & Davis, K. M. (2000). Relation of the therapeutic alliance with outcome and other variables: A meta-analytic review. *Journal of Consulting and Clinical Psychology, 68,* 438–450.

Marziali, E. (1984). Three viewpoints on the therapeutic alliance: Similarities, differences, and associations with psychotherapy outcome. *Journal of Nervous and Mental Disease, 172,* 417–423.

Meissner, W. W. (2007). Therapeutic alliance: Themes and variations. *Psychoanalytic Psychology, 24*(2), 231–254.

Messer, S. B., & Abbass, A. A. (2010). Evidence-based psychodynamic therapy with personality disorders. In J. Magnavita (Ed.), *Evidence-based treatment of personality dysfunction: Principles, methods, and processes* (pp. 79–111). Washington, DC: American Psychological Association.

Muran, J. C., Safran, J. D., Samstag, L. W., & Winston, A. (2005). Evaluating an alliance-focused treatment for personality disorders. *Psychotherapy: Theory, Research, Practice, Training, 42,* 532–545.

Nuetzel, E. J., Larsen, R. J., & Prizmic, Z. (2007). The dynamics of empirically derived factors in the therapeutic relationship. *Journal of the American Psychoanalytic Association, 55,* 1321–1353.

Piper, W. E., Azim, H. F. A., Joyce, A. S., & McCallum, M. (1991). Transference interpretations, therapeutic alliance, and outcome in short-term individual psychotherapy. *Archives of General Psychiatry, 48,* 946–953.

Piper, W. E., Boroto, D. R., Joyce, A. S., McCallum, M., & Azim, H. F. A. (1995). Pattern of alliance and outcome in short-term individual psychotherapy. *Psychotherapy: Theory, Research, Practice, Training, 32,* 639–647.

Puschner, B., Wolf, M., & Kraft, S. (2008). Helping alliance and outcome in psychotherapy: What predicts what in routine outpatient treatment? *Psychotherapy Research, 18,* 167–178.

Richards, A. D., & Lynch, A. A. (2008). The identity of psychoanalysis and psychoanalysts. *Psychoanalytic Psychology, 25*(2), 203–219.

Safran, J. D., & Muran, J. C. (2000). *Negotiating the therapeutic alliance: A relational treatment guide.* New York: Guilford Press.

Sandler, J., Dare, C., & Holder, A. (1992). *The patient and the analyst: The basis of the psychoanalytic process* (2nd ed.). Madison, CT: International Universities Press.

Saunders, S. M. (2000). Examining the relationship between the therapeutic bond and the phases of treatment outcome. *Psychotherapy: Theory, Research, Practice, Training, 37,* 206–218.

Siefert, C. J., Hilsenroth, M. J., Weinberger, J., Blagys, M. D., & Ackerman, S. J. (2006). The relationship of patient defensive functioning and alliance with therapist technique during short-term psychodynamic psychotherapy. *Clinical Psychology and Psychotherapy, 13,* 20–33.

Stein, M. H. (1981). The unobjectionable part of the transference. *Journal of the American Psychoanalytic Association, 29,* 869–892.

Sterba, R. (1934). The fate of the ego on analytic therapy. *International Journal of Psycho-Analysis, 15,* 117–126.

Stiles, W. B., Agnew-Davies, R., Hardy, G. E., Barkham, M., & Shapiro, D. A. (1998). Relations of the alliance with psychotherapy outcome: Findings in the Second Sheffield Psychotherapy Project. *Journal of Consulting and Clinical Psychology, 66,* 791–802.

Stone, L. (1961). *The psychoanalytic situation: An examination of its development and essential nature.* New York: International Universities Press.

Strachey, J. (1934). The nature of the therapeutic action of psycho-analysis. *International Journal of Psycho-Analysis, 15,* 127–159.

Strachey, J. (1937). Symposium on the theory of the therapeutic results of psychoanalysis. *International Journal of Psychoanalysis, 18,* 139–145

Wallerstein, R. S. (1986). *Forty-two lives in treatment: A study of psychoanalysis and psychotherapy.* New York: Guilford Press.

Wallerstein, R. S. (2003). Psychoanalytic therapy research: Its coming of age. *Psychoanalytic. Inquiry, 23,* 375–404.

Zetzel, E. R. (1956). Current concepts of transference. *International Journal of Psycho-Analysis, 37,* 369–375.

Zetzel, E. R. (1966). The analytic situation. In R. E. Litman (Ed.), *Psychoanalysis in the Americas* (pp. 86–106). New York: International Universities Press.

Zuroff, D. C., & Blatt, S. J. (2006). The therapeutic relationship in the brief treatment of depression: Contributions to clinical improvement and enhanced adaptive capacities. *Journal of Consulting and Clinical Psychology, 74,* 130–140.

CHAPTER 7

■ ■ ■ ■ ■

An Interpersonal Perspective on Therapy Alliances and Techniques

Lorna Smith Benjamin
Kenneth L. Critchfield

Freud initially used Breuer's method of suggestion to treat symptoms, but soon gave it up because results were not lasting. He switched from "superimposing something" to trying to "bring out something," namely the pathogenic ideas that had been repressed and were supporting resistance to change. The technique was complex, he warned, and required the physician to minimize intrusion so that the patient was free to focus primarily on his or her own mental processing (Freud, 1904/1959, pp. 252–257). Rogers (1951) emphasizes relationship more than technique and proposed that three effective components for any psychotherapy are empathy, unconditional positive regard, and congruence. He pierced the veil of secrecy in psychotherapy by recording sessions, opening the door to therapy process research. Rogers's studies (e.g., 1954), rarely cited now, were the first to establish theoretically effective relational aspects of treatment as they affected outcome. Subsequent research on the therapy relationship has directly benefited from Rogers's legacy.

In 1965, within psychoanalysis itself, Greenson made the stunning proposal that a working alliance is as important as analyzing the transference neurosis. Bordin (1979) elevated the working alliance even more, claiming that across therapies "the effectiveness [is] in part, if not entirely, a function of the strength of the alliance" (p. 253). Bordin defined the alliance in terms of a collaboration between therapist and patient while engaged in a series of tasks designed to lead toward agreed-upon goals; in that process, a bond develops that supports the patient's capacity for hopeful and trustful states. Two American Psychological Association task forces (Norcross, Beutler, & Levant, 2006, p. 5) reviewed empirical studies of the connections between selected aspects of the therapy relationship and outcome. A variety of definitions of alliance and relationship have shown robust associations with treatment outcome. The variations led Horvath (2006) to call for "a clearer definition of the alliance; ... consensus about the alliance's relation to other elements in the therapeutic relationship; [and] more clearly specifying the role and function of the alliance in different phases of treatment" (p. 258).

Given the demonstrated power of the alliance in determining outcome, it is surprising that in practice today technique is assumed to account for therapy change. Editors, grant reviewers, American Psychological Association training program certifiers, and insurance administrators who decide which treatments to reimburse all agree that acceptable psychotherapy approaches must be certified as effective according to the empirically supported treatment (EST) paradigm. A therapy that qualifies as an EST meets these standards: the treatment method (technique) is detailed specifically enough to be taught by a manual; has been applied to a specific problem (i.e., diagnosis; symptom group) within a specific population; and is shown superior to an appropriate contrast group in a randomized controlled trial (RCT). Results should be replicated at more than one site (Chambless & Ollendick, 2001). In sum, effective treatments are classified by technique, with the impact of relationship present implicitly only as a supporting factor.

There have been many articles critical of the EST paradigm (an early, still relevant, example is Goldfried & Woolf, 1996). Nonetheless, ignoring evidence that the therapy alliance has a direct link to outcome as well as the fact that therapy technique has not often been linked,[1] the gatekeepers of professional norms have chosen the EST paradigm. Manualized sets of therapy techniques that pass the $p < .05$ test in an RCT are the assumed agents of change. There was an attempt to "manualize" the therapy relationship

---

[1]Crits-Christoph, Cooper, and Luborsky (1988) made a good beginning in showing that the accuracy of interpretation was associated with outcome in a psychodynamic treatment. But Imber et al. (1990) reported negative results in a large multisite study of different approaches funded by the National Institute of Mental Health. The paucity of information about technique–outcome associations might be attributable in part to editorial policies against publishing negative findings (*Science News*, October 10, 2009).

itself (Crits-Christoph et al., 2006), but to date, no manual of "effective relating"[2] has reached the status of an EST.

The credibility of the EST design rests on the fact that it was imported from medical protocols for testing the effectiveness of drugs. The assumption of comparability between a particular psychotherapy and a particular drug overlooks the fact that in drug studies the purity of the treatment is assured; there is nothing comparable in most EST studies of psychotherapy. Moreover, the literature shows that, even with the proliferation of ESTs, there are substantial numbers of patients who have not responded to any treatments, EST or otherwise. These people are known as treatment-resistant or nonresponsive, and we discuss them later in this chapter.

Fortunately, there recently has been renewed concern about adherence to treatment models in psychotherapy research. Perepletchikova, Hilt, Chereji, and Kazdin (2009, p. 212) wrote:

> Treatment integrity refers to implementing interventions as intended. Treatment integrity is critically important for experimental validity and for drawing valid inferences regarding the relationship between treatment and outcome. Yet, it is rarely adequately addressed in psychotherapy research.

Barber (2009) also has recently addressed the technique/alliance controversy, as he emphasized the need for better understanding of what causes therapy change. Barber, Connolly, Crits-Christoph, Gladis, and Siqueland (2009) remind researchers that cause is identified only by sequential measures and provide evidence suggesting that the alliance does cause change. Since most people show immediate symptom relief when starting therapy, these investigators statistically adjusted successive measures of alliance scores for prior symptom change. The adjusted alliance scores then predicted subsequent symptom change independently of initial enthusiasm and the symptom relief often observed when starting therapy. This sort of model could truly begin to identify mechanisms of change in psychotherapy.

INTERPERSONAL STUDIES OF THE ALLIANCE

The present review of social interactive aspects of the therapy alliance begins with a glimpse at research results from measures based on factor analysis.

---

[2]There is a manual for parent–child training that touches on relationship skills relevant to therapy. These include reflective listening, recognizing and responding to children's feelings, therapeutic limit setting, building children's self-esteem, and structuring sessions with selected vehicles for learning (Bratton, Landreth, Kellam, & Blackard, 2006).

Then, a description of Structural Analysis of Social Behavior (SASB; Benjamin, 1979, 1987, 1996) is followed by examples of how SASB provides interpersonal descriptions useful in addressing alliance problems when treating individuals with personality disorders. A range of SASB-based research studies of the alliance are reviewed. Finally, we describe interpersonal reconstructive therapy (IRT; Benjamin, 2003), which evolved over three decades of using SASB methods in practice and research. IRT is an integrative approach that is used successfully in treating CORDS (comorbid, often rehospitalized, dysfunctional, suicidal) individuals who are *screened out of EST protocols* because of their prior nonresponsiveness, high levels of comorbidity, danger, diagnoses (e.g., drug and alcohol abuse often is ruled out), and difficulty in staying on protocol. A view of the alliance in relation to technique will be followed by an example of an alliance breach and repair in a complex CORDS case. Finally, our method of establishing connections between treatment integrity and outcome is described.

Interpersonal Studies of the Therapy Alliance, Using Measures Derived via Factor Analysis

In the interpersonal research literature, personality typically is defined by profiles based on factor analysis of data from representative populations. Examples are the Minnesota Multiphasic Personality Inventory (Hathaway et al., 2000) and the five-factor model (e.g., Costa & McCrae, 1992). Their reliability and concurrent validity are well established. There is a related interpersonal literature based on the single circumplex, which originally reflected an attempt to simplify factor-analytic descriptions. When descriptions of personality are reduced to just two dimensions, it is easy to plot a graph that locates individuals (or variables) in the underlying two-space. In the interpersonal research literature, two dimensional models usually are drawn as an interpersonal circle (IPC; Freedman, Leary, Ossorio, & Coffey, 1951; Leary, 1957). The two dimensions usually are Love versus Hate on the horizontal and Dominate versus Submit on the vertical. Wiggins (1982) reviewed these circles and their derivatives and offered an updated, geometrically "perfect" version of the IPC (Wiggins, Trapnell, & Phillips, 1988).

Of special current interest is Horowitz's (1988) *Inventory of Interpersonal Problems* (IIP), which plots individuals' responses to a checklist of interpersonal problems, weighting their scores by using factor loadings that define the two dimensions of the IPC. Research shows that individuals with more interpersonal problems are more likely to have a poor alliance (Pavio & Bahr, 1998). Some patients who begin with poorer alliances (cold, detached subtype) can improve alliance-related behavior during treatment (Hersoug, Hogland, Havik, von der Lippe, & Monsen, 2009). Puschner,

Bauer, Horowitz, and Kordy (2005) studied the alliance and IIP in 714 patients and reported:

> Interpersonal problems were most prevalent in the octants "introverted," "submissive," "exploitable," and "overly nurturant." Interpersonal problems were related to the helping alliance in different ways: "Too hostile" patients reported relatively poor initial helping alliance whereas "too friendly" patients rated more favorably the relationship to the therapist. However, interpersonal problems at intake did not predict the therapeutic alliance one-and-a-half years later. The results indicate that a poor initial helping alliance might be reversed during the course of treatment. (p. 415)

Research with measures derived by factor analysis consistently show that there are patient and therapist personality characteristics that can interfere with or enhance the alliance (Barber, 2009, p. 3). Results based on these methods begin and end with empirical findings. They are derived by factor analysis and tested for validity by factor analysis. Then, the measures are correlated with diagnoses, symptoms, and/or other variables. For example, Agreeableness, Openness, and Extraversion from the five-factor model are associated with a good therapy alliance (Coleman, 2006). While they make good intuitive sense in many cases, these examples of concurrent validity have not yet provided an integrative theoretical perspective that can produce testable constructs that separate alliance from technique or that explain mechanisms of change.

Structural Analysis of Social Behavior

SASB is similar to the IPC except that it includes a third dimension (focus) and its vertical axis ranges from enmeshment (control/submit) to differentiation (emancipate/separate) rather than from control to submit. SASB can be applied to a wide variety of interpersonal and intrapsychic patterns, whether of the therapy relationship, of loved ones from the present or past, or even of hallucinations (Benjamin, 1989). A central feature of IRT (Benjamin, 2003) is that SASB Intrex questionnaires provide operationalized assessments of internalized representations, mental templates for interaction that were described by Bowlby (1977) as "internal working models." A parallel objective observer coding system allows comparison of self ratings on the SASB Intrex questionnaires and objective observer opinions in the same metric.[3] Items that assess SASB were first constructed on the basis

---

[3]SASB ratings are processed by software available from the University of Utah (email: *Intrex@ psych.utah.edu*).

of dimensional ratings of item content by using samples of naïve raters. After dimensional ratings demonstrated that the content of items was as hypothesized, the validity of the items was then tested with factor analysis in which subjects applied the items to themselves. The conceptual advantages of using one method to write the items and another to test their validity when the goal is to palpate "the nature of nature" are discussed in Benjamin (in press-a).

The one-word cluster (i.e., simplified[4]) version of the SASB model appears in three sections indicated by three types of print in Figure 1. These three domains represent the dimension of focus. The **bolded** part shows transitive action directed toward another person (focus on other) and are prototypically parentlike. The underlined print shows intransitive reaction to another (focus on self) and are prototypically childlike. The *italicized* part represents what Sullivan (1953) called introjection, and it shows transitive action turned inward (introject).

For each of these types of focus, the horizontal dimension ranges from hate to love, shown in Figure 7.1 as **Attack**/Recoil/*Self-Attack* on the left and **Active Love**/Reactive Love/*Active Self-Love* on the right. The general name for the horizontal dimension is Affiliation. The general name for the vertical axis is Interdependence. For parentlike (transitive) focus, the range is from **Control** to **Emancipate**. For childlike (intransitive) focus, the range is from Submit to Separate. While the IPC opposes **Control** with Submit, SASB opposes **Control** with **Emancipate**, as suggested by Schaefer (1965). The matched points at the lower pole of the vertical dimension (**Control**/Submit) describe Enmeshment, while the matched points at the upper pole (**Emancipate**/Separate) describe Differentiation.

Predictive Principles

Any given point on the model is defined by the three dimensions of focus, affiliation, and interdependence. For example, the position Trust involves intransitive focus on self that is about 50% Reactive Love and 50% Submit. Its vector is (+4.5, −4.5) on the 9-point scales used for the full model. The predictive principles of the SASB model relate any given point to specific other points by variations in sign of the horizontal or vertical dimensions as well as by shifts in focus. Predictive principles are not expected to apply in every situation because they can be affected by other variables like gender, developmental age, social context, and more.

---

[4]There also is a two-word cluster model (Benjamin, 1987). In many of the citations that follow, the two-word version was used. The full model (Benjamin, 1979) provides even more informative detail about the interpersonal space depicted in Figure 7.1.

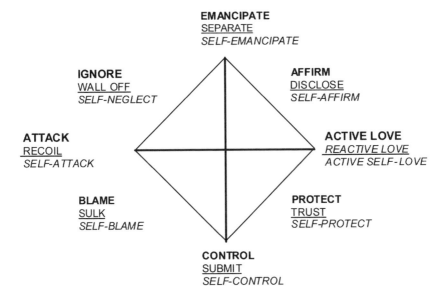

FIGURE 7.1. Simplified SASB cluster model. Focus on other, self, or introject are respectively indicated by **bold**, <u>underlined</u>, and *italic* fonts. From Benjamin (1996). Copyright 1996 by The Guilford Press, Reprinted by permission.

INTROJECTION

Introjection, shown in italicized print in Figure 7.1, describes *X* treating self as *X* has been treated. If mother **Protects** Susie, Susie likely will introject mother's protective behavior and engage in *Self-Protection*. If mother **Ignores** Susie, Susie will be more likely to *Self-Neglect*.

COMPLEMENTARY SETS

Complementary sets describe matches between persons *X* and *Y*. They are represented in Figure 7.1 by adjacent **bold** and <u>underlined</u> points. Coordinates for Complements are identical in sign and value on the affiliation and interdependence axes but differ in focus. For example, the complement of <u>Trust</u> is **Protect**. If Susie <u>Trusts</u> Ted, and Ted **Protects** Susie, they are in a complementary relationship, shown at the same geometric place on the model. Each is composed of about 50% friendliness and 50% enmeshment (+4.5, –4.5). Although their focus is "different," both are focusing on the same person. For example, if Ted focuses on Susie, and Susie focuses on herself, both are focused on Susie. The shared attentional focus with matching components on both axes means complementary pairs are likely to form a stable dyad.

SIMILARITIES

Predictions of similarity mean that persons X and Y show exactly the same patterns. If Susie Trusts her sister and her sister Trusts her, they have identical locations. Similarity is maximally unstable. For example, if two people both show friendly dependency, the relationship is likely to be unstable unless one moves to the complement, **Protect**.

OPPOSITES

The focus remains the same, but the signs of affiliation and interdependence are reversed. If Susie **Blames** Ted, both are focused on Ted, but Susie has switched to the exact opposite of **Affirm**. Instead of extending loving autonomy (+4.5, +4.5), she engages in hostile control (−4.5, −4.5).

ANTITHESES

Everything that can be changed is changed for antitheses. They differ in focus, affiliation, and interdependence; thus, an antithesis is the opposite of a complement. For example, the antithesis of **Blame** is Disclose (focus on other, −4.5, −4.5; focus on self, +4.5, +4.5). According to the principle of antithesis, if Susie **Blames** Ted, the antithesis is for Ted to Disclose: "I feel like leaving when you accuse me of being so terrible." This response has a chance of prompting Susie to **Affirm** his perspective instead of escalating the attack.

COMPLEX CODES

A useful feature of SASB, especially when working with severe disorders, is the ability to unpack complex messages. They are not unusual in therapy, as therapists may unwittingly include a hostile component in a seemingly friendly message like "Why couldn't you just do the therapy homework?" said in a warm way (Henry, Schacht, & Strupp, 1990). Depending on context, there may be merely the appearance of a friendly inquiry embedded in an implicit accusation (**Affirm** + **Blame**).

SASB and Therapy Goals

The origin of the SASB model was primate behavior, and its goal is to palpate "the nature of nature" (Benjamin, in press-a). Darwin's evolutionary theory was based on the idea of natural selection, and from that perspective "normal" can be defined by what is adaptive for a herd animal. Calling attention to the role of group behavior in survival makes it clear why attachment is so powerful in shaping human primate behavior. One consequence of the theoretical commitment to the primacy of attachment in human behavior is that therapy goal behaviors can be defined in positive qualitative terms related to survival rather than in negative and/or relativistic terms (i.e., through appeal to normative ratings/experience, with normality defined as the absence of "pathology"). In IRT, positive therapy goals are described by "goals speeches" at the beginning of treatment and by using everyday language. Therapy goal behavior (shown on the right side of Figure 7.1) consists of an interpersonal baseline of friendliness, moderate enmeshment, moderate differentiation, and a balance of focus. Affects predicted to accompany these friendly and balanced interpersonal positions are pleasant; parallel cognitive styles are functional. Although the positive goal patterns are predetermined in a global sense by the SASB model, the particular forms are chosen by each patient as his or her "healing image." In IRT, pathological behaviors also are listed and tagged for reduction. These are defined by the hostile regions of the SASB model; by extreme enmeshment or differentiation (poles of the vertical axis); and by an imbalance of focus. They are paralleled by uNPLeasant affects and dysfunctional cognitive styles.

The assumptions are supported empirically by the fact that friendly baselines are endorsed by normal samples while hostile patterns are more characteristic of patient samples. The proposal that extremes of enmeshment or differentiation also characterize psychopathology is less well supported but holds in some contexts (Benjamin, Wamboldt, & Critchfield, 2006).

SASB and Studies of the Alliance

In therapy approaches that focus on interpersonal interactions, it can be difficult to draw firm lines between relationship, alliance, and technique. Skillfully relating to patients could be seen as technique, particularly if, for example, some aspects of the therapy relationship are incorporated into the patient's self-concept. Evidence from SASB studies suggests that the therapy relationship, including the alliance, does have a more integral role in change than simply providing facilitative conditions for change. The general relevance of SASB to studies of relationship in therapy was marked by Rudy, McLemore, and Gorsuch (1985), who studied 42 patients and 11 therapists and found that "SASB scores can predict at least 65% of the reported progress variance, lending credence to claims that 'reflexive social behavior' and 'the relationship' are important determinants of certain aspects of therapeutic outcome" (p. 264).

PATIENT CONTRIBUTIONS TO THE ALLIANCE

Patient Friendliness. Patient friendliness enhances the alliance. Coady and Marziali (1994) noted that clients who showed more SASB-coded friendliness in sessions received higher alliance ratings from their therapist as well as from judges rating the alliance. Friendliness measured by SASB can be considered part of the therapy bond; it also is a necessary part of collaboration.

Patient Self-Directed Hostility. Patient self-directed hostility can be destructive to the alliance. Dunkle and Friedlander (1996) found that self-directed hostility (SASB introject) interferes with the alliance while perceived social support and a large degree of comfort with attachment enhance it. The same researchers report that the destructive effect of self-directed hostility appears particularly strong for the bond component of the alliance, suggesting that helping patients to address self-hatred could improve the alliance. Patient hostility in the therapy process can also appear in different forms at different times. For example, Dunkle and Friedlander (1996) showed that walling off and avoiding (hostile withdrawal) early in therapy predict a poor alliance, while later in therapy sulking and appeasing are associated with poorer alliance. This pattern suggests that the alliance can be improved if patient disengagement is addressed early in therapy, while resentful compliance might be of greater concern later in the therapy process.

Personality Disorders. Individuals with personality disorders (defined in the DSM-IV, American Psychiatric Association, 1994) often undermine the working alliance. For example, an individual with schizotypal personality disorder[5] probably will be sensitive to humiliation and tend to leave therapy for safety. The patient may be angry but not able or willing to talk about it. The therapist may be the target of irrational attributions involving mind reading. Individuals with passive–aggressive personality disorder may ask for therapy-related structure, agree to it, and then resist it ("I forgot; I was too busy; too upset by the session; didn't understand it when I got home"). Individuals with obsessive–compulsive personality disorder may try to control the therapy process in maladaptive ways. For example, they might be outwardly concerned about perfect compliance with therapy procedures and they take notes on everything the therapist says, to be sure to get it right—all without experiencing and participating in the therapy process itself.[6]

---

[5]This is one of the descriptors of the illustrative case cited later in this chapter.

[6]That would be described by a complex SASB code, Trust + Wall Off.

SASB codes of the criteria for each of the DSM-IV personality disorders, as well as prototypical relational histories, provide interpersonal descriptions for each disorder (Benjamin, 1996). These interpersonal patterns can alert clinicians to likely alliance problems. The SASB-based descriptions have been confirmed in a small number of research studies. Klein, Wonderlich, and Crosby (2001) estimated multiple partial correlations between personality disorder scales and SASB descriptions of the introject ($n = 366$) and reported: "Although there was some overlap between categories, most were associated with fairly distinct patterns of self-concept. The disorders also clustered together in meaningful ways along the major axes of Benjamin's interpersonal model of the self-concept" (p. 150).

Transference. Patient distortions of therapist behavior or therapy process can interfere with the alliance. Connolly et al. (1996) tested the psychoanalytic idea that transference problems should be the focal point of treatment. They used the QUAINT, a coding system that describes each person's Core Conflict Relationship Themes (CCRTs) in terms of Relationship Episodes (REs). The CCRT has 3 components: Responses of Others; Responses of Self; Wishes about Others. Each RE has a profile expressed in terms of categories mostly represented by SASB codes. Connolly et al. analyzed 35 patient QUAINT profiles describing the relationship with the therapist as well as with people mentioned in the therapy narrative. The existence of several clusters suggests that, for most patients, more than one profile was needed to describe his or her different ways of relating. For any given person, the profile that described the relationship with his or her therapist "was not necessarily the most pervasive pattern." In other words, transference exists but does not reflect all of a patient's patterns of relating. Patient relationship problems extend beyond transference problems that appear in therapy process.

Discrepancies between Patient and Therapist Views of the Therapy Process. Discrepancies between patient and therapist views of the therapy process mark problems in the alliance. Hartkamp and Schmitz (1999) used a nonlinear sequential analysis with successive SASB ratings of a patient's introject as well as his or her view of the therapy relationship; the therapist also made successive ratings of the therapy relationship. Among other things, they concluded:

> A divergence between the therapist and the patient views concerning their therapeutic relationship ... might indicate that both parties have different ideas of how the mutual relation should "function" or "work." At worst the therapist ... believes the patient capacity for disclosing himself and for

expressing his inner feelings to be the multivariate dominating variable. (p. 211)

By contrast, the patient's view in this study was that <u>trusting and relying</u> was the dominant variable. Speculating, it seems that the therapist might not have attended to the patient's feelings of dependency (seeking out complementary nurturance), instead interpreting the patient as simply sharing feelings. Such misreadings might interfere with the therapy alliance.

THERAPIST CONTRIBUTIONS TO THE ALLIANCE

Therapist Friendliness. Therapist friendliness enhances the alliance. Studies of therapy process typically show that therapist baseline codes reflect friendly focus on other (**Affirm** and **Protect**), while clients typically take the complementary position of friendly focus on self (<u>Disclose</u> and <u>Trust</u>) (e.g., Critchfield, Henry, Castonguay, & Borkovec, 2007). The friendly stance of each participant enhances bonding and the collaborative components of the therapy alliance.

Therapist Hostility. Therapist hostility is destructive to the alliance. Dunkle and Friedlander (1996) and Pavio and Bahr (1998) showed hostile therapist introjects are destructive to the alliance in general and the bond in particular. In addition, hostility in a therapist's interpersonal history, measured by SASB questionnaires, can leak into therapy process and interfere with the alliance (Hilliard, Henry, & Strupp, 2000). This idea is further supported by a study linking poor outcome to "negative complementarity," that is, therapist behavior that matches patient hostility rather than providing its friendly opposite (Henry, Schact, & Strupp, 1986). von der Lippe, Monsen, Ronnestad, and Eilertsen (2008) showed the same effect in delayed form. Lagged correlations suggested that therapists usually responded to patient hostility with immediate friendliness but then introduce hostility into later therapy exchanges. The authors suggest that this approach reflects a "subtly hostile therapeutic climate." Such findings support the need for therapists to be aware of and able to contain personal vulnerabilities. The too-common tendency to be hostile threatens both the therapy alliance and outcome.

Repairing Alliance Ruptures. Perceived hostility from the therapist is likely to be associated with a rupture[7] in the therapy alliance. Safran and Muran (1996) offered a model for repairing rupture in the therapy alli-

---

[7]A rupture is defined as patients reporting after sessions that they experienced tension, problems, misunderstanding, conflict, or disagreement. The SASB codes of these concepts all include some version of hostility.

ance. Neutral or hostile intransitive responses (SASB codes of <u>deferring &</u> <u>submitting</u>, <u>sulking & appeasing</u>, or <u>walling off & avoiding</u>) marked the beginning of ruptures.[8] The therapist should (1) notice the rupture and call for discussion of it; (2) find out what the rupture felt like; (3) explore the patient's response to it; and (4) help the patient say what he or she has to say about it (even if angry with the therapist). After the therapist validates (acknowledges, accepts, and supports) the patient's perspective, apologizing if appropriate, the breach is likely to have been repaired and the alliance restored. Other studies have confirmed the generality of this method of preserving the alliance (Muran et al., 2009).[9]

Therapist Focus on the Patient. Therapists are supposed to focus on the patient. The focus dimension of the SASB model constitutes a very important but frequently overlooked aspect of interpersonal relationships. Typically, in SASB studies of therapy process, therapists focus on patients and patients focus on themselves. In a small sample ($n = 9$), Coady and Marziali (1994) showed that the alliance is diminished if there is role reversal as the therapist focuses on him- or herself.[10] In a much larger sample ($n = 42$), Rudy, McLemore, and Gorsuch (1985) used SASB to assess both therapist and patient views of self and other and found "therapist ratings of *clients* as 'helping or protecting,' which suggest role reversal, were negatively associated with symptom amelioration" (p. 264).

Countertransference. Psychoanalysts formally recognize the possibility that therapists' personal reactions to the client can find their way into the therapy process. Traditionally that was seen as a problem due to incomplete analysis of the therapist. However, in more recent years, countertransference has been said potentially to be a proper basis for giving feedback about the patient's impact (e.g., "This is what makes people angry at you."). Whether constructive or destructive, countertransference does exist. Hamilton and Kevlignan (2009, p. 312) established that therapists' CCRTs affected judgment of patient CCRTs—especially the wish component. This trend was "moderated by therapeutic experience and receipt of personal therapy."

---

[8]Codes at the pole of extreme hostility have never been made in SASB-based psychotherapy studies.

[9]SASB is no longer used in assessing rupture repair, but the Wisconsin Personality Disorders Inventory (WISPI; Smith, Klein, & Benjamin, 2003) is a measure of outcome. The WISPI is based directly on SASB codes (interpersonal translations) of the DSM-IV descriptions of personality disorders (Benjamin, 1996).

[10]There was a negative correlation between therapist <u>disclosing and expressing</u> and the alliance.

Interactions, Contexts, and Contingencies

Content of the therapy narrative provides important context for interpreting therapy process, and therefore SASB studies that jointly study process and content can be especially informative. Karpiac and Benjamin (2004) provide a useful paradigm for attending to content of the narrative in relation to the alliance components: bonding and focus on the therapy goal. They identify instances in which the therapist was coded as <u>Affirming and Understanding</u> in a sample of treatment with cognitive-behavioral therapy (CBT) as well as another sample that used time-limited dynamic therapy (TLDP; Strupp & Binder, 1984). Whatever the patients did immediately after the therapist affirmed was classified into one of seven categories: interpersonal-adaptive, interpersonal-maladaptive, interpersonal-neutral, symptom-adaptive, symptom-maladaptive, symptom-neutral, and other. In both groups patients were more likely to continue talking about any topic after it was affirmed. In CBT, affirmations of goal behaviors were clearly associated with better outcomes (symptom reduction). In TLDP, affirmation of adaptive statements[11] improved outcome in the relationship with a significant other, assessed at termination and at 12 months posttreatment. Data show that therapist affirmation reinforces whatever is being said at the time. If affirming statements follow descriptions of goal behaviors, outcome is improved. This version of operant conditioning may depend on the therapy bond and may constitute a mechanism of change embedded in the therapy relationship.

On the basis of clinical observations, Benjamin (1996) noted that when confronted with a dilemma patients sometimes say, "What would [therapist's name] say or do?" Recalling the therapy discussion, they are able to implement new patterns of self management and more adaptive behaviors. Similarly, SASB introject theory, based on Sullivan's ideas, suggests that therapist friendliness enhances patient friendliness toward self. Quintana and Meara (1990) documented internalization of the therapist by asking 48 clients from two counseling centers to rate the therapy relationship and their own introjects on the SASB long-form questionnaires at the beginning and end of a brief treatment, concluding that clients internalized dispositions they perceived counselors held toward them.

Summary of SASB Studies of the Alliance

This review identified a number of patient and therapist attributes as well as aspects of therapist patient interactions that affect alliance and outcome,

---

[11]Changes in self-concept in TDLP showed an unexpected reverse effect: the affirmation of maladaptive statements regarding the significant other was associated with better SASB introject ratings at the end of treatment. The difference between therapies might be related to clarity in the definitions of goals. Alternatively, it might be attributable to the fact that some people feel better about themselves if affirmed after complaining about someone else, perhaps their significant other person.

showing that they carry significant outcome variance. Findings extend beyond the idea that the alliance simply increases hope and provides support for work on therapy tasks and goals. Patterns in the therapy relationship can provide a basis for more effective internal working models of self (introject) and other (relationship with significant others). On the other hand, hostile self-concepts and relational patterns in both patients and therapists can interfere with alliance and outcome.

INTERPERSONAL RECONSTRUCTIVE THERAPY

Although the incorporation of therapist positivity is important in therapy change, more is needed for maximal effect. This is particularly true when working with CORDS patients, who have already failed to improve with multiple trials of medications and versions of psychotherapy. Interpersonal reconstructive therapy (IRT) grew from SASB-based findings and theory as they applied to Benjamin's clinical practice primarily with personality disordered individuals. IRT is an integrative approach that explicitly combines principles from psychodynamic, cognitive-behavioral, client-centered, and existential humanist psychotherapies. Its case formulation method reflects a theory of psychopathology that relies heavily on the idea that primate social learning happens mostly through imitation or copying of loved ones, much like information about structure and function in the body is passed between generations by copying DNA. IRT explicitly seeks to address the focal point of pathology, just as internal medicine marks ways to contain a bacterium that causes a particular infectious disease. In IRT, the core psychopathogen is the Gift of Love (GOL), described below. Basic principles and methods of IRT are described in Benjamin (2003). Several recent enrichments of both theory and practice presented here are contained in Benjamin (in press-b).

IRT Case Formulation[12]

Presenting symptoms are linked to personality patterns that have evolved in relation to loved ones. The mechanism for developing personality patterns (in interaction with temperament) is imitation manifest as one or more of three copy processes: be like him or her (identification), act as you did with him or her (recapitulation), or treat yourself as you were treated

---

[12]Kenneth L. Critchfield and Kathleen Levenick, MD, have independently developed case formulations from video of the IRT consultative interview with their respective trainees. Formulations from eight cases were compared within and between sites for rater agreement about key figures, copy process, and links to symptoms. Strong reliability was observed for each comparison type, ranging from 71 to 95% agreement (Hawley, Critchfield, Dillinger, & Benjamin, 2005).

(introjection). For example, if a husband saw his father constantly criticize his mother and now constantly criticizes his own wife, he has identified with his father. If he complied resentfully with whatever his father wanted and now does that with his wife, he recapitulates his relationship with his father. If his father blamed him a lot and he blames himself, he is introjecting his relationship with his father. He is very likely to be depressed because he will continue to feel disappointed (if he is critical of everything) or oppressed (if he feels criticized and pushed around), helpless (to make others change or to have others treat him better) and self-critical. Copy processes reflect the SASB predictive principles[13] and have been supported by data in inpatient and outpatient populations, correcting for base rates (Critchfield & Benjamin, 2008). In our CORDS population, people will continue maladaptive copy process even after seeing the connections or receiving instruction in assertion. "Insight" and "instruction" is not enough. The case formulation provides a road map; the trip has to be taken experientially.

According to IRT, the reason such maladaptive and "unreasonable" patterns continue is that they are supported by GOL. These reflect loyalty to the rules and values of *the internalized representations* of loved ones (family in the head) whose affirmation and love still is deeply desired (e.g., the father in the preceding examples of copy process). The persistence is due to the fact that primates are hardwired to attach to whoever is in proximity during the early, vulnerable years. Modeling by those to whom we attach early on is powerful and permanent, probably because finding safety and avoiding threat are so basic to survival. The ideal parenting figure, described by Bowlby, provides a secure base. This identification fosters development of the "birthright self," which is characterized by the SASB descriptions of normal behavior and IRT goals previously described. Bowlby noted that a secure base allows the developing child to have the courage to go out and explore the world and develop an independent self. Harlow confirmed Bowlby's description of the "dance between dependence and independence" in laboratory experiments with rhesus monkeys (Harlow, 1958). If the parenting figure, the secure base by default, also poses threat, there is severe affective dysregulation because the reflexes appropriate to safety are mixed with reflexes appropriate to threat. The effect is that children abused by caregivers learn to see safety in threat. Examples of threat-based messages from caregivers include "Don't do better than your brother" or "I wish you had never been born." Children who hear things like that get the idea they should fail, not exist, and the like, depending on what the message was. Trying to please others who seem to wish you ill leads to intractable

---

[13]Identification reflects similarity. Recapitulation often reflects complementarity. Introjection remains as it was.

self-sabotage. Loyalty to the destructive rules and values in the hope of ulti-mate love from the family in the head typically invokes an implicit "time machine" that operates in the primitive mind to convince the patient it is possible to relive childhood again, this time with lots of love and support for self-actualization.

Complexity in personality is reflected in the IRT concepts of a Regres-sive Loyalist (Red) and a Growth Collaborator (Green). Red reflects self-sabotaging patterns connected through copy process to key figures via the GOL. Red patterns involve hostility, extremes of enmeshment/differentia-tion, and/or an imprecise focus, and these naturally correlate with symp-toms (Benjamin et al., 2006). Green patterns reflect the birthright self and are paralleled by therapy goal affects, behaviors, and cognitions. Everyone, therapists included, has copy processes, and some are Red and others Green. Differences between normality and pathology are found in what is copied.

IRT Treatment Model

IRT therapy interventions are described by a core algorithm that has these directives: convey accurate empathy; support Green patterns more than Red ones; use the case formulation; elicit detail about input, response, and impact on self; elicit parallel affects, cognitions, and behaviors associated with each incident under discussion; and follow the five steps, which are (1) collaborate, (2) learn about patterns (where they come from and what they are for), (3) block maladaptive patterns, (4) engage the will to change, and (5) learn new patterns. The ultimate challenge is to work toward confrontation of the impos-sibility of reliving childhood "as it should have been" and to grieve all the asso-ciated losses that have come from life choices in the service of GOL. Freedom from the past depends on (friendly) differentiation (*separation*) from the inter-nalized representations of key GOL figures whose approval is sought through self-sabotage. Moving forward depends on confronting new models of relating and rewiring affective circuits through extended practice and patience.

IRT Case Example: Jenn

The case of Jenn, treated in our IRT clinic first by a trainee and later by Ken-neth L. Crutchfield (KLC), illustrates the main features of IRT in relation to the alliance. Interestingly, the alliance-related points in each of the studies reviewed above appear in this case in one form or another.

Presenting problems

Jenn is a 50-year-old woman functioning at a high level as she manages a nursing home. She had been in a long and difficult divorce the year that preceded this, her third psychiatric hospitalization. She suffered from panic attacks, flashbacks of childhood trauma, and severe depression. She felt deeply humiliated and faulted herself for being "selfish"—causing her husband to leave—while at the same time she was enraged at his "unfair" actions. A suicide plan to "fix" her situation was supported by Jenn's belief that her deceased parents beckoned to her with promises of comfort in the afterlife. Her Axis I diagnoses of record included Bipolar Disorder and PTSD; she also had SCID-II diagnoses of borderline, paranoid, and schizotypal personality disorders.

Presenting Problems in the Context of Jenn's Early History

Jenn's childhood was dominated by recurrent, violent, and humiliating physical and sexual abuse by two older brothers. The brothers threatened to kill her if she told, and they backed up their threat with demonstrations, including one in which they nearly buried her alive. She chose to endure and be silent. Jenn was often publicly humiliated by her father, who would praise and admire her, only to become sarcastic and mock her later on for her trusting response. He said she was "weak" and "not like my boys." Her mother's response to complaints about the abuse was simply "Boys will be boys," seeming to go along with the father's degrading treatment of Jenn. She recalls crying loudly in her room for hours, hoping that her mother would come in to ask what was wrong and comfort her. Instead, she was either ignored or told to take care of one of her younger brothers. Having needs and feelings of one's own were "selfish" and "bad." Hugs for her were rare. She learned that the only path to acceptance was to be "strong" and seemingly unaffected by abuse, neglect, and humiliation. Jenn applied these rules and values as she chose a profession dedicated to serving and helping others. She had several long-term relationship partners who were beneficiaries of her service and caring. Her pattern with her husband was recapitulating a longer pattern of service to exploiters and critics dating back to her earliest years.

Copy Process and the GOL

Jenn's pattern of serving abusive and exploitative males recapitulates the relationships with her brothers and her father. She also continues to live the pattern of introjecting blame for whatever goes wrong, using self-talk that echoes the words used by her father and brothers. Her mother did not rescue her or provide solace, and so Jenn now neglects herself and does not recognize—much less attend to—her own needs (introjection of neglect as self-neglect). She expects and even enables the courts to treat her unfairly by not seeking counsel. Following the rules of the family in her head seals her fate as a highly functional "server" who can be used and dismissed until needed again. All this is supported by the conscious wish that she will join her parents in death and at last be loved by them (GOL). From time to time, as these scenarios recur, she becomes panicked, exhausted, and dangerously suicidal.

A Promising Beginning to Treatment

Jenn began treatment with an IRT trainee who offered empathy and validation. A very positive therapy alliance developed, and Jenn began to talk about forbidden stories and feelings. This openness made her extremely anxious. For all IRT patients, Red punishes defiance of the old rules,[14] including doing and feeling well. This inclination reliably shows up in self-talk and action to destroy a promising therapy. When that happened, the trainee used IRT techniques to help Jenn discover that after productive sessions she "heard" her father's voice mocking her for "being weak" and "telling too much." In addition, after a good session, Jenn would sometimes hear her mother's voice urging her to drive her car off the road and finally be soothed in the afterlife. With the help of the trainee, Jenn eventually began to "talk back" to the internalized representations of her mother and father. When she was able to do this, Jenn saw participating in the therapy process as healthy (Green) rather than "selfish" (Red). She began to think that staying alive might be preferable to dying solely in order to meet her mother in the afterlife. She was approaching ever more closely accepting the therapy goal, namely, her birthright self. The treatment was adherent in that it was using the case formulation to help her stop self-sabotaging herself after working toward the goal of a good life. The technique of discussing copy process helped Jenn reframe her view of the family in her own head and to begin to differentiate from it. Patterns of self-care emerged, and suicidality diminished. After several posttherapy conversations with the angry family in her head, the therapy alliance became even stronger, and Jenn seemed to be gaining strength from her secure therapy base. She was introjecting the therapist's caring to take better care of herself, incorporating the therapy relationship in her psychic structure.[15]

Some months later, Jenn discussed the early abuse by her brothers in fuller detail and again became extremely anxious and suicidal. Session frequency was increased to enhance the security of the therapy base. Jenn and

---

[15]Jenn's ratings of self-treatment (using the SASB Intrex questionnaires) clearly supported this expectation.

[14]This is an explanation for the saying "Things will get worse before they get better." Using adherence scales that reflect the interaction of process and content, we can account for—and even predict—ups and downs in symptoms.

the therapist agreed to stop talking about the trauma because the reactiva-tion of affects was not well controlled. For reasons unknown at the time, Jenn began to withhold information from her therapist and to call suicide hotlines instead. Rather than recognize the withdrawal (implying the thera-pist was perceived as engaging in complementary **Ignoring**) and take steps to repair the breach, the trainee focused on crisis management and safety contracts. Two emergency room visits and hospitalization followed. The trainee was overwhelmed and frustrated. Jenn unilaterally terminated IRT, saying she felt unsupported.

Several weeks later, Jenn called the IRT clinic, asking to resume treat-ment. As the trainee had chosen to leave the clinic, KLC met with Jenn to debrief her and explore the possibility of resuming therapy. Jenn explained that the discussion of trauma was not the problem per se (although this topic was very difficult for her). Instead, she felt that her therapist had withdrawn emotionally after discussing the abuse so concretely (confirming the predic-tion of complementarity mentioned previously). Our guess is that the trainee may have been withdrawing subtly, at least in part because all the extra ses-sions and the high stakes were wearing her out.[16] The trainee received extra supervisory sessions to parallel the increase in sessions for Jenn, but nonethe-less Jenn saw emotional withdrawal—as would be expected from her case formulation. Perceived (or actual) hostility begets hostility, and outcome is worsened, just as the research shows. Jenn was asking for understanding and support on a topic that had been expressly denied a hearing when she was a child. Crying about the outrageous abuse and her pain had been for-bidden. Instead of feeling heard and supported in the way she needed, in the context of suicidal threats, the emphasis had been on safety contracts and limits, perceived by Jenn as further rejection. Moreover, taking inordinate responsibility as always, Jenn thought she had hurt her therapist somehow. In sum, Jenn was primed to see her therapist as agreeing with her internal-ized family, and we had a full-blown old-fashioned negative transference (or recapitulation, in IRT terms).

This breach might have been less likely if the IRT rule "If things go wrong, check the therapy relationship first" had been emphasized along with the safety contracts. The SASB codes of Jenn's distress calls to the cri-sis lines and the repeated ER visits suggested she was not getting what she needed from IRT; so, exploring Jenn's feelings as well as the trainee's feel-ings about the therapy process likely would have helped. These appropriate interventions did happen later, as KLC met with Jenn and acknowledged our failure to help her understand and talk about the abuse and explored

---

[16]In fact, the trainee cared very much, and that may have added to the overload factor in explaining why she felt overwhelmed by the nonresponsiveness of the crisis behaviors.

how she felt about the subsequent therapy process. As is appropriate after repairing a breach, Jenn was ready to resume IRT, this time with KLC as her therapist.

As therapy continued, Jenn had dreams that KLC would act like family, but they discussed these incidents as they occurred, maintained the alliance, and continued the work on differentiation from family "in the head" to become free to move on toward the goal of rescuing the birthright self. Eventually Jenn learned to recognize her distortions in the therapy relationship and maintain the alliance without reminders from KLC. Again, the technique of working with copy process helped her keep perspective, whether she struggled with trusting KLC and distinguishing him from her ex-husband or struggled with other traumatic figures from her past. KLC's function as a secure base is best illustrated by the fact that Jenn decided to take an "imaginary KLC" with her to a difficult hearing in her long, drawn-out divorce process. Thinking of him being there with her calmed her greatly, and she did very well in asserting herself in behalf of her own needs! She also continued to work on differentiating from the destructive rules of the "family in the head." She had imaginary "two-chair" conversations with her father, speaking now from her "birthright self." This imaginary process, as always, became very real. In the middle of it, she announced, "He does not like you." KLC replied, "Of course not," reminding her indirectly of how Red dislikes progress and hope, and the conversation continued. Slowly, she approached the core task of revising her hopes that interactions with her family *could have been* different (GOL). This process was accompanied by deep grief over realization that they *never will have loved her* and that loyalty to old rules had cost her dearly in her life choices up to then. As she began to accept these nonlinear but compelling truths, Jenn began focusing even more on caring for herself more in the present and coping with current problems with new therapy goal behaviors. She became better able to resist the "call of the Red" to regress and increased her efforts to choose new patterns in friendship. She even began to date a very kind man. The final IRT step of learning new patterns was under way. Many Red attacks were to follow, which is always the case. If both patient and therapist hold steady on behalf of the birthright self, profound change can occur (Benjamin, in press-b).

Alliance and Technique

Bordin's definition of an alliance can cover all treatments for mental disorder, including delivering medications. Indeed, even the placebo group in the National Institute of Mental Health Collaborative Study of Depression had a significant alliance/outcome effect (Krupnick et al., 1996). To review: If there is a working alliance, patient and therapist agree on the problems to be solved, goals to be reached, and procedures to be used to try to reach the goals. In the process, a bond develops. If the various therapies all have alliances of this sort, *then technique would distinguish therapies primarily by descriptions of the goal, procedures used to reach the goal, and the mechanisms that explain how techniques achieve the goal.* In a drug treatment, the goal is symptom relief, and the patient and physician collaborate to identify and administer optimal drugs in optimal doses. In CBT, the patient would seek symptom relief and collaborate with the therapist in learning and practicing more adaptive cognitive styles. The mechanism is partially understood by assuming that affects parallel cognitions, and so if you *willfully* change cognitions you can change related affects (depression, anxiety, anger). In IRT, the goal is to develop optimal attachment behaviors that reduce symptoms. The method involves transforming the internal working models that affirm self-sabotage to models that support the birthright self. SASB questionnaires and codes of process and content of sessions are crucial in assessing changes in internal working models relative to in-session changes and those reported in everyday life.

Mechanisms of change, according to IRT, start with the hypothesis that pathology arises when copy processes are associated with symptoms and supported by allegiance to internalized representations of caregivers who offered both safety and threat. Self-sabotage is manifest as the patient seeks safety via compliance with perceived rules and values of the not-so-safe secure base. The SASB studies reviewed earlier showed that introjection and imitation[17] of therapist interactions contribute significantly to the alliance and the outcome. IRT theory would interpret that result to mean that the therapy bond enhances attachment (alliance and outcome) because it provides a benign template for building a new secure base consisting of internalized representations of normative relationships. Call the effects of the installation of this more benign template "the structural impact of the alliance." This happens naturally, whether or not it is discussed in therapy. The structural impact of the alliance likely is transtheoretical, with some therapy approaches maximizing the effect more than others. For example, given the view of the human being as a herd animal, it is highly likely that *well-managed* group treatments can have a large structural impact via the alliance by installing a *powerful benevolent introject* of "the group."

As in other therapies, the alliance in IRT supports the willingness to engage in the therapy and has the structural impact just described. Also, like other therapies, IRT techniques offer instruction in adaptive ways of behaving and managing affect and cognitive style. If support of such new learning

---

[17]Additional copy processes likely are involved. With SASB they could be measured across types of therapy.

plus structural change from the alliance suffices, well and good. However, if those factors fail to be helpful enough, which always is the case in our CORDS, more is needed. Here, the more unique factors associated with IRT technique (the use of case formulation's applications of copy process and GOLs that support pathological patterns) become especially important. Mechanisms of change inhere in the technique of consistently addressing the motivation (GOL) that supports the self-sabotaging behaviors that *actively interfere with new learning*. IRT technique continually focuses on the task of becoming free of wishes based in the past that support self-sabotage as well as of the need to maintain a vision of therapy goal behaviors. Jenn's progress in IRT clearly illustrates how difficult the shift is from old wishes to new goals. As positive change emerged, Red loyalties sought to destroy the therapy alliance. Good sessions reliably elicited attacks on her, the therapist, and the therapy. Call this a "dynamic breach" to mark the fact that it results from Red internal processes reacting to progress and to distinguish it from a breach (described by Safran and Muran) that results from therapist error (e.g., misunderstanding; or therapist Red showing up as subtle hostility). A dynamic breach is repaired if the therapist provides an adequately secure base; uses IRT technique to motivate distance from old loyalties by reminding the patient of the interpersonal basis of instructions to self-destruct; reactivates the patient's own vision of the Green goal; and, most importantly, elicits collaboration in setting up concrete, realistic, effective counterstrategies to the Red attacks. New flow charts for techniques that help Green prevail in the struggle with Red appear in Benjamin (in press-b).

Effectiveness of IRT

For practical as well as ideological reasons, we favor intensive small-*n* effectiveness research that involves reliable definitions of the presumed active ingredients of the treatment model and connecting them to progress. We developed an adherence scale that assesses each element of the IRT core algorithm by using concrete behavioral anchors from the negative extreme of egregious violations to the positive end that describes full implementation of the element being rated (Critchfield, Davis, Gunn, & Benjamin, 2008). The ability clearly to identify errors as well as to correct interventions and to relate them directly to symptom change (as in Jenn's case) is vital to the goal of having a valid science of psychotherapy. A pilot study of seven treatment-resistant personality disordered cases in our IRT clinic has yielded a significant correlation between progress with the Gift of Love (an important part of adherence) and residualized change in symptoms. Separate inspection of scales with a different sampling of cases suggests that collaboration and engaging the will to change (via use of GOL concepts) contributes maximally to successful therapy completion (versus dropout) in highly comorbid, severely personality-disordered patients who have long, well-documented histories of much treatment and little or no prior change.

REFERENCES

American Psychiatric Association. (1994). *Diagnostic and statistical manual of mental disorders* (4th ed.). Washington, DC: Author.

Barber, J. P. (2009). Toward a working through of some core conflicts in psychotherapy research. *Psychotherapy Research, 19*, 1–12.

Barber, J. P., Connolly, M. B., Crits-Christoph, P., Gladis, L., & Siqueland, L. (2000). Alliance predicts patients' outcome beyond in-treatment change in symptoms. *Journal of Consulting and Clinical Psychology, 68*(6), 1027–1032.

Benjamin, L. S. (1979). Structural analysis of differentiation failure. *Psychiatry: Journal for the Study of Interpersonal Processes, 42*, 1–23.

Benjamin, L. S. (1987). Use of the SASB dimensional model to develop treatment plans for personality disorders: I. Narcissism. *Journal of Personality Disorders, 1*, 43–70.

Benjamin, L. S. (1989). Is chronicity a function of the relationship between the person and the auditory hallucination? *Schizophrenia Bulletin, 15*, 291–310.

Benjamin, L. S. (1996). *Interpersonal diagnosis and treatment of personality disorders*. New York: Guilford Press.

Benjamin, L. S. (2003). *Interpersonal reconstructive therapy: Promoting change in nonresponders*. New York: Guilford Press. (Paperback edition 2006, with subtitle *An integrative personality based treatment for complex cases*)

Benjamin, L. S. (in press-a). SASB and the nature of nature. In S. Strack & L. Horowitz (Eds.), *Handbook on interpersonal psychology: Theory, research, assessment, and therapeutic interventions*. New York: Wiley.

Benjamin, L. S. (in press-b). *Interpersonal Reconstructive Therapy (IRT) for anger, anxiety and depression*. Washington, DC: American Psychological Association.

Benjamin, L. S., Wamboldt, M. Z., & Critchfield, K. L. (2006). Defining relational disorders and identifying their connections to Axes I and II. In S. R. H. Beach, M. Wamboldt, N. Kaslow, R. E. Heyman, M. E. First, L. E. Underwood, & D. Reiss (Eds.), *Relational processes and DSM-V: Neuroscience, assessment, prevention and intervention*. Washington, DC: American Psychiatric Association.

Bordin, E. S. (1979). The generalizability of the psychoanalytic concept of the working alliance. *Psychotherapy, Theory, Research, and Practice, 16*, 252–260.

Bowlby, J. (1977). The making and breaking of affectional bonds. *British Journal of Psychiatry, 130*, 201–210.

Bratton, S. C., Landreth, G. L., Kellam, T., & Blackard, S. R. (2006). *Child–Parent Relationship Therapy (CPRT) treatment manual: A 10-session filial therapy model for training parents*. New York: Routledge/Taylor & Francis.

Chambless, D. L., & Crits-Christoph, P. (2006). What should be validated? In J. C. Norcross, L. E. Beutler, & R. F. Levant (Eds.), *Evidence-based practices in mental health: Debate and dialogue on the fundamental questions*. Washington, DC: American Psychological Association.

Chambless, D. L., & Ollendick, T. H. (2001). Empirically supported psychological interventions: Controversies and evidence. *Annual Review of Psychology, 52,* 685–716.

Coady, N. F., & Marziali, E. (1994). The association between global and specific measures of the therapeutic relationship. *Psychotherapy, 31,* 17–27.

Coleman, D. (2006). Client personality, working alliance and outcome: A pilot study. *Social Work in Mental Health, 4,* 83–98.

Connolly, M. B., Crits-Christoph, P., Demorest, A., Azarian, K., Muenz, L., & Chittams, J. (1996). Varieties of transference patterns in psychotherapy. *Journal of Consulting and Clinical Psychology, 64,* 1213–1221.

Costa, P. T., & McCrae, R. R. (1992). Normal personality assessment in clinical practice: The NEO-5 Inventory. *Psychological Assessment, 4,* 5–13.

Critchfield, K. L., & Benjamin, L. S. (2008). Internalized representations of early interpersonal experience and adult relationships: A test of copy process theory in clinical and nonclinical populations. *Psychiatry: Interpersonal and Biological Processes, 71,* 71–92.

Critchfield, K. L., Davis, M. J., Gunn, H. E., & Benjamin, L. S. (2008, June). *Measuring therapist adherence in Interpersonal Reconstructive Therapy (IRT): Conceptual framework, reliability, and validity.* Poster presented to the International Society for Psychotherapy Research, Barcelona, Spain.

Critchfield, K. L., Henry, W. P., Castonguay, L. G., & Borkovec, T. D. (2007). Interpersonal process and outcome in variants of cognitive-behavioral psychotherapy. *Journal of Clinical Psychology, 63*(1), 31–51.

Crits-Christoph, P., Connolly Gibbons, M. B., Crits-Christoph, K., Narducci, J., Schamberger, M., & Gallop, R. (2006). Can therapists be trained to improve their alliances?: A pilot study of Alliance-Fostering Therapy. *Psychotherapy Research, 13,* 268–281.

Crits-Christoph, P., Cooper, A., & Luborsky, L. (1988). The accuracy of therapists' interpretations and the outcome of dynamic psychotherapy. *Journal of Consulting and Clinical Psychology, 56,* 490–495.

Dunkle, J. H., & Friedlander, M. L. (1996). Contribution of therapist experience and personal characteristics to the working alliance. *Journal of Consulting Psychology, 43,* 456–460.

Freedman, M. B., Leary, T. F., Ossorio, A. G., & Coffey, H. S. (1951). The interpersonal dimensions of personality. *Journal of Personality, 20,* 143–161.

Freud, S. (1904/1959). On psychotherapy. Reprinted in *Sigmund Freud Collected Papers, Volume 1.* New York: Basic Books.

Goldfried, M. R., & Woolf, B. E. (1996). Psychotherapy practice and research: Repairing a strained alliance. *American Psychologist, 51,* 1007–1016.

Greenson, R. R. (1965). The working alliance and the transference neurosis. *Psychoanalytic Quarterly, 34,* 155–179.

Hamilton, J., & Kevlignan, D. M. (2009). Therapists' projection: The effects of therapists' relationship themes on their formulation of clients' relationship episodes. *Psychotherapy Research, 19,* 312–322.

Harlow, H. F. (1958). The nature of love. *American Psychologist, 13,* 673–685.

Hartkamp, H., & Schmitz, H. (1999). Structures of introject and case study of inpatient psychotherapy therapist–patient interaction in a single case study of inpatient psychotherapy. *Psychotherapy Research*, 9, 199–215.

Hathaway, S. R., McKinley, J. C., Meehl, P. E., Drake, L. E., Welsh, G. S., MacAndrew, C., et al. (Ed.). (2000). *Basic sources on the MMPI-2*. Minneapolis: University of Minnesota Press.

Hawley, N., Critchfield, K. L., Dillinger, R. J., & Benjamin, L. S. (2005). *Case formulation in Interpersonal Reconstructive Therapy: Using SASB and copy process theory to reliably track repeating interpersonal themes*. Poster presented to the International Society for Psychotherapy Research, Toronto, Canada

Henry, W. P., Schacht, T. E., & Strupp, H. H. (1986). Structural analysis of social behavior: Application to a study of interpersonal process in differential psychotherapeutic outcome. *Journal of Consulting and Clinical Psychology*, 54, 27–31.

Henry, W. P., Schacht, T. E., & Strupp, H. H. (1990). Patient and therapist introject, interpersonal process, and differential therapy outcome. *Journal of Consulting and Clinical Psychology*, 58, 768–774.

Hersoug, A. G., Hoglend, P., Havik, O., von der Lippe, A., & Monsen, J. (2009). Therapist characteristics influencing the quality of alliance in long-term psychotherapy. *Clinical Psychology and Psychotherapy*, 216, 100–110.

Hilliard, R. B., Henry, W. P., & Strupp, H. H. (2000). An interpersonal model of psychotherapy: Linking patient and therapist developmental history, therapeutic process and types of outcome. *Journal of Consulting and Clinical Psychology*, 68, 125–133.

Horowitz, L. M. (1988). Inventory of Interpersonal Problems: Psychometric properties and clinical applications. *Journal of Clinical and Consulting Psychology*, 56, 885–892.

Horvath, A. (2006). The alliance in context: Accomplishments, challenges, and future directions. *Psychotherapy: Theory, Research, Practice, Training*, 43, 258–263.

Imber, S. D., Pilkonis, P. A., Sotsky, S. M., Elkin, I., Watkins, J. T., Collins, J. F., et al. (1990). Mode-specific effects among 3 treatments for depression. *Journal of Consulting and Clinical Psychology*, 58, 352–359.

Karpiak, C. P., & Benjamin, L. S. (2004). Therapist affirmation and the process and outcome of psychotherapy: Two sequential analytic studies. *Journal of Clinical Psychology*, 60, 659–676.

Klein, M. H., Wonderlich, S. A., & Crosby, R. (2001). Self-concept correlates of the personality disorders. *Journal of Personality Disorders*, 15, 150–156.

Krupnick, J. L., Sotsky, S. M., Simmens, S., Moyer, J., Elkin, I., Watkins, J., et al. (1996). The role of the therapeutic alliance in psychotherapy and pharmacotherapy outcome: Findings in the National Institute of Mental Health Treatment of Depression Collaborative Research program. *Journal of Consulting and Clinical Psychology*, 64, 532–539.

Leary, T. (1957). *Interpersonal diagnosis of personality: A functional theory and methodology for personality evaluation*. New York: Ronald Press.

Luborsky, L. (1984). *Principles of psychoanalytic psychotherapy: A manual for supportive–expressive treatment*. New York: Basic Books.

Muran, J. C., Safran, J. D., Gorman, B. S., Samstag, L. W., Eubanks-Carter, C.,

& Winston, A. (2009). The relationship of early alliance ruptures and their resolution to process and outcome in three time-limited psychotherapies for personality disorders. *Psychotherapy Theory, Research, Practice, Training, 46,* 233–248.

Norcross, J. C., Beutler, L. E., & Levant, R. F. (Eds.). (2006). *Evidence-based practices in mental health: Debate and dialogue on the fundamental questions.* Washington, DC: American Psychological Association.

Pavio, S. C., & Bahr, L. M. (1998). Interpersonal problems, working alliance, and outcome in short-term experiential therapy. *Psychotherapy Research, 8,* 392–407.

Perepletchikova, F., Hilt, L. M., Chereji, E., & Kazdin, A. E. (2009). Barriers to implementing treatment integrity procedures: Survey of treatment outcome researchers. *Journal of Consulting and Clinical Psychology, 77,* 212–218.

Puschner, B., Baue, S., Horowitz, L. M., & Kordy, H. (2005). The relationship between interpersonal problems and the helping alliance. *Journal of Clinical Psychology, 61,* 415–429.

Quintana, S. M., & Meara, N. M. (1990). Internalization of therapeutic relationships in short-term psychotherapy. *Journal of Counseling Psychology, 37,* 123–130.

Rogers, C. R. (1951). *Client-centered therapy.* Cambridge MA: Riverside Press.

Rogers, Carl R., & Dymond, R. F. (Eds.) (1954). *Personality and psychotherapy change.* Chicago: University of Chicago Press.

Rudy, J. P., McLemore, C. W., & Gorsuch, R. L. (1985). Interpersonal behavior and therapeutic progress: therapists and clients rate themselves and each other. *Psychiatry: Journal for the Study of Interpersonal Process, 48,* 264–281.

Safran, J. D., & Muran, J. C. (1996). The resolution of ruptures in the therapeutic alliance. *Journal of Consulting and Clinical Psychology, 64,* 447–458.

Schaefer, E. S. (1965). Configurational analysis of children's reports of parent behavior. *Journal of Consulting Psychology, 29,* 552–557.

Smith, L. T., Klein, M. H., & Benjamin, L. S. (2003). Validation of the Wisconsin Personality Disorders Inventory-IV with the SCID-II. *Journal of Personality Disorders, 17,* 173–187.

Strupp, H. H., & Binder, J. L. (1984). *Psychotherapy in a New Key: A Guide to Time-Limited Dynamic Psychotherapy.* New York: Basic Books.

Sullivan, H. S. (1953). *The interpersonal theory of psychiatry.* New York: Norton.

von der Lippe, A. L., Monsen, J. T., Ronnestad, M. H., & Eilertsen, D. E. (2008). Treatment failure in psychotherapy: The pull of hostility. *Psychotherapy Research, 18,* 420–432.

Wiggins, J. S. (1982). Circumplex models of interpersonal behavior in clinical psychology. In P. C. Kendall & J. N. Butcher (Eds.), *Handbook of research methods in clinical psychology.* New York: Wiley.

Wiggins, J. S., Trapnell, P., & Phillips, N. (1988). Psychometric and geometric characteristics of the Revised Interpersonal Adjective Scales (IAS-R). *Multivariate Behavioral Research, 23,* 517–530.

CHAPTER 8

■ ■ ■ ■ ■

The Therapeutic Alliance in Cognitive-Behavioral Therapy

Louis G. Castonguay
Michael J. Constantino
Andrew A. McAleavey
Marvin R. Goldfried

The nature and role of the therapeutic relationship in cognitive and behavioral therapies (CBTs) has long been discussed and debated. Although cognitive-behavioral therapists have from the beginning recognized the importance of the therapeutic relationship in the change process, it has only relatively recently been given considerable attention in the CBT research literature as the operationalized construct of the alliance. Although its conceptual roots are in psychodynamic therapy, the alliance is now considered an integral part of virtually all psychotherapies, including CBTs. Presently commonly viewed as a transtheoretical common factor, the alliance has been deemed "the quintessential integrative variable" (Wolfe & Goldfried, 1988). While controversy continues to exist, especially as to whether or not the alliance contributes causally to symptomatic outcomes (cf. Barber, 2009; Barber, Connolly, Crits-Christoph, Gladis, & Siqueland, 2000; Crits-Christoph, Connolly Gibbons, & Hearon, 2006; DeRubeis, Brotman, & Gibbons, 2005), the alliance has risen to prominence in empirical, theoretical, and clinical writing. The primary purpose of this chapter is to explore the evolution of the alliance construct and its determinants in the CBT literature.

CBTs (and treatments heavily influenced by these approaches) focus on the direct reduction of psychopathological symptoms and ascribe to the belief that therapy should (and good therapy does) provide clients with coping skills with which they can approach their daily lives in the absence of a therapist (Barber & DeRubeis, 1989; Castonguay, Newman, Borkovec, Grosse Holtforth, & Maramba, 2005). CBTs have been developed for numerous disorders including, but not limited to, depression, phobias, panic disorder and agoraphobia, posttraumatic stress disorder, social anxiety disorder, obsessive–compulsive disorder, bipolar disorder, eating disorders, borderline personality disorder, and substance abuse (see Barlow, 2008). Moreover, cognitive and behavioral therapies have become very popular theoretical orientations among practicing clinicians (Norcross, Karpiak, & Santoro, 2005). Many CBTs are empirically supported (Nathan & Gorman, 2002), reflecting the epistemological outlook and historical strength of CBTs in establishing, relying on, and encouraging scientific research.

Interestingly, it may be that CBTs' foundation on learning and conditioning is the main reason why the therapeutic relationship went for years as an underrecognized factor in most of these treatments. Although the pioneers of behavior therapy highlighted the importance of the relationship, many described it as strictly context for learning to take place. As Wilson and Evans (1977) postulated, " 'Relationship' is not easily defined operationally, unlike contingencies of social attention. Not only could these social contingencies be defined and measured, but they could also be altered, and with them the client's behavior" (p. 545). In this paradigm, it makes sense that CBT techniques have historically received the bulk of attention, considering it took time to operationalize the relationship and to subject it to experimental manipulation. Once empirical evidence supported the operationalization and valid measurement of the relationship as well as its correlation with outcome in CBTs, proponents of this approach have more readily accepted the alliance as a *potentially* potent treatment factor in its own right.

In the remaining pages, we explore the historical, theoretical, and empirical treatment of the alliance within CBTs. First, we describe what can be considered the "traditional" behavioral, cognitive, and cognitive-behavioral approach to the relationship: those qualities of the relationship put forth by CBT pioneers such as Wolpe, Goldfried and Davison, Wilson, and Beck that distinguish a CBT relationship from other therapies. Next, we explore the ways in which CBTs have fostered and maintained this orientation-specific ideal relationship. Then we will examine several pieces of empirical evidence regarding the role of the alliance in CBTs as it is practiced and offer some conclusions regarding the way CBTs actually make use of the relationship. Finally, we examine how developments within CBTs led to different ways to conceptualize and use the alliance.

NATURE AND FUNCTION OF THE ALLIANCE IN CBTs

When behavior therapy was developing during the 1950s and '60s, there was little empirical support for the effectiveness of relationship variables outside of the Rogerian constructs of therapist empathy, warmth, and genuineness (Rogers, 1951, 1957). However, given the substantial influence of Rogers's work, early behaviorally oriented theorists noted the clinical importance of such relational qualities even in behavior therapy, often directly crediting these contributions to other orientations. Wolpe (1958), for instance, noted that many of his clients who appeared to like him early in treatment showed noticeable improvement before specific treatment methods were used.

Later, Goldfried and Davison (1976), in one of the first full chapters devoted to the therapeutic relationship from a CBT perspective, made the bold statement "Any behavior therapist who maintains that principles of learning and social influence are all one needs to know in order to bring about behavior change is out of contact with clinical reality" (p. 55), going on to state that "the truly skillful behavior therapist ... interacts in a warm and empathic manner with his client" (p. 56). Similarly, Brady suggested that the therapist should seek to be perceived as an "honest, trustworthy, and decent human being with good social and ethical values" (Brady et al., 1980). Beck, Rush, Shaw, and Emery (1979), in describing a cognitive approach to therapy, also emphasized the similarity between orientations, noting that "cognitive and behavior therapies probably require the same subtle therapeutic atmosphere that has been described explicitly in the context of psychodynamic therapy" (p. 50). Further, they went on to discuss warmth, accurate empathy, and genuineness as important characteristics of cognitive and behavioral therapists.

The statements and quotes above are characteristic of the way that the relationship was treated by behavior therapists early on (and often currently as well): brief descriptions of warm relationships without explicit elaboration or specification. Such unelaborated descriptions are likely attributable to the fact that CBTs historically considered the alliance to be a "nonspecific" variable, that is, a nontechnical, noninstrumental, and essentially interpersonal factor that is auxiliary to the specific variables (technical procedures) that actually produce change (Castonguay, 1993). Wolpe and Lazarus (1966) famously concluded that a client's positive emotional reaction toward a therapist would engender "nonspecific reciprocal inhibition," meaning that the presence of the therapist reduces anxiety and therefore facilitates the aim of specific desensitization through behavioral techniques. Nonspecific factors, historically including the placebo effect, demand characteristics, suggestion, empathy, expectation, and rapport, were treated for some time in the literature as undefined (and possibly indefinable) variables in therapy, with effects that are assumed to be good, yet somehow tangential to therapy.

However, in keeping with the epistemological foundation of CBT, Wilson and Evans (1977) attempted to specify and observe the constituents of the therapeutic relationship. Drawing on Bandura's (1969) social cognitive theory, they offered a nuanced and advanced operationalization of the relationship in behavior therapy. As these authors wrote:

> Social influence processes such as persuasion, expectancy, attitude change, and interpersonal attraction are integral features of behavior modification thus conceived. Within this expanded context, the reciprocal influence processes which define the therapist–client relationship are viewed as being of the utmost importance to the understanding and effective use of behavioral treatment methods. (Wilson & Evans, 1977, p. 546)

These authors suggested that the relationship is not a diffuse effect but rather an amalgam of many different factors that are endemic to social learning theory. To Wilson and Evans, the relationship provides social reinforcement, elicits client behavior in session, increases therapist influence by improving client attraction to the therapist, allows the therapist to serve as a role model, and fosters therapeutic expectancies.

Thus, CBTs have a long history of recognizing relationship variables as significant contributors to the therapeutic process, generally in the same ways that other orientations defined the relationship. Of course, the alliance in CBTs is different (at least theoretically) in some ways from the types of alliances formed in other orientations. The primary distinction is that a CBT alliance emphasizes collaboration and teamwork more than most other therapies do—especially those that are less directive (Raue & Goldfried, 1994). The model of "collaborative empiricism" has emerged primarily from (Beck et al., 1979, p. 6) and continues to be central to cognitive therapy (e.g., Young, Rygh, Weinberger, & Beck, 2008), with proponents of recent behavioral therapies (e.g., Dimidjian, Martell, Addis, & Herman-Dunn, 2008) and CBTs (e.g., Fairburn, Cooper, Shafran, & Wilson, 2008; Turk, Heimberg, & Magee, 2008) using the construct of a collaborative relationship extensively. In a collaborative relationship, clients and therapists work together to identify the central problems clients face and to identify possible solutions. While all therapists seek to identify central client problems, a sense of collaboration is eschewed in some treatments. For example, from their Gestalt therapy perspective, Perls, Hefferline, and Goodman (1977) tellingly state, "We employ a method of argument that at first sight may seem unfair, but that is unavoidable" (p. 286). In client-centered therapy, the power for change is theoretically deferred to the client (Rogers, 1951). In contrast, when describing empiricism (which seeks to move past distorted perception and toward verifiable observation), Beck et al. (1979) used the analogy of two scientists who must work together, one providing the "raw data" and the other guiding the research questions.

Another important difference in the way CBTs and other orientations have treated the alliance underscores the role that this treatment factor is assumed to play in the change process. Specifically, as with many directive therapies, CBTs are primarily concerned with orientation-specific techniques that can demonstrably produce change on their own. Therefore, the alliance has typically been treated as a factor that facilitates the use of and adherence to specific techniques not as a change mechanism itself. That is, the main purpose of the therapeutic relationship is to foster engagement in the specific techniques of therapy, and a collaborative relationship is ideally suited for this purpose. Simply put, cognitive and behavioral therapists have generally seen the alliance as a necessary, but not sufficient, therapeutic change factor (Beck et al., 1979; DeRubeis et al., 2005; Friedberg & Gorman, 2007; Wolpe & Lazarus, 1966).

Raue and Goldfried (1994) used a particularly evocative metaphor illustrating this stance:

> From a cognitive-behavioral vantage point, the alliance plays an important role in the change process in much the same way that anesthesia is needed during surgery. The implementation of certain surgical procedures requires an adequate and appropriate level of anesthesia. Great care is taken to ensure that an effective anesthesia is in place before surgery begins. Once surgery is underway, the primary concern is with the effective implementation of the surgical procedures—the primary reason the patient entered the treatment setting. (p. 135)

Just as the anesthetic is not necessarily valuable in and of itself, but because it allows the surgeon to perform complex procedures that directly improve the patient's health, the alliance allows the therapist's use of CBT technical interventions (e.g., identifying automatic thoughts, searching for alternative attributions, systematic desensitization). Linehan (1993) has echoed this sentiment in a more modern CBT treatment (dialectical-behavioral therapy; DBT): "Not much in DBT can be done before [a strong positive] relationship is developed" (p. 98; also see further discussion of the relationship in DBT below).

DEVELOPING AND MAINTAINING
A THERAPEUTIC ALLIANCE:
GOALS AND TECHNIQUES IN CBT

As summarized above, there are essentially two reasons that CBT thera-pists seek to have a good relationship with their clients. First, a strong rela-tionship is indirectly beneficial by providing a facilitative context for the specific techniques, and, second, the relationship can be used more or less directly as a vehicle for promoting therapeutic learning, such as by provid-ing empathic responding as a social reinforcer (Krasner, 1962). These two basic functions have led to developing methods that should foster a strong alliance.

Beck et al. (1979), echoing earlier calls from behavior therapy (e.g., Goldfried & Davison, 1976), emphasized relationship variables such as basic trust and rapport, which are now widely valued in CBTs. Basic trust requires that the client have faith in the therapist acting in his or her best interest. Rapport is defined as an interactive experience between therapist and client involving a secure, comfortable, sensitive, and empathic exchange. It has been said that certain populations and treatments may differentially require trust and rapport to be successful. For instance, in working with trauma victims, Hembree, Rauch, and Foa (2003) have noted that trust is an absolutely essential element of the therapeutic relationship in prolonged exposure (PE) therapy, because of the difficult and distressing nature of the PE process. Linehan (1993) suggested that a good relationship, which is high in rapport, is essential to treating clients with borderline personality disorder because these individuals may be unable to fully utilize any other form of reinforcement to change behavior.

Moreover, Beck et al. (1979) argued that the use of CBT techniques in a collaborative manner is in itself relationship building and good for treatment. The main goal of using specific CBT techniques in a collabora-tive way is to increase client expectancies of succeeding in behavior change. To this end, several authors (e.g., Goldfried & Davison, 1976; Wilson & Evans, 1977) have advanced the importance of the therapist clearly explain-ing the treatment rationale, structure, and case conceptualization in order to demonstrate an understanding of the client's problems and how they link with plausible solutions. In a sense, what these authors have suggested (and what clinical experience often bears out) is that by focusing on the tasks and goals of therapy and by using the CBT techniques that are designed to produce change, the therapist can develop a sound working alliance without spending valuable time in session explicitly devoted to "just" the relation-ship. These relationship variables may be seen as direct manipulating sev-eral common factors of treatment—particularly Frank's (1961) suggestion about providing a "myth" that links the cause of a problem and a possible solution—as well as encouraging clients' expectations of change.

As in any other form of psychotherapy, problems in developing or maintaining an alliance occur in CBTs. Such alliance ruptures can occur in many forms and degrees of severity. For example, clients may lack trust in the therapist, may fail to attend sessions regularly, may outright argue or disagree with the therapist, and so on (see Samstag, Safran, & Muran, 2004). Many traditional views (such as Beck et al., 1979; Goldfried & Davison, 1976) on relationship problems in CBTs entail essentially two options, both of which assume that the problem can best be addressed by focusing on the client's problems: first, try to identify the client's symptoms (e.g., maladaptive automatic thoughts or avoidance patterns) that are contributing to the impasse, and work directly on those by using the typical CBT techniques; second, attempt to reengage the client in treatment by directly manipulating his or her expectancies for treatment success. The latter option is primarily achieved in CBT by reiterating the rationale of the approach, providing realistic time courses for therapy gains, and challenging the client's expectations with rational collaborative empiricism. These traditional approaches to problems with the relationship remain popular in the CBT literature (e.g., J. S. Beck, 1995). It has also been noted that problems in therapy may arise not owing to client factors but to therapist or technique factors (such as improper diagnosis or conceptualization, unskilled application of therapeutic procedures, etc.). As discussed below, cognitive and behavioral therapists have often been encouraged to reconsider their case formulations and assumptions about the client when therapeutic alliance breaks occur (e.g., Goldfried & Davison, 1976; Persons, 1989). Thus, the standard techniques of CBT can be used to address the relationship directly and have been used in this way for many years.

EMPIRICAL EVIDENCE FOR THE ALLIANCE IN CBTs

As described above, the relationship in CBTs has often been conceptualized as a secondary factor contributing to therapeutic change by increasing social influence, instilling hope for change in the client, and providing a context within which to make use of techniques. Underscoring the ameliorative primacy of techniques, some CBT clinicians have endorsed a view of the alliance as a *consequence* of good therapeutic technique rather than a constituent of productive therapeutic process (e.g., DeRubeis et al., 2005). However, from the beginning, evidence has suggested that the therapeutic relationship may be used in different ways and have more power to create change than the historical CBT theories suggest.

Breger and McGhaugh (1965) offered a detailed analysis of therapist-reported case studies in behavioral treatments, finding many more similarities between behavioral and psychodynamic therapy than were typically acknowledged at the time. Relationship variables were among those prominently observed in the behavioral therapies, including clients' emotional attachment to therapists and therapist empathy. Observations like these have been fairly common over the years. For instance, Brown (1967) published a detailed description of J. Wolpe's therapeutic practice following 2 years of direct observation. Brown's description included a number of therapist–client relationship variables and client cognitions that were not highlighted in systematic desensitization theory, and Brown suggested that these may act as important mediators of the change process. As Brown noted: "The behavior therapy of Joseph Wolpe is a multifaceted therapeutic tool consisting of his personality, his rapport with his patients, his skilled verbal responses, and his specific behavior techniques. To concentrate on the last factor alone produces a disturbing bias" (p. 857).

Klein, Dittmann, Parloff, and Gill (1969), with the cooperation of Wolpe and Lazarus, conducted a similar clinical observation study and concluded that the therapeutic relationship in behavioral therapy directly increases client expectancies and motivation for treatment, beyond the traditional stance of behavior therapists. Marmor (1971) examined the relationship factors present in three major behavioral therapy approaches of the time (including systematic desensitization, aversive conditioning of homosexuality, and Masters and Johnson's techniques for sexual impotence and frigidity), in each case highlighting infrequently noticed aspects of the relationships that may well have been operative in producing therapeutic change.

Since these initial clinical observations, there have been numerous studies comparing relationship variables among orientations. Much of this literature has been reviewed elsewhere (see Lejuez, Hopko, Levine, Gholkar, & Collins, 2006; Morris & Magrath, 1983; Raue & Goldfried, 1994; Waddington, 2002; Wright & Davis, 1994); so, we instead discuss only selected works here. In a classic study, Sloane, Staples, Cristol, Yorkston, and Whipple (1975) found that behavior therapists displayed significantly more empathy, genuineness, and interpersonal contact, as well as comparable warmth, than did psychoanalysts. This finding, obviously counter to the idea of behavior therapists as simply dry conduits for techniques, was highly unexpected, though these differences in ratings were not associated with outcome. Brunink and Schroeder (1979) studied verbal utterances of expert therapists in psychoanalytic, Gestalt, and behavioral therapies, finding no differences in empathy, rapport, or structure of the session. Notably, however, behavior therapists were more supportive than the other therapists, likely a result of their emphasis on positive reinforcement.

Raue and colleagues (Raue, Castonguay, & Goldfried, 1993; Raue,

Putterman, Goldfried, & Wolitzky, 1995) conducted two studies on psychodynamic-interpersonal therapy and CBTs. In the first study using CBT-trained coders, the authors found that CBT therapists were rated as significantly higher on the alliance measure than psychodynamic therapists (Raue et al., 1993). However, repeating the study with psychodynamically trained coders yielded different results: not only did the psychodynamic coders rate the alliances universally lower than the CBT coders, but also they did not find any difference in alliance quality according to therapy type (Raue et al., 1995). While there are many possible explanations for these conflicting findings, they (as well as others, e.g., McMain, Guimond, Links, & Burckell, 2009; Salvio, Beutler, Wood, & Engle, 1992) nevertheless suggest that CBT-oriented therapists can be rated as high or higher than therapists in other orientations on alliance scores.

Along with such observational evidence, phenomenologically both patients and therapists report that the relationship is one of the most important factors influencing therapy success and failure in cognitive therapies, behavioral therapies, and CBTs. For example, in a study of behavioral therapy, Ryan and Gizynski (1971) found that the proportion of behavioral therapy techniques used did not correlate with outcome judgments by clients, therapists, or experimenters. Further, therapists emphasizing techniques during treatment was correlated with client reports indicating less liking of the therapist, viewing the therapist as less competent, and experiencing the techniques as less pleasant.

In contrast, a number of studies during the 1970s that used retrospective self-reports of clients in behavioral therapies suggested that clients believe relationship factors play a key role in these treatments. In the Sloane et al. study (1975) introduced above, the authors found that successful patients of both behavioral therapy and psychodynamically oriented therapy identified many of the same factors as being most important to their treatment. Nearly all of these factors were closely related to relationship variables such as encouragement and reassurance. Mathews et al. (1976) found that agoraphobic patients in behavioral therapy rated therapist encouragement and sympathy as being more important to the success of their treatment than such factors as behavioral practice and learning to cope with panic. Rabavilas, Boulougouris, and Perissaki (1979) found that at 1 year posttreatment, client reports of therapists' understanding, interest, and respect all correlated positively with outcome among phobic and obsessive–compulsive patients of flooding techniques. Studies like these suggested what was already known in other psychotherapies (e.g., Feifel & Eells, 1963), namely, that clients in behavioral therapy consistently report relationship variables as central processes in producing therapeutic gains while therapists frequently put less emphasis on the same variables.

Such self-report studies, though obviously limited, provided consistent support for a link between relationship variables (broadly defined) and outcome in psychotherapy in general and CBTs in particular. In an attempt to further substantiate this link, Persons and Burns (1985) studied single sessions of cognitive therapy to uncover the relative contributions of cognitive change in session and relationship variables on mood change. The authors found that client-reported relationship quality and changes in the strength of automatic thoughts (a specific mechanism of change in this orientation) made independent contributions to mood changes from pre- to postsession. That is, relationship quality explained additional variance of change in mood over and above change in automatic thoughts. The authors suggested that "training therapists to handle interpersonal issues skillfully is as important in cognitive therapy as in any other form of psychological or medical treatment" (p. 548).

Similarly, Burns and Nolen-Hoeksema (1992) investigated therapist empathy and symptom severity in CBTs for depression. The authors found that not only did therapist empathy have a substantial effect on depression when controlling for homework compliance (which also showed an effect on depression scores), but also the corresponding effect of depression change on empathy ratings was small by comparison. This study was among the first to attempt to separate the effects of therapeutic relationship on symptom outcome from the reciprocal effect of symptomatic improvement on relationship quality ratings in any orientation. While this does not definitively establish the direction of causality, it provides support for the notion of the alliance as an important piece of the therapy process in CBTs.

Further correlational studies on relationship variables and outcome in CBTs are numerous and have been detailed elsewhere (see Waddington, 2002). While some studies have failed to find a positive correlation between outcome and relationship factors (notably DeRubeis & Feeley, 1990; Feeley, DeRubeis, & Gelfand, 1999), the majority have (e.g., Castonguay, Goldfried, Wiser, Raue, & Hayes, 1996; Muran et al., 1995; Raue, Goldfried, & Barkham, 1997; Stiles, Agnew-Davies, Hardy, Barkham, & Shapiro, 1998).

While these findings are all suggestive (as correlational studies cannot truly answer questions of causality), researchers have been attempting for years to address these questions with rigorously controlled experimental studies. Morris and Suckerman (1974) conducted an experimental study in which they compared the effects of automated systematic desensitization when delivered in a warm versus cold manner. This study found that not only did participants in the warm condition show better outcomes, but also participants in the cold therapist condition were not significantly improved at posttreatment as compared to a no-treatment control. Though perhaps using relatively crude methodology, this study highlights the potential role of relationship factors even in such well-developed behavioral techniques as systematic desensitization. It should be noted that Morris and Magrath (1983), however, found that a colder therapist had better outcomes than a warm therapist in using contact desensitization, and other studies on balance have been inconclusive, some finding clear support for warmth in CBT and others, especially earlier studies, finding the opposite. The reasons for this inconsistency (especially in the early years of CBTs) may be related to the specific behavioral techniques implemented, study design, population sampled, or many other factors (see Morris & Magrath, 1983, for further discussion). Generally speaking, however, therapist warmth and empathy are empirically supported as facilitative variables in most contemporary therapies (see Burns & Auerbach, 1996; Castonguay & Beutler, 2005).

The alliance, of course, is only one possible mechanism for change in CBTs, and research into other mechanisms has been prominent as well. A number of studies have suggested that specific techniques prescribed in cognitive therapies (e.g., homework) are predictive of outcome (e.g., Burns & Spangler, 2000; DeRubeis & Feeley, 1990). Yet, over the past several years, evidence has emerged that suggests that the orientation-specific techniques of any psychotherapy, including CBTs, account for a much smaller percentage of outcome variance than initially thought. For instance, Ilardi and Craighead (1994) reviewed the temporal sequencing of symptomatic changes in cognitive therapy for depression and concluded that much of the therapeutic effect is achieved prior to the introduction of cognitive restructuring techniques, suggesting that these technical variables cannot account for the changes nearly so well as "nonspecific" factors.

Taking all of this evidence (and more) into account, several authors have developed theoretical extensions of CBTs, which may help account for the rather large role that the therapeutic relationship, and the alliance in particular, appears to play in these treatments. We now turn our attention to strategies that seek to improve the CBT approach to the therapeutic alliance.

DEVELOPMENTS AND VARIATIONS OF CBTs: THERAPEUTIC RELATIONSHIP VARIABLES AND TECHNIQUES FROM THEORETICAL AND CLINICAL PERSPECTIVES

Based in part on research findings on the alliance in CBTs, several advances have taken place under the umbrella of CBTs with the aim of improving the way that therapists understand and use the therapeutic relationship. In large part, these efforts have involved the assimilation of theory and technique from other orientations, especially relying on psychodynamic–interpersonal and humanistic techniques. These contributions have come largely in two changes to CBT practice and conceptualization: identifying new ways to resolve alliance ruptures and reevaluating the theoretical role of the alliance itself.

Resolving Alliance Ruptures

Several authors have examined ways of handling alliance ruptures in CBTs (e.g., Safran & Muran, 1996). What does a therapist do when there is an obvious impasse in treatment because the relationship is suffering? In broad terms, two approaches to an alliance rupture can be distilled from the literature.

First, if the therapist determines that there is a therapy process variable or therapist effect that might be contributing to the alliance break, the therapist has historically been advised to use the rupture as an opportunity to reconsider the case conceptualization and treatment plan in a collaborative way and to realign client and therapist shared goals (e.g., Beck 1996; Beck et al., 1979; Goldfried & Davison, 1976; Persons & Mikami, 2002). Ideally, this opportunity is used to encourage client reengagement in therapy. However, it has a major downside that makes it difficult to implement in practice: sometimes the client resists treatment, against his or her best interests. If the therapist blindly concedes the case conceptualization and treatment plan when clients do not want to, or are ambivalent about, change, it is possible that treatment itself will stall (though the client may be more comfortable in the short term). In addition, ruptures may not be attributable to the choice of treatment or intervention use per se, but rather to the way that the treatment is conducted.

Alternatively, if the therapist determines that the rupture is a manifestation of a problem or symptom the client is experiencing, the therapist is advised to attempt to directly address that problem. This possibility may at times be accurate. Clients who are depressed, for example, may have an inaccurate view of the therapist's skills (or genuine empathy) and/or possess a pessimistic prognosis about the therapy's ability to reduce depression; in this case, the client's inaccurate beliefs may contribute directly to the relationship problem, and addressing these automatic thoughts about the relationship may be a fruitful intervention. Yet, if CBT therapists automatically assume that their clients' reluctance to engage in therapy is primarily the result of distorted thoughts, then they may not be fully aware of how they are contributing to the alliance rupture. This shortcoming, in turn, may lead therapists to adhere too blindly and rigidly to the prescribed techniques and lose sight of another, more pressing, problem in the relationship, such as an empathic failure (Burns & Auerbach, 1996) or a case formulation based on incomplete or outdated information (see Beck et al., 1979; Persons, 1989).

Such rigid patterns of interactions have been observed in different approaches (Henry, Schacht, & Strupp, 1986, 1990; Piper et al., 1999; Schut et al., 2005), including cognitive therapies. For example, Castonguay et al. (1996) found that, when confronted with alliance rupture, cognitive therapists frequently increased their attempts to persuade clients of the validity of the cognitive therapy rationale and/or the beneficial impact of the cognitive therapy techniques. This increased adherence, however, did not appear to repair the alliance breach and may have actually exacerbated it by creating a vicious cycle of misattunement to the client's experiences.

A number of CBT therapists have made valuable contributions toward more skillfully resolving alliance ruptures. For example, Burns (1989; Burns & Auerbach, 1996) developed a set of "listening skills" to address client disagreement or disengagement from therapy. First, therapists invite the client to express his or her present emotional and subjective state, particularly inviting disclosure of perceived therapeutic failures. Second, therapists empathically relate to the client's response, hopefully making the client feel validated and understood. Finally, using the "disarming" technique, therapists explicitly validate the client's negative feelings or criticisms of treatment (and/or the therapist) by finding some truth in them (even if the reaction is seemingly excessive). According to Burns, doing so signals to the client that the he or she is respected and that the therapist is willing to assume equal— if not more—blame for the relationship problems.

Similarly, Safran and colleagues (Safran & Muran, 1996; Safran & Segal, 1990) have developed methods of alliance rupture repair that start with the therapist's recognizing his or her contribution to the problem. This technique, which is similar to Burns's (1989) disarming, is then used as the catalyst to encourage clients to share their own feelings about treatment. Further, the goal is to encourage clients to discuss their own contribution to the therapeutic impasse and, by extension, to interpersonal problems outside of therapy. Also like Burns's disarming technique, Linehan's (1993) "techniques of acceptance" involve the therapist's ability to see reasonableness in the client's dysfunctional behaviors, accept the client's hostile affect, and recognize his or her own mistakes. Like Burns and Safran, Linehan has argued that alliance problems are frequent and that their resolution can lead to the client's acquiring skills that can be used in interpersonal difficulties outside the sessions.

The techniques of addressing alliance ruptures developed by Burns and Safran have been associated with some empirical support. For example, Safran, Muran, and colleagues (e.g., Muran et al., 2009; Safran, Crocker, McMain, & Muran, 1990; Safran & Muran, 1996; Safran, Muran, & Samstag, 1994) have found that the in-session exploration of the experiences of both the therapist and client facilitates rupture resolution and contributes to treatment outcome. The researchers have also developed brief relational therapy (BRT; Muran, Safran, Samstag, & Winston, 2005), which as a stand-alone alliance-based treatment has been shown to produce lower dropout from and higher engagement in treatment than short-term psychodynamic and cognitive and behavioral therapies (Muran, Safran, Samstag, & Winston, 2005; Safran, Muran, Samstag, & Winston, 2005). Assimilating the rupture repair techniques directly into a more traditional cognitive therapy, Castonguay et al. (2004) developed integrative cognitive therapy (ICT) for depression. ICT has performed well in two preliminary trials. In a comparison to a wait-list control involving 21 outpatients, ICT achieved a pre–post effect size of $d = 1.91$ on the Beck Depression Inventory (BDI; Beck, Ward, Mendelsohn, Mock, & Erbaugh, 1961), more than twice the size of comparable studies of traditional cognitive therapies (Castonguay et al., 2004). In a second study, ICT was compared to standard cognitive therapy with 11 clients in each group, and results favored ICT with a medium effect size, $d = 0.50$, also on the BDI (Constantino et al., 2008). In the latter study, the ICT clients not only evidenced greater posttreatment improvement than the CT clients but also reported higher alliance and therapist empathy ratings across treatment. Taken together, these findings suggest (albeit preliminarily) that alliance ruptures can be effectively addressed in the context of specifically relational therapies as well as more traditional cognitive therapies, and that such rupture resolution strategies might have a positive impact on treatment engagement and outcome. Indeed, many additional authors have described ways of managing problems in the therapeutic relationship in CBTs as essential skills with numerous therapeutic benefits (e.g., Leahy, 1993; Newman, 1998; Persons, 1989; Young, 1999).

The Corrective Role of the Alliance in CBTs

Several authors have suggested that therapists would be wise to foster strong alliances not just as indirect facilitation of but also as part of a theoretically cohesive system of CBT designed to achieve a direct path toward changing cognitions, changing interpersonal behavior, and providing corrective experiences to clients (e.g., Arnkoff, 1981; Goldfried, 1985; Goldfried & Padawer, 1982; Grosse Holtforth & Castonguay, 2005; Safran & Segal, 1990). This postulation is in line with Linehan's (1993) argument that the therapeutic relationship is "of value in its own right, apart from any changes that the patient makes as a result of therapy" (p. 98).

Arnkoff (1981) wrote a detailed clinical and theoretical chapter on ways of expanding cognitive therapy, including a section on incorporating the relationship itself. In this, she provided a series of case studies illustrating, for example, that the relationship can provide much the same information in cognitive therapies as it does in a transference-focused psychodynamic therapy. Goldfried and Davison (1976) have also suggested that behavior in-session, including the relationship, can be viewed as a sample of behavior of the client itself, likely very relevant to the way the client behaves in nontherapy situations. Taking this a step further, Goldfried (1985) has suggested that cognitive and behavior therapists can conceptualize interventions focused on the relationship as *in vivo* interventions: "We know that in vivo interventions are much more powerful than imaginal or described ones. So if we can look at the person's actions right at the time—when they are being upset about something, or when they are being inhibited and cannot act in a given way or say something within the session itself—we have broadened our therapeutic focus" (p. 143). Using this conceptualization, a CBT therapist might be able to address important events in the therapy sessions with the ultimate goal of identifying and altering major interpersonal patterns that affect not only the therapy relationship but the client's other relationships as well. These techniques also lend themselves to the development of corrective experiences, which may be the central common factor of therapy (Goldfried, 1980).

Kohlenberg and colleagues (Kanter et al., 2009; Kohlenberg & Tsai, 1991; Tsai, Kohlenberg, & Kanter, Chapter 9, this volume) have also developed CBT treatments that use the therapeutic relationship extensively and that are based largely on research into *in vivo* interventions. Young (1999), in an influential work on cognitive therapy for personality disorders, suggests that therapists use references to the therapy relationship to better activate schemata, and indicates that this technique is very similar to using transference in psychoanalysis (p. 34).

Hayes and colleagues, in developing acceptance and commitment therapy (ACT), have also incorporated a view of the relationship that is simultaneously an independent positive force promoting client change while also functioning in the background of the more specific technical and theoretical influences. Thus, Hayes, Strosahl, and Wilson (1999) suggest that, while the relationship is not the end purpose of therapy, it is curative inasmuch as it is based on love, acceptance, respect, and openness toward oneself and others (p. 279). This perception suggests that the relationship between therapist and client can—if predicated on and conducted according to the right conditions—serve as an important learning event and corrective experience for the client, a position frequently cited over the years (e.g., Safran & Segal, 1990).

CONCLUSION

The therapeutic relationship has been an integral part of behavioral and cognitive therapies for decades, despite the fact that this orientation has frequently been described as mechanical. Although relationship factors have been traditionally viewed in this approach as secondary to learning and cognitive techniques, the therapeutic alliance has consistently been regarded as necessary for successful therapy. And while many CBT scholars (e.g., DeRubeis, Brotman, & Gibbons, 2005) have referred to relationship variables as nonspecific (i.e., not yet clearly defined or fully understood), some leaders of this orientation have offered detailed descriptions (based on basic research and social learning theory) and even developed a new construct (collaborative empiricism) to explain the role of the therapeutic relationship in the change process as well as to provide guidelines on how to enhance the relationship for the sake of implementing behavioral and cognitive interventions (Beck et al., 1979; Wilson & Evans, 1977). Over the years, clinical observations and empirical investigation (including clients' perceptions of helpful elements of therapy) have provided support for the role of relationship variables in CBTs. In particular, studies on the working alliance have found that, as a whole, the quality of the bond and the level of collaboration between client and therapist are robust predictors of clients' improvement in CBTs. Furthermore, based in part on this empirical evidence as well as on clinical experience, scholars and therapists have developed and/ or integrated within their general CBT framework a number of interventions aimed at resolving treatment impasses as well as fostering the curative impact that the alliance is believed (at least by some) to have.

There are, however, important questions that remain to be addressed. For example, one of the most important debates in the field is whether or not the alliance contributes causally to client change or, rather, whether its predictive quality is mostly an epiphenomenon (see Barber, Khalsa, & Sharpless, Chapter 2, this volume). As argued elsewhere, while some research has begun to address the direction and nature of the alliance impact on the outcome, it is likely that if a consensus is achieved it is not going to reflect an "either–or" answer. In our view, the process of change "involves interdependent, non-orthogonal, and/or synergistic relationships between different variables" (Castonguay, Constantino, & Grosse Holthforth, 2006, p. 274). Another crucial question is whether interventions that have been recently integrated into CBTs may be necessary for all clients. For example, a substantial number of clients do benefit from the standard cognitive therapies for depression, and, as such, the treatment progress of these individuals may not require the addition of techniques aimed at repairing alliance ruptures. It will therefore be important for future research not only to determine whether or not the addition of such techniques can improve cognitive therapies in general but also to identify the clients for whom these techniques may be particularly indicated. Such research, especially if guided by theoretical models attending to complex interactions between technical, relationship, and participants variables (Castonguay & Beutler, 2005), are likely to further improve the beneficial impact of CBTs on psychological suffering.

REFERENCES

Arnkoff, D. B. (1981). Flexibility in practicing cognitive therapy. In G. Emery, S. D. Hollon, & R. C. Bedrosian (Eds.), *New directions in cognitive therapy* (pp. 203–223). New York: Guilford Press.

Bandura, A. (1969). *Principles of behavior modification*. New York: Holt, Rinehart, & Winston.

Barber, J. P. (2009). Toward a working through of some core conflicts in psychotherapy research. *Psychotherapy Research, 19*, 1–12.

Barber, J. P., Connolly, M. B., Crits-Christoph, P., Gladis, P., & Siqueland, L. (2000). Alliance predicts patients' outcome beyond in-treatment change in symptoms. *Journal of Consulting and Clinical Psychology, 68*, 1027–1032.

Barber, J. P., & DeRubeis, R. J. (1989). On second thought: Where the action is in cognitive therapy for depression. *Cognitive Therapy and Research, 13*(5), 441–457.

Barlow, D. H. (Ed.). (2008). *Clinical handbook of psychological disorders: A step-by-step treatment manual* (4th ed.). New York: Guilford Press.

Beck, A. T., Rush, J. J., Shaw, B. F., & Emery, G. (1979). *Cognitive therapy of depression*. New York: Guilford Press.

Beck, A. T., Ward, C. H., Mendelsohn, M., Mock, J., & Erbaugh, J. (1961). An inventory for measuring depression. *Archives of General Psychiatry, 4*, 561–571.

Beck, J. S. (1995). *Cognitive therapy: Basics and beyond*. New York: Guilford Press.

Brady, J. P., Davison, G. C., Dewald, P. A., Egan, G., Fadiman, J., Frank, J. D., et al. (1980). Some views on effective principles of psychotherapy. *Cognitive Therapy and Research, 4*, 271–306.

Breger, L., & McGhaugh, J. L. (1965). Critique and reformulation of "learning theory" approaches to psychotherapy and neurosis. *Psychological Bulletin, 63*, 338–358.

Brown, B. M. (1967). Cognitive aspects of Wolpe's behavior therapy. *American Journal of Psychiatry, 124*(6), 162–167.

Brunink, S. A., & Schroeder, H. E. (1979). Verbal therapeutic behavior of expert psychoanalytically oriented, gestalt, and behavior therapists. *Journal of Consulting and Clinical Psychology, 47*, 567–574.

Burns, D., & Auerbach, A. (1996). Therapeutic empathy in cognitive-behavioral therapy: Does it really make a difference? In P. Salkovskis (Ed.), *Frontiers of cognitive therapy*. New York: Guilford Press.

Burns, D. D. (1989). *The feeling good handbook: Using the new mood therapy in everyday life*. New York: William Morrow.

Burns, D. D., & Nolen-Hoeksema, S. (1992). Therapeutic empathy and recovery from depression in cognitive-behavioral therapy: A structural equation model. *Journal of Consulting and Clinical Psychology, 60*, 441–449.

Burns, D. D., & Spangler, D. L. (2000). Does psychotherapy homework lead to improvements in depression in cognitive-behavioral therapy or does improvement lead to increased homework compliance? *Journal of Consulting and Clinical Psychology, 68*(1), 46–56.

Castonguay, L. G. (1993). "Common factors" and "non-specific variables:" Clarification of the two concepts and recommendations for future research. *Journal of Psychotherapy Integration, 3,* 267–286.

Castonguay, L. G., & Beutler, L. E. (Eds.). (2005). *Principles of therapeutic change that work.* New York: Oxford University Press.

Castonguay, L. G., Constantino, M. J., & Grosse Holtforth, M. (2006). The working alliance: Where are we and where should we go? *Psychotherapy: Theory, Research, Practice, and Training, 43,* 271–279.

Castonguay, L. G., Goldfried, M. R., Wiser, S., Raue, P. J., & Hayes, A. M. (1996). Predicting the effect of cognitive therapy for depression: A study of unique and common factors. *Journal of Consulting and Clinical Psychology, 64,* 497–504.

Castonguay, L. G., Newman, M. G., Borkovec, T. D., Grosse Holtforth, M., & Maramba, G. G. (2005). Cognitive-behavioral assimilative integration. In J. C. Norcross & M. R. Goldfried (Eds.), *Handbook of psychotherapy integration* (2nd ed., pp. 241–260). New York: Oxford University Press.

Castonguay, L. G., Schut, A. J., Aikins, D., Constantino, M. J., Laurenceau, J. P., Bologh, L., et al. (2004). Repairing alliance ruptures in cognitive therapy: A preliminary investigation of an integrative therapy for depression. *Journal of Psychotherapy Integration, 14,* 4–20.

Constantino, M. J., Marnell, M., Haile, A. J., Kanther-Sista, S. N., Wolman, K., Zappert, L., et al. (2008). Integrative cognitive therapy for depression: A randomized pilot comparison. *Psychotherapy, 45,* 122–134.

Crits-Christoph, P., Connolly Gibbons, M. B., & Hearon, B. (2006). Does the alliance cause good outcome?: Recommendations for future research on the alliance. *Psychotherapy: Theory, Research, Practice, Training, 43*(3), 280–285.

DeRubeis, R. J., Brotman, M. A., & Gibbons, C. J. (2005). A conceptual and methodological analysis of the nonspecifics argument. *Clinical Psychology: Science & Practice, 12,* 174–183.

DeRubeis, R. J., & Feeley, M. (1990). Determinants of change in cognitive therapy for depression. *Cognitive Therapy Research, 14,* 469–482.

Dimidjian, S., Martell, C. R., Addis, M. E., & Herman-Dunn, R. (2008). Behavioral Activation for Depression. In D. H. Barlow (Ed.), *Clinical handbook of psychological disorders: A step-by-step treatment manual* (4th ed., pp. 328–364). New York: Guilford Press.

Fairburn, C. G., Cooper, Z., Shafran, R., & Wilson, G. T. (2008). Eating disorders: A transdiagnostic protocol. In D. H. Barlow (Ed.), *Clinical handbook of psychological disorders: A step-by-step treatment manual* (4th ed., pp. 578–614). New York: Guilford Press.

Feeley, M., DeRubeis, R., & Gelfand, L. (1999). The temporal relation of adherence and alliance to symptom change in cognitive therapy for depression. *Journal of Consulting and Clinical Psychology, 67,* 578–582.

Feifel, H., & Eells, J. (1963). Patients and therapists assess the same psychotherapy. *Journal of Consulting Psychology, 27*(4), 310–318.

Frank, J. D. (1961). *Persuasion and healing.* Baltimore: Johns Hopkins University Press.

Friedberg, R. D., & Gorman, A. A. (2007). Integrating psychotherapeutic processes with cognitive behavioral procedures. *Journal of Contemporary Psychotherapy*, *37*, 185–193.

Goldfried, M. R. (1980). Toward the delineation of therapeutic change principles. *American Psychologist*, *35*(11), 991–999.

Goldfried, M. R. (1985). In vivo intervention or transference? In W. Dryden (Ed.), *Therapists' dilemmas*. London: Harper & Row.

Goldfried, M. R., & Davison, G. C. (1976). *Clinical behavior therapy*. New York: Holt, Rinehart, & Winston.

Goldfried, M. R., & Padawer, W. (1982). Current status and future directions in psychotherapy. In M. R. Goldfried (Ed.), *Converging themes in psychotherapy* (pp. 3–49). New York: Springer.

Grosse Holtforth, M., & Castonguay, L. G. (2005). Relationship and techniques in cognitive-behavioral therapy—a motivational approach. *Psychotherapy: Theory, Research, Practice, Training*, *42*(4), 443–455.

Hayes, S. C., Strosahl, K. D., & Wilson, K. G. (1999). *Acceptance and commitment therapy: An experiential approach to behavior change*. New York: Guilford Press.

Hembree, E. A., Rauch, S. A. M., & Foa, E. B. (2003). Beyond the manual: The insider's guide to prolonged exposure therapy for PTSD. *Cognitive and Behavioral Practice*, *10*, 22–30.

Henry, W. P., Schacht, T. E., & Strupp, H. H. (1986). Effectiveness of targeting the vulnerability factors of depression in cognitive therapy. *Journal of Consulting and Clinical Psychology*, *64*, 623–627.

Henry, W. P., Schacht, T. E., & Strupp, H. H. (1990). Patient and therapist introject, interpersonal process, and differential psychotherapy outcome. *Journal of Consulting and Clinical Psychology*, *58*, 768–774.

Ilardi, S., & Craighead, W. (1994). The role of non-specific factors in cognitive-behavior therapy for depression. *Clinical Psychology: Science and Practice*, *1*, 138–155.

Kanter, J. W., Rusch, L. C., Landes, S. J., Holman, G. I., Whiteside, U., & Sedivy, S. K. (2009). The use and nature of present-focused interventions in cognitive and behavioral therapies for depression. *Psychotherapy: Theory, Research, Practice, Training*, *46*, 220–232.

Klein, M. H., Dittmann, A. T., Parloff, M. B., & Gill, M. M. (1969). Behavior therapy: Observations and reflections. *Journal of Consulting and Clinical Psychology*, *33*, 259–266.

Kohlenberg, R. J., & Tsai, M. (1991). *Functional analytic psychotherapy: A guide for creating intense and curative therapeutic relationships*. New York: Plenum Press.

Krasner, L. (1962). The therapist as a social reinforcement machine. In H. H. Strupp & L. Luborsky (Eds.), *Research in psychotherapy* (vol. II). Washington, DC: American Psychological Association.

Leahy, R. (1993). *Overcoming resistance in cognitive therapy*. New York: Guilford Press.

Lejuez, C. W., Hopko, D. R., Levine, S., Gholkar, R., & Collins, L. M. (2006). The therapeutic alliance in behavior therapy. *Psychotherapy: Theory, Research, Practice, Training*, *42*, 456–468.

Linehan, M. M. (1993). *Cognitive-behavioral treatment of borderline personality disorder*. New York: Guilford Press.

Marmor, J. (1971). Dynamic psychotherapy and behavior therapy: Are they irreconcilable? *Archives of General Psychiatry, 24*, 22–28.

Mathews, A. M., Johnston, D. W., Lancashire, M., Munby, M., Shaw, P. M., & Gelder, M. G. (1976). Imaginal flooding and exposure to real phobic situations: Treatment outcome with agoraphobic patients. *British Journal of Psychiatry, 129*, 362–371.

McMain, S., Guimond, T., Links, P., & Burckell, L. (2009, August). *The therapy alliance as a mechanism of change in the treatment of persons with borderline personality disorder*. Paper presented at the 11th International Society for the Study of Personality Disorders Congress. New York.

Morris, R. J., & Magrath, K. H. (1983). The therapeutic relationship in behavior therapy. In M. J. Lambert (Ed.), *Psychotherapy and patient relationships* (pp. 154–189). Homewood, IL: Dow Jones-Irwin.

Morris, R. J., & Suckerman, K. R. (1974). Therapist warmth as a factor in automated systematic desensitization. *Journal of Consulting and Clinical Psychology, 42*, 244–250.

Muran, J. C., Gorman, B. S., Safran, J. D., & Twining, L., Samstag, L. W., & Winston, A. (1995). Linking in-session change to overall outcome in short-term cognitive therapy. *Journal of Consulting and Clinical Psychology, 63*, 651–657.

Muran, J. C., Safran, J. D., Gorman, B. S., Samstag, L. W., Eubanks-Carter, C., & Winston, A. (2009). The relationship of early alliance ruptures and their resolution to process and outcome in three time-limited psychotherapies for personality disorders. *Psychotherapy: Theory, Research, Practice, Training, 46*(2), 233–248.

Muran, J. C., Safran, J. D., Samstag, L. W., & Winston, A. (2005). Evaluating an Alliance-Focused Treatment for Personality Disorders. *Psychotherapy, 42*, 532–545.

Nathan, P. E., & Gorman, J. M. (2002). *A guide to treatments that work* (2nd ed.). New York: Oxford University Press.

Newman, C. F. (1998). The therapeutic relationship and alliance in cognitive therapy. In J. D. Safran & J. C. Muran (Eds.), *The therapeutic alliance in brief psychotherapy* (pp. 95–122). Washington, DC: American Psychological Association.

Norcross J. C., Karpiak C. P., & Santoro S. O. (2005). Clinical psychologists across the years: The division of clinical psychology from 1960 to 2003. *Journal of Clinical Psychology, 61*, 1467–1483.

Perls, F., Hefferline, R. F., & Goodman, P. (1977). *Gestalt therapy: Excitement and growth in the human personality* (rev. ed.). New York: Bantam Books.

Persons, J. B. (1989). *Cognitive therapy in practice: A case formulation approach*. New York: Norton.

Persons, J. B., & Burns, D. D. (1985). Mechanisms of action of cognitive therapy: The relative contributions of technical and interpersonal interventions. *Cognitive Therapy and Research, 9*, 539–551.

Persons, J. B., & Mikami, A. Y. (2002). Strategies for handling treatment failure successfully. *Psychotherapy: Theory, Research, Practice, Training, 39*(2), 139–151.

Piper, W. E., Joyce, A. S., Rosie, J. S., Ogrodniczuk, J. S., McCallum, M., O'Kelly, J. G., et al. (1999). Prediction of dropping out in time-limited interpretive individual psychotherapy. *Psychotherapy, 36,* 114–122.

Rabavilas, A. D., Boulougouris, J. C., & Perissaki, C. (1979). Therapist qualities related to outcome with exposure in vivo in neurotic patients. *Journal of Behavior Therapy and Experimental Psychiatry, 10,* 293–294.

Raue, P., Goldfried, M., & Barkham, M. (1997). The therapeutic alliance in psychodynamic–interpersonal and cognitive-behavioral therapy. *Journal of Consulting and Clinical Psychology, 65,* 582–587.

Raue, P., Putterman, J., Goldfried, M. R., & Wolitzky, D. (1995). Effect of rater orientation on the evaluation of therapeutic alliance. *Psychotherapy Research, 5*(4), 337–342.

Raue, P. J., Castonguay, L. G., & Goldfried, M. R. (1993). The working alliance: A comparison of two therapies. *Psychotherapy Research, 3,* 197–207.

Raue, P. J., & Goldfried, M. R. (1994). The therapeutic alliance in cognitive-behavior therapy. In A. O. Horvath & L. S. Greenberg (Eds.), *The working alliance: Theory, research and practice* (pp. 131–152). New York: Wiley.

Rogers, C. (1957). The necessary and sufficient conditions of therapeutic personality change. *Journal of Consulting and Clinical Psychology, 22,* 95–103.

Rogers, C. R. (1951). *Client-centered therapy: Its current practice, implications and theory.* Boston: Houghton Mifflin.

Ryan, V. L., & Gizynski, M. N. (1971). Behavior therapy in retrospect: Patients' feelings about their behavior therapies. *Journal of Consulting and Clinical Psychology, 37,* 1–9.

Safran, J. D., Crocker, P., McMain, S., & Murray, P. (1990). Therapeutic alliance rupture as a therapy event for empirical investigation. *Psychotherapy, 27*(2), 154–165.

Safran, J. D., & Muran, J. C. (1996). The resolution of ruptures in the therapeutic alliance. *Journal of Consulting and Clinical Psychology, 64*(3), 447–458.

Safran, J. D., Muran, J. C., & Samstag, L. W. (1994). Resolving therapeutic alliance ruptures: A task analytic investigation. In A. O. Horvath & L. S. Greenberg (Eds.), *The working alliance: Theory, research, and practice* (pp. 225–255). New York: Wiley.

Safran, J. D., Muran, J. C., Samstag, L. W., & Winston, A. (2005). Evaluating alliance-focused intervention for potential treatment failures: A feasibility study and descriptive analysis. *Psychotherapy, 42,* 512–531.

Safran, J. D., & Segal, Z. V. (1990). *Interpersonal process in cognitive therapy.* New York: Basic Books.

Salvio, M., Beutler, L. E., Wood, J. M., & Engle, D. (1992). The strength of the therapeutic alliance in three treatments for depression. *Psychotherapy Research, 2*(1), 31–36.

Samstag, L. W., Muran, J. C., & Safran, J. D. (2004). Defining and identifying alliance ruptures. In D. P. Charman (Ed.), *Core processes in brief psychodynamic psychotherapy: Advancing effective practice* (pp. 187–214). Mahwah, NJ: Erlbaum.

Schut, A. J., Castonguay, L. G., Flanagan, K. M., Yamasaki, A. S., Barber, J. P.,

Bedics, J. D., et al. (2005). Therapist interpretation, patient–therapist interpersonal process, and outcome in psychodynamic psychotherapy for avoidant personality disorder. *Psychotherapy: Theory, Research, Practice, Training, 42*(4), 494–511.

Sloane, R. B., Staples, F. R., Cristol, A. H., Yorkston, N. J., & Whipple, K. (1975). *Psychotherapy versus behavior therapy.* Cambridge, MA: Harvard University Press.

Stiles, W. B., Agnew-Davies, R., Hardy, G., Barkham, M., & Shapiro, D. A. (1998). Relations of the alliance with psychotherapy outcome: Findings in the second Sheffield psychotherapy project. *Journal of Consulting and Clinical Psychology, 66,* 791–902.

Turk, C. L., Heimberg, R. G., & Magee, L. (2008). Social anxiety disorder. In D. H. Barlow (Ed.), *Clinical handbook of psychological disorders: A step-by-step treatment manual* (4th ed., pp. 123–163). New York: Guilford Press.

Waddington, L. (2002). The therapy relationship in cognitive therapy: A review. *Behavioural and Cognitive Psychotherapy, 30,* 179–191.

Wilson, G. T., & Evans, I. M. (1977). The therapist–client relationship in behavior therapy. In A. S. Gurman & A. M. Razin (Eds.), *Effective psychotherapy: A handbook of research* (pp. 309–330). New York: Pergamon Press.

Wolfe, B. E., & Goldfried, M. R. (1988). Research on psychotherapy integration: Recommendations and conclusions from an NIMH workshop. *Journal of Consulting and Clinical Psychology, 56*(3), 448–451.

Wolpe, J. (1958). *Reciprocal inhibition therapy.* Stanford, CA: Stanford University Press.

Wolpe, J., & Lazarus, A. (1966). *Behavior therapy techniques.* New York: Pergamon Press.

Wright, J. H., & Davis, D. (1994). The therapeutic relationship in cognitive-behavioral therapy: Patient perceptions and therapist responses. *Cognitive and Behavioral Practice, 1*(1), 25–45.

Young, J. E. (1999). *Cognitive therapy for personality disorders: A schema-focused approach* (3rd ed.). Sarasota, FL: Professional Resource Press.

Young, J. E., Rygh, J. L., Weinberger, A. D., & Beck, A. T. (2008). Cognitive therapy for depression. In D. H. Barlow (Ed.), *Clinical handbook of psychological disorders: A step-by-step treatment manual* (4th ed., pp. 250–305). New York: Guilford Press.

CHAPTER 9

■ ■ ■ ■ ■

A Functional Analytic Psychotherapy (FAP) Approach to the Therapeutic Alliance

Mavis Tsai
Robert J. Kohlenberg
Jonathan W. Kanter

The therapeutic alliance is one of the few factors consistently found to be predictive of therapeutic outcome (e.g., Barber, Connolly, Crits-Christoph, Gladis, & Siqueland, 2000; Horvath, 2001; Martin, Garske, & Davis, 2000). This predictive property holds across a wide range of treatment approaches (Safran & Muran, 1998). Thus, therapeutic alliance is a candidate for being a "common factor" (Klein, 1996; Lambert & Bergin, 1994) hypothesized to underlie psychotherapy efficacy. Accordingly, over the past 30 years there has been a great deal of interest in this construct, resulting in an extensive empirical and conceptual literature. In reviewing the current status of the concept, Safran and Muran (2006) assert that the main contribution of the therapeutic alliance construct is in bringing the "therapeutic relationship into focus" (p. 289).

Recent work on empirically supported therapy relationships further substantiates the idea that the therapeutic relationship plays a significant role in the outcome of therapy (Norcross, 2001). Formed in reaction to the movement on evidence-based practices that they deemed to represent therapy as the disembodied manualized treatment of Axis I disorders, the

American Psychological Association Division 29 Task Force on Empirically Supported Therapy Relationships asserted that to separate the interpersonal dimension of behavior from the instrumental may be a fatal flaw if the aim is to extrapolate from research results to clinical practice. Its conclusions, based on a review of empirical research, were as follows: (1) the therapy relationship is crucial to outcome independent of the specific type of treatment; (2) treatment guidelines should explicitly address therapist behaviors that promote a facilitative therapy relationship; (3) effective therapy takes into account the strength of the therapy relationship, acting in concert with discrete interventions, patient characteristics, and clinician qualities; and (4) customizing both discrete methods and relationship stances on a patient-by-patient or moment-to-moment basis enhances the effectiveness of treatment. The task force stated unequivocally that the most responsible mode of therapy practice pays special attention to the nuances and quality of the therapist–patient relationship.

Although it is clear that the therapeutic relationship is important and is related to treatment outcome, this assertion raises two main questions of interest to theorists and clinicians. First, what is the mechanism of change that underlies the curative properties of the therapeutic relationship? Second, exactly what should therapists do to facilitate this process? With few exceptions (B. S. Kohlenberg, 2000; B. S. Kohlenberg, Yeater, & R. J. Kohlenberg, 1998; Lejuez & Hopko, 2005), a behaviorally informed perspective is underrepresented in addressing these questions. We believe that viewing the therapeutic alliance from a behavioral standpoint can point to phenomena and interventions that may be useful to all therapists and researchers, regardless of their orientation. As we have argued before, behaviorism has considerable potential to cross theoretical boundaries and serve as a basis for psychotherapy integration (R. J. Kohlenberg & Tsai, 1994).

Thus, our goal in this chapter is to discuss our view of the therapeutic relationship from a behaviorally informed approach, specifically from the perspective of functional analytic psychotherapy (FAP; R. J. Kohlenberg & Tsai, 1991; Tsai et al., 2008). We describe the principles and rules of FAP that specify the (1) mechanism of action operating within the therapeutic relationship that is responsible for client change and (2) therapist interventions used in the process. We also discuss empirical findings that support (1) our approach to understanding how the therapeutic relationship produces change and (2) our recommended therapeutic interventions.

FUNCTIONAL ANALYTIC PSYCHOTHERAPY

FAP uses behavioral principles to create a sacred space of awareness, courage, and love where the therapeutic relationship is the primary vehicle for client healing and transformation (R. J. Kohlenberg & Tsai, 1991; Tsai et al., 2008). We sought to explain the transformative powers of therapist–client relationships by using a radical behavioral analysis (Skinner, 1953, 1974) of the psychotherapeutic process that emphasized each individual's unique history. FAP is an interpersonal therapy based on the assumption that, because the major causes of psychopathology are intimately related to problems in relationships (Horowitz, 2004), a relational treatment can be particularly potent.

At the core of FAP is its hypothesized mechanism of clinical change—contingent responding by the therapist to *in vivo* client problems and improvements as they are occurring in session. Given that the terms "behavioral," "radical behavioral analysis," "contingent responding," and "Skinner" might give some readers a distorted view of what FAP is all about, we say at the outset that FAP embraces the notion that effective treatment often involves an intensive, in-depth, and emotional therapeutic relationship as well as a therapist who is willing to become aware of his or her own feelings and explore their relevance to the therapeutic process. While remaining true to the fundamentals of behaviorism and functional analysis, FAP deals with the full range of interpersonal relating and is fully at ease with such notions as "intimacy," "an open heart," and "therapeutic love."

The behavioral theory and the proposed mechanism of change upon which FAP is built are deceptively simple—consisting in "you and I and our clients act the way we do because of the contingencies of reinforcement we have experienced in past relationships" (although less relevant to the therapeutic process, the complete behavioral account also includes the contingencies of survival and genetic influences). Clinical improvements or therapeutic change also involve, based on this theory, contingencies of reinforcement that occur in the relationship between the client and therapist.

Reinforcement

The term "reinforcement" is used here in its generic sense, referring to all consequences or contingencies that affect (increase or decrease) the strength of behavior, including positive and negative reinforcement and punishment. From our perspective, reinforcement is ubiquitous and usually occurs at an unconscious level in our daily lives, and is the ultimate and fundamental cause of action. Complete explanations for behavior necessarily involve identifying the relevant reinforcement history. One asks for water not because reinforcement will occur and the water will be received in that instance but rather because asking the question has been reliably reinforced with water in the past. A client may say he yelled at his spouse because he was angry. As a behavioral explanation this response is incomplete, however, and requires information about past contingencies that account for both the actions of getting angry and yelling. That is, not every spouse gets angry under those circumstances, nor, even if angry, do all spouses yell. A complete explanation addresses these issues in addition to the individual's internal states and current situation. Two aspects of reinforcement particularly relevant to the psychotherapy situation are natural versus contrived reinforcers and within-session contingencies.

Natural versus Contrived Reinforcers

Unfortunately, simply saying "good" or offering a tangible reward to a client for behaving as the therapist wants are typical images that come to mind when the term "reinforcement" is mentioned. These images not only are technically erroneous but also exemplify contrived reinforcement. The distinction between natural and contrived reinforcement is especially important in the change process (Ferster, 1967; Skinner, 1982). Natural reinforcers are typical and reliable in daily life, whereas contrived ones generally are not. For example, giving a child candy for putting on a coat is contrived, whereas getting chilled for remaining coatless is a natural reinforcer. Similarly, fining a client a nickel for not making eye contact is contrived, while the spontaneous wandering of the therapist's attention when the client is looking away is natural.

Within-Session Contingencies

A well-known feature of reinforcement is that the closer in time and place a consequence is to the behavior, the greater the effect of that consequence. It follows, then, that treatment effects will be stronger if clients' problem behaviors and improvements occur during the session, where they are closest in time and place to the available reinforcement. For example, if a female client states that she has difficulty trusting others, the therapy will be much more powerful if her distrust actually manifests itself in the therapeutic relationship where the therapist can react immediately rather than just talking about such incidents that occur in between sessions. Significant therapeutic change results from the contingencies that occur during the therapy session within the client–therapist relationship.

Thus, natural reinforcement contingent on the goal behavior is the primary change agent available in the therapeutic situation. If the therapist attempts to purposely "use" the existing natural reinforcers, however, they may lose their effectiveness, induce countercontrol, and produce a manipulative treatment. The dilemma is obviated, however, when the therapy is structured so that the genuine reactions of the therapist to client behavior naturally reinforce improvements as they happen. More specifically, because the dominant aspect of psychotherapy is interactional, the immediate natural reinforcement of client improvements is most likely when the client–therapist relationship naturally evokes the client's presenting problems, such as when a caring relationship evokes feelings of lack of self-worth or fears of eventual abandonment.

Clinically Relevant Behaviors

Central to the implementation of FAP's "here-and-now" approach and relationship focus is the concept of clinically relevant behaviors (CRBs)—the clients' interpersonal daily life problems that also occur with the therapist during the therapy session. Two types of clinically relevant client behavior of central importance to the therapy process can occur during the session.

CRB1s: Client Problems That Occur in Session

CRB1s are in-session occurrences of client repertoires that have been specified as problems according to the client's goals for therapy and the case conceptualization. There should be a correspondence between specific CRB1s and particular daily life problems. In successful FAP, CRB1s should decrease in frequency over the course of therapy. Typically, CRB1s are under the control of aversive stimuli and consist of avoidance (often emotional avoidance), but CRB1s are by no means restricted to problematic avoidance repertoires. Examples of CRB1s, that is. in-session instances of presenting clinical problems, may include: (1) a woman who has no friends and "does not know how to make friends" avoids eye contact, answers questions by talking at length in an unfocused and tangential manner, has one "crisis" after another, demands to be taken care of, gets angry at the therapist for not having all the answers and frequently complains that the world "shits" on her and that she gets an unfair deal; and (2) a depressed man who feels controlled by his wife shows up session after session with nothing to contribute to the therapy agenda and passively accepts and is compliant with whatever the therapist suggests.

CRB2s: Client Improvements That Occur in Session

CRB2s are in-session improvements, which should increase in frequency over the course of successful FAP. During the early stages of treatment CRB2 behaviors are rare and of low strength when an instance of the clinical problem, CRB1, occurs. For example, consider a client whose problem is withdrawal and accompanying feelings of low self-esteem when "people don't pay attention" to him during conversations and in other social situations. This client may show similar withdrawal behaviors when the therapist does not attend to what he is saying or interrupts him. Possible CRB2s for this situation might include repertoires of assertive behavior that try to direct the therapist back to what the client was saying, or the ability to discern the therapist's waning interest before the therapist actually proceeds to the point of interrupting him.

From a FAP standpoint, client change is facilitated by the therapist's awareness of and contingent responding to the client's clinically relevant behaviors. Explicitly, it is important for the therapist to extinguish CRB1s (in-session problem behaviors) and naturally reinforce CRB2s (in-session improvements). In order to effectively implement these core principles of discrimination and contingent responding, it is essential to do a functional analysis of the historical and current variables controlling the client's behavior, to understand the true function of a behavior rather than just looking at its topography.

Functional Analysis

Functional analysis answers the question "What is a behavior's function?" and requires understanding each client's unique history. This understanding allows us to define topographically similar behaviors according to different functions. For example, to say that the individual has an alcohol drinking problem is not sufficient. This is simply a description of the topography of the behavior—what it looks like. We prefer descriptions such as "the problem functions to alleviate anxiety," to numb depression, to gain benefits from lowered social inhibition, or that "the problem has multiple functions." The important point for now is that, as behaviorists, we define behavior *according to its function*. A functional analysis is often facilitated by asking the client questions to discern the potential functions of a behavior. Client reactions to the therapist are also an important source of information to aid functional analysis.

In terms of CRBs related to therapeutic alliance, it appears that when therapeutic alliance is operationalized, it tends to focus on the topography of the client's behavior, that is, what the behavior looks like rather than its function. In contrast, a FAP conceptualization of in-session behavior would focus on how a particular client behavior functions for the client, not whether it looks like a preconceived notion of how a client would act if there were therapeutic alliance. For instance, Adler (1980) noted that behavior that appeared topographically to be associated with alliance building in session may in fact function as compliance—in other words, a CRB1 or problem that should not be reinforced for a particular client. Consider the example of an unassertive male client who dutifully does his assigned homework but feels like he is not getting anything out of it. Again, what looks like a positive alliance behavior in this case is a CRB1, an in-session example of problematic behavior where he is not expressing his feelings and thoughts about what works and what does not. If this client were to state doubts about the validity of the homework, topographically it may look like alliance-disrupting behavior, but functionally it is an improvement and will lead to a strengthening of the therapeutic alliance if the client's concerns are taken seriously by the therapist. On the other hand, if compliant behavior were assessed to be a CRB2 (e.g., in the case of a client who is excessively critical of any ideas that are not his own), then it would be interpreted by a FAP therapist to be alliance-building behavior, and stating doubts about the validity of homework would indeed be CRB1. Thus, it is important to functionally assess client behaviors for their clinical relevance in alliance building rather than looking at just the form, or topography, of a behavior. In addition, a FAP perspective allows us to explain and predict how an alliance would be forged near the beginning of therapy as the result of general contingent reinforcement by the therapist of client CRB2s (Callaghan, Naugle, & Follette, 1996).

It should be pointed out that we are not saying that therapists who focus on the therapeutic alliance are likely to make such countertherapeutic errors. For example, the clinical examples given in Safran and Muran's (2000) book on negotiating the therapeutic alliance illustrate exceptionally skilled and nuanced therapeutic interventions that are consistent with FAP. We suspect these examples were provided by competent and experienced therapists who are intuitively sensitive to the CRB1–CRB2 distinction. For less experienced therapists, however, the FAP approach explicitly addresses this issue, does not rely on intuition, and thus could help reduce errors and improve outcome.

Clinical Interventions: How to Focus on the Therapeutic Relationship

FAP provides a set of five guidelines or rules specifying ways for therapists to notice, evoke, and naturally reinforce CRBs so that positive changes that take place in session can generalize to clients' daily lives (Tsai et al., 2008). Our goal is to point to phenomena and interventions that could be useful to all therapists and researchers regardless of their orientation.

Rule 1: Watch for CRBs (Be Aware)

This rule forms the core of FAP, and its implementation can lead to a stronger therapeutic alliance and interpersonally oriented treatment. The key question for therapists to answer is "How do the client's issues show up in this therapeutic relationship?"

A therapist's personal reactions to a client can be a valuable marker for identifying CRBs. Questions one can ask oneself include:

- What are the ways your client has a negative impact on you?
- Does your attention wander because you experience him as droning on and on?
- Is she avoidant of your questions?
- Does he frustrate you because he procrastinates with respect to his homework assignments?
- Does she say one thing and do another?
- Is he mean or unreasonable with you?
- Is she late with her payments?
- Is he critical of your every intervention?
- Does she shut down when you are warm?
- Does he pull away when the two of you have had a close interaction?
- Does she seem to have no interest or curiosity about you as a person?

A major concern is knowing when one's own responses to a client are representative of how others in the client's life might respond or, rather, are idiosyncratic. In other words, one's own reactions are an accurate guide to client CRBs to the extent that these responses are similar to the responses of those in the client's life. It is important, therefore, when using one's own reactions as a guide, to have some understanding of the other important people in the client's life and how they might respond. Overtly, this requirement may involve nothing more than asking, "I'm having [x] reaction to you right now—how would your significant other (or boss, coworker, family member, friend) react?" This approach, however, also requires a continual effort over time to truly and deeply understand the consequences that have shaped and maintained the client's behavior in the outside world.

It also is imperative that therapists continually engage in the personal work necessary to address their own deficits, promote their target behaviors, and ensure that any negative reactions to their clients are not based on personal issues. At a minimum, ongoing peer consultation helps to evaluate whether negative reactions toward clients are representative of how others in the client's daily life might respond. As therapists take advantage of therapeutic opportunities to evoke and reinforce CRB2s, their positive reactions are by definition a barometer of client improvement.

In many ways, CRBs and Rule 1 relate to Safran and Muran's (1996) approach to ruptures in the therapeutic alliance. According to Safran and Muran, ruptures are interpersonal markers "indicating critical points in therapy for exploration" (p. 447). We would rephrase this observation as a rule directing that therapists should "watch for and be aware of these markers." For the FAP therapist, CRBs are also interpersonal markers providing special opportunities that become the focus of treatment. Although therapeutic alliance ruptures are usually CRBs, the latter concept is broader and includes client interpersonal behavior other than alliance ruptures.

Rule 2: Evoke CRBs (Be Courageous)

From a FAP standpoint, the ideal client–therapist relationship evokes CRB1s, which in turn are the precursors for the development and nurturing of CRB2s. CRBs are idiographic or pertain to the unique circumstances and histories of individual clients, and thus the ideal therapeutic relationship will depend on what a particular client's daily life problems happen to be. If a client is anxious, depressed, or has difficulty committing to a course of action, then almost any type of psychotherapy has the potential to evoke CRBs. FAP, however, also focuses on relationship and intimacy issues such as the ability to deeply trust others, take interpersonal risks, be authentic, and give and receive love. Thus, FAP calls for therapists to be present and to structure their therapy in a manner not typically found in other behavior therapies.

Implementing the steps necessary to create an evocative therapeutic relationship requires therapists to take risks and push their own intimacy boundaries. Such risks involve being courageous and having the mental or moral strength to venture, to persevere, and to withstand the fear of difficulty. When therapists are doing FAP well, they are most likely stretching their limits and venturing beyond their comfort zone.

Therapists can evoke CRBs in three major ways:

1. Structure a therapeutic environment that evokes significant CRBs. From the very first contact, therapists can prepare clients for an intense and evocative therapy that focuses on *in vivo* interactions via the therapeutic rationale that is given. For example, this is something we typically would say to a depressed client:

> "I understand that you are seeking treatment for depression. One reason why people get depressed might be that they find it hard to express what they feel and to assert what they want from important individuals. Do you find that this is true for you? [The answer is usually "Yes."] Well, one focus of our therapy will be on how you can become a more powerful person, someone who can speak your truth compassionately and go after what you want. [The response is typically "That sounds good."] The most effective way for you to develop into a more expressive person is to start right here, right now, with me, to tell me what you are thinking, feeling, needing, even if it feels scary or risky. If you can bring forth your best self with me, then you can transfer these behaviors to other people in your life. How does that sound?"

2. Use evocative therapeutic methods. FAP is an integrative therapy and calls for varied techniques that no single therapeutic orientation would predict, depending on what will evoke client issues and what will be naturally reinforcing of client target behaviors. What is important is not the theoretical origin of a specific technique but rather its function with the client. To the extent that a technique—any technique—functions to evoke CRBs, it is potentially useful to FAP. Methods such as free association, writing exercises, empty chair work, mindfulness, cognitive restructuring, evoking emotion by focusing on bodily sensations, and hypnotherapy have all been used in FAP (Kanter, Tsai, & Kohlenberg, 2010; Tsai, Kohlenberg, Kanter, & Waltz, 2008). What these techniques have in common is that they can create contexts that may help clients access and express to the therapist avoided thoughts and feelings.

3. Use oneself as an instrument of change. To the extent that therapists can allow themselves to be who they really are, a more powerful and unforgettable relationship can be created. Giving some thought to the following questions may help you as a therapist to increase your potency as an agent of change:

• What are your unique qualities that make you distinctive as a person and as a therapist? How can you use your distinctiveness to your clients' advantage?

• Do any of your client's interests match yours? Consider disclosing this mutual interest. Similarly, do you have comparable life experiences, such as growing up Catholic, birth order, moving around a lot as a child, or being a member of a minority group? A major factor to take into account in making a decision to disclose is whether such disclosure will facilitate clients having greater contact with their issues or whether it will take them away from their own focus. Other considerations include whether the disclosure will engender more closeness from the client and whether the disclosure is problem behavior or a target behavior for the therapist.

• What is your experience of your client? What do you see as really special about this person, how does this person positively impact you, and how evocative would it be for you to mirror back to this client what is most special about him or her? Clients are often only in touch with their flaws and shortcomings; thus, for you to consistently tell them how you experience their positive characteristics is an experience they may not have had before, creating a turning point in self-perception.

• What are the ways in which you care about your client? Anyone can say the words "I care about you," but it is far more impactful to describe your behaviors that indicate caring. For example, you can talk about the ways clients affect you outside of the therapy hour, such as, "I had a dream about you," "I was thinking the other day about what you said to me," or "I saw a movie and thought at the time, 'I've got to tell you about this movie because you would really like it,'" or "I went to a workshop on art therapy with you in mind because I thought the techniques would be really helpful in our work together." Statements such as these are likely to be both evocative (Rule 2) and naturally reinforcing (Rule 3).

- How can you take risks to deepen your therapeutic relationship in ways that serve the client's best interests? Are there topics you avoid addressing with your clients (e.g., his lateness, her behaviors that push you away, wanting him to say what he is feeling underneath his façade) because your discomfort would match your clients'? Are there ways you can ask your clients to be more present and open with you?

These kinds of questions facilitate exploration of how one can become a more compassionate and transparent change agent through disclosing one's own thoughts, reactions, and personal experiences. Such strategic disclosures can enhance the therapeutic relationship, normalize clients' experiences, model adaptive and intimacy-building behavior (Goldfried, Burckell, & Eubanks-Carter, 2003), demonstrate genuineness and positive regard for clients (Robitschek & McCarthy, 1991), and equalize power in the therapeutic relationship (Mahalik, Van Ormer, & Simi, 2000). From a FAP perspective, the most important effect is that such behavior may evoke CRBs, block CRB1s, and encourage and nurture (reinforce) CRB2s. Thus, disclosure should be undertaken strategically with an awareness for how it may evoke, reinforce, or punish CRBs for a particular client (Vandenberghe, Coppede, & R. J. Kohlenberg, 2006).

Rule 3. Reinforce CRB2s Naturally (Be Therapeutically Loving)

This rule is somewhat enigmatic in that FAP is based on the assertion that reinforcement is the primary mechanism of change, and yet deliberate efforts to reinforce run the risk of producing contrived or arbitrary, rather than natural, reinforcement. We emphasize that naturally reinforcing behaviors are "therapeutically loving." Therapeutic love is ethical, is always in the client's best interests, and is genuine. Loving clients does not necessarily mean using the word "love" with them, but it does mean fostering an exquisite sensitivity and benevolent concern for the needs and feelings of clients, and caring deeply. Factors that determine whether therapists' reactions are likely to be therapeutically loving and naturally reinforcing include (1) responding to CRB1s effectively—it is best to address CRB1s only after a client has experienced sufficient natural positive reinforcement and a solid therapeutic alliance has formed, and after a client has given permission for the therapist to address the CRB1s; (2) being governed by clients' best interests and reinforced by their improvements; (3) having clients' goal repertoires—a therapist who is avoidant of intimacy will be less effective in facilitating intimacy building behaviors in his or her clients; and (4) matching one's expectations with clients' current repertoires—it is important to have reasonable expectations and to be tuned into successive approximations or nuances of improvement.

Rule 4: Observe the Potentially Reinforcing Effects of Therapist Behavior in Relation to Client CRBs (Be Aware of One's Impact)

Rule 4 highlights the importance of paying attention to client reactions and the therapist's observing his or her effect on the client. By definition, the client has experienced therapeutic reinforcement only if his or her target behavior is strengthened. Therefore, it is essential that therapists assess the degree to which their behaviors that were intended to reinforce actually functioned as reinforcers. By continuing to pay close attention to the function of one's own behavior, the therapist can adjust his or her responding, as needed, to maximize the potential for reinforcement. It also is important for therapists to focus on the role of T1s (therapist in-session problem behaviors) and T2s (therapist in-session target behaviors), because an increased awareness of oneself goes hand in hand with an increased awareness of one's impact on clients. We recommend that therapists set aside time to explore questions such as the following:

- What do you tend to avoid addressing with your clients?
- How does this avoidance affect the work that you do with these clients?
- What do you tend to avoid dealing with in your life (e.g., tasks, people, memories, needs, feelings)?
- How do your daily life avoidances affect the work that you do with your clients?
- What are the specific T2s you want to develop with each client, based on the case conceptualization?

Rule 5: Provide Functionally Analytically Informed Interpretations and Implement Generalization Strategies (Interpret and Generalize)

A functional analytically informed interpretation includes a history that accounts for how it was adaptive for clients to act in the ways they do and how to generalize progress in therapy to daily life. Implementing Rule 5 emphasizes "out-to-in parallels" when common daily life events are suggested by in-session experiences or situations and "in-to-out parallels" when in-session experiences have useful implications for common daily life events (Tsai, R. J. Kohlenberg, Kanter, & Waltz, 2008). Both are important, and a good FAP session may involve considerable weaving between daily life and in-session content through multiple in-to-out and out-to-in parallels. One example might involve a client's pulling away from her therapist's expressing caring (out-to-in parallel), versus relaxing into this caring and allowing it to happen in her daily life (in-to-out parallel). Provision of homework is also important to Rule 5; the best homework assignments are when a client has engaged in a CRB2 and the assignment is for the client to then take the improved behavior "on the road" and test it with significant others.

In sum, when these five rules are applied well, we hypothesize that the process leads to an increased focus on the therapeutic relationship that entails heightened awareness and appropriate risking and involvement by both clients and therapists, thus maximizing therapeutic outcome.

EFFECTS OF FOCUSING ON CRBs: EMPIRICAL FINDINGS

In essence, FAP's focus on the therapeutic relationship involves watching for, noticing, and responding to CRBs, and it is our contention that adding in such a focus may improve the intensity and power of psychotherapy, broadly defined. While converging lines of evidence exist from a variety of literature sources in support of some of FAP's basic principles (Baruch et al., 2008), the question remains: What are the effects of such therapist focus on CRBs, both in FAP-specific therapy relationships and in other therapy relationships? We have attempted to gather data on this question in several ways, all focused on measuring therapist behavior (and sometimes client behavior) in session and exploring relations between in-session therapist behavior and indicators of client outcomes.

Our first study explored the impact of adding in FAP's focus on CRBs with a set of experienced cognitive therapists (R. J. Kohlenberg, Kanter, Bolling, Parker, & Tsai, 2002). In this study four experienced research cognitive therapists first did cognitive therapy with 15 depressed patients. Then, while receiving training and supervision in FAP, they saw an additional 23 patients, continuing to do cognitive therapy, but with an added emphasis on noticing and using CRBs. This latter treatment was termed FAP-enhanced cognitive therapy (FECT). Outcome analyses suggested that FECT improved several indices of interpersonal functioning and the durability of treatment as compared to cognitive therapy alone.

In the FECT study (R. J. Kohlenberg et al., 2002), we were particularly interested in measuring what therapists did in FECT sessions and whether the specific focus on CRBs was predictive of acute treatment outcomes and session-by-session indicators of improvement. Videotapes of therapy sessions were coded by using an adherence scale developed for the purposes of the study that measured traditional cognitive therapy interventions (such as focusing on inaccurate cognitions in daily life), a focus on CRBs, and when both occurred simultaneously. An example of both cognitive therapy and a focus on CRBs occurring simultaneously would be the therapist's attending to the client's inaccurate beliefs and cognitions about the therapist or the therapeutic relationship. Results indicated that therapists focused on CRBs significantly more frequently when performing FECT as compared to traditional cognitive therapy and that the combined CT-CRB interventions significantly predicted improvements in interpersonal functioning at the end of treatment, as measured by the Social Avoidance and Distress Scale (Watson & Friend, 1969).

One limitation of this analysis was that only a small number of sessions were coded, owing to the training burden of the adherence measure. To explore this issue more thoroughly, a simpler coding scheme was employed (Kanter, Schildcrout, & R. J. Kohlenberg, 2005). This analysis involved coding every client and therapist's turn at speech during each of the treatment sessions in the FECT study. In contrast to the use of the labor-intensive but more precise adherence scale mentioned above (with some 40 categories of therapist interventions), these turns were simply rated as either an *in vivo* hit or not. An *in vivo* hit occurred when the therapist referred to working on client problems that occurred in therapy in relation to the therapy process, the therapy relationship, or anything else having to do with therapy, such as "I've noticed that you don't look at me when we are discussing sensitive issues," "What's so important about whether I like you or not?," and "Do you feel responsible for coming up with something to say every time we set the agenda?"

Of course, not all *in vivo* hits mean that a CRB was noticed by the therapist. On the other hand, the absence of a therapist comment involving a relational statement would mean that no CRBs were noticed. Thus *in vivo* hits include noticing CRB as well as other aspects of the therapist–client relationship that may not be related to the client's presenting problem. It is of interest to point out that *in vivo* hits would also include those instances in which the therapist attended to ruptures (Kanter, Rusch, Landes, Holman, Whiteside, & Sedivy, 2009).

As shown in Figure 9.1, training therapists to focus on CRBs appeared to increase the number of *in vivo* hits, with the cumulative number of *in vivo* hits in FECT and cognitive therapy appearing to separate at about Session 4 or 5 of 20 sessions for the study therapists. Log linear (Poisson) regression analysis established that the relative rate of *in vivo* hits was 2.8 times higher

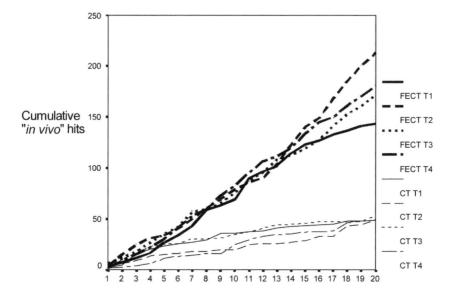

FIGURE 9.1. Cumulative record of "*in vivo*" hits for each therapist (T1, T2, T3, T4) for CT and FECT sessions.

in FECT as compared with cognitive therapy (95% confidence interval [CI] = 2.2–3.6, p < .001).

In order to assess whether a therapist's attending to the therapy relationship (an *in vivo* hit) had beneficial effects on session-by-session indicators of outcome, Kanter et al. (2005) evaluated the relationship between the number of *in vivo* hits in a session and both overall progress and relationship-specific improvements reported by the client for the week following the session. The client's weekly report was made before the next therapy session, placed in a sealed envelope, and not shown to the therapist. Results indicated a statistically significant relationship between *in vivo* hit rates per session and whether or not clients reported that the session was helpful in making progress with their problems (odds rates [OR] = 1.32, 95% CI = 1.11–1.58, p < .001). There also was a trend showing a relationship between *in vivo* hits in a session and relationship improvements in the week following that session (OR = 1.10, 95% CI = 0.98–1.22, p = .10). The turn-at-speech analysis supports the notion that for every five *in vivo* hits that are added by therapists in a session there is an increment in outcome. Our explanation for this finding is that an increased number of *in vivo* hits is consistent with a therapist following FAP Rule 1 namely, "Watch for CRBs."

Several researchers have taken these coding schemes one step further and have demonstrated the utility of turn-by-turn coding of specific FAP client and therapist behaviors. Basically, coders are taught to identify, on a turn-by-turn basis, specific instances of client CRBs based on individual case conceptualizations, as well as specific instances of therapist application of the primary FAP rules. In this way, a comprehensive description of the session, in terms of the flow of client and therapist behavior into and out of FAP-relevant themes, is possible. The first attempt at such detailed process coding, by Callaghan, Summers, and Weidman (2003), involved segments of four sessions of a client with personality disorder not otherwise specified successfully treated with FAP. Results demonstrated that coders could reliably identify client CRBs and therapist contingent responses to CRBs with this system and that client CRB1s decreased and CRB2s increased over the course of therapy in response to therapist contingent responses. Next, Busch, Callaghan, Kanter, Baruch, and Weeks (2010) replicated this result with a client diagnosed with borderline personality disorder successfully treated with FAP.

These early results using intensive turn-by-turn coding were limited because the clients coded were case studies that did not systematically control exactly what the therapist did in session to rule out alternative hypotheses. This shortcoming was remedied by Busch et al. (2009) on a client with comorbid depression and histrionic personality disorder. This client was successfully treated with FECT by using a within-subject design that allowed for the effects of focusing on CRBs to be isolated from the effects of cognitive therapy alone (Kanter et al., 2006). This client demonstrated large and sudden improvements when the therapist began focusing on CRBs, and turn-by-turn coding of every session of this case by Busch et al. demonstrated a clear link between focusing on (observing, evoking, and responding to) CRBs and client improvements, both in and out of session.

This research focusing on CRBs is still in its infancy. Nevertheless, taken together, there is accumulating support for the specific mechanism of action in the therapy relationship, according to FAP. We should note that this research does not indicate that FAP's proposed mechanism is the only active way the therapeutic relationship may positively impact clients, but it does appear to be one such way. Essentially, FAP's behavioral approach to the psychotherapy relationship, by focusing on specific client and therapist behaviors and their impact on each other, has facilitated a process research agenda that has provided a window into exactly what a therapist may do in session to create a powerful, intense relationship that has measurable positive effects on client relational problems, defined individually for each client.

CONCLUSION

The construct of therapeutic alliance has led to an increased focus on the therapeutic relationship as a means of improving psychotherapy outcome. FAP utilizes basic learning principles to explain how the focus on the therapeutic relationship leads to change. FAP not only proposes that the therapist–client relationship is important because it lies at very heart of the change process, but also it offers specific behaviorally defined therapist guidelines to help clients establish intimacy skills that are transferred to their daily lives Our behavioral approach takes into account the client's unique history and, as called for by the American Psychological Association Division 29 Task Force on Empirically Supported Relationships (Norcross, 2001), tailors both discrete methods and relationship stances on a patient-by-patient or moment-to-moment basis. We hope that FAP offers an inspiring and conceptually clear framework that crosses theoretical boundaries and provides additional ways to focus on the therapeutic relationship as a means of facilitating meaningful client change.

REFERENCES

Adler, G. (1980). Transference, real relationship, and alliance. *International Journal of Psychoanalysis, 61*, 547–558.

Barber, J. P., Connolly, M. B., Crits-Christoph, P., Gladis, L., & Siqueland, L. (2000). Alliance predicts patients' outcome beyond in-treatment change in symptoms. *Journal of Consulting and Clinical Psychology, 68*(6), 1027–1032.

Baruch, D. E., Kanter, J. W., Busch, A. M., Plummer, M. D., Tsai, M., Rusch, L. C., et al. (2008). Lines of evidence in support of FAP. In M. Tsai, R. J. Kohlenberg, J. W. Kanter, B. Kohlenberg, W. C. Follette, & G. M. Callaghan, (Eds.), *A guide to functional analytic psychotherapy: Awareness, courage, love, and behaviorism* (pp. 21–36). New York: Springer.

Busch, A. M., Callaghan, G. M., Kanter, J. W., Baruch, D. E., & Weeks, C. E. (2010). The Functional Analytic Psychotherapy Rating Scale: A replication and extension. *Journal of Contemporary Psychotherapy, 40*, 11–19.

Busch, A. M., Kanter, J. W., Callaghan, G. M., Baruch, D. W., Weeks, C. E., & Berlin, K. S. (2009). A micro-process analysis of Functional Analytic Psychotherapy's mechanism of change. *Behavior Therapy, 40*, 280–290.

Callaghan, G. M., Naugle, A. E., & Follette, W. C. (1996). Useful constructions of the client–therapist relationship. *Psychotherapy, 33*(3), 381–390.

Callaghan, G. M., Summers, C. J., & Weidman, M. (2003). The treatment of histrionic and narcissistic personality disorder behaviors: A single-subject demonstration of clinical effectiveness using Functional Analytic *Psychotherapy*. *Journal of Contemporary Psychotherapy, 33*, 321–339.

Ferster, C. B. (1967). Arbitrary and natural reinforcement. *The Psychological Record, 22*, 1–16.

Goldfried, M. R., Burckell, L. A., & Eubanks-Carter, C. (2003). Therapist self-disclosure in cognitive-behavior therapy. *Journal of Clinical Psychology*, *59*(5), 555–568.

Horowitz, L. M. (2004). *Interpersonal foundations of psychopathology*. Washington, DC: American Psychological Association.

Kanter, J. W., Landes, S. J., Busch, A. M., Rusch, L. C., Brown, K. R., Baruch, D. E., et al. (2006). The effect of contingent reinforcement on target variables in outpatient psychotherapy for depression: A successful and unsuccessful case using Functional Analytic Psychotherapy. *Journal of Applied Behavior Analysis*, *39*, 463–467.

Kanter, J. W., Rusch, L. C., Landes, S. L., Holman, G. I., Whiteside, U., & Sedivy, S. K. (2009). The use and nature of present-focused interventions in cognitive and behavioral therapies for depression. *Psychotherapy: Research, Theory, Practice, Training*, *46*, 220–232.

Kanter, J. W., Schildcrout, J. S., & Kohlenberg, R. J. (2005). In vivo processes in cognitive therapy for depression: Frequency and benefits. *Psychotherapy Research*, *15*(4), 366–373.

Kanter, J. W., Tsai, M., & Kohlenberg, R. J. (Eds.). (2010). *The practice of functional analytic psychotherapy*. New York: Springer.

Klein, D. F. (1996). Preventing hung juries about therapy studies. *Journal of Consulting and Clinical Psychology*, *64*(1), 81–87.

Kohlenberg, B. S. (2000). Emotion and the relationship in psychotherapy: A behavior analytic perspective. In M. J. Dougher (Ed.), *Clinical Behavior Analysis* (pp. 271–289). Reno, NV: Context Press.

Kohlenberg, B. S., Yeater, E., & Kohlenberg, R. J. (1998). Functional analysis, therapeutic alliance, and brief psychotherapy. In J. D. Safran & J. C. Muran (Eds.), *The therapeutic alliance in brief psychotherapy* (pp. 64–94). Washington, DC: American Psychological Association.

Kohlenberg, R. J., Kanter, J. W., Bolling, M. Y., Parker, C., & Tsai, M. (2002). Enhancing cognitive therapy for depression with functional analytic psychotherapy: Treatment guidelines and empirical findings. *Cognitive and Behavioral Practice*, *9*(3), 213–229.

Kohlenberg, R. J. & Tsai, M. (1991). *Functional analytic psychotherapy: Creating intense and curative therapeutic relationships*. New York: Plenum Press.

Kohlenberg, R. J., & Tsai, M. (1994). Functional analytic psychotherapy: A radical behavioral approach to treatment and integration. *Journal of Psychotherapy Integration*, *4*(3), 175–201.

Lambert, M. J., & Bergin, A. E. (1994). The effectiveness of psychotherapy. In A. E. Bergin & S. L. Garfield (Eds.), *Handbook of psychotherapy and behavior change* (4th ed., pp. 143–189). Oxford, UK: Wiley.

Lejuez, C. W., & Hopko, D. R. (2005). The therapeutic alliance in behavior therapy. *Psychotherapy*, *42*(4), 456–468.

Mahalik, J. R., Van Ormer, E. A., & Simi, N. L. (2000). Ethical issues in using self-disclosure in feminist therapy. In M. Brabeck (Ed.), *Practicing Feminist Ethics in Psychology* (pp. 189–201). Washington, DC: American Psychological Association.

Martin, D. J., Garske, J. P., & Davis, M. K. (2000). Relation of the therapeutic alliance with outcome and other variables: A meta-analytic review. *Journal of Consulting and Clinical Psychology, 68*(3), 438–450.

Norcross, J. D. (Ed.). (2001). Empirically supported therapy relationships: Summary Report of the Division 29 Task Force. *Psychotherapy, 38*(4), 495–497.

Robitschek, C. G., & McCarthy, P. R. (1991). Prevalence of counselor self-reference in the therapeutic dyad. *Journal of Counseling and Development, 69*(3), 218–221.

Safran, J. D., & Muran, J. C. (1996). The resolution of ruptures in the therapeutic alliance. *Journal of Consulting and Clinical Psychology, 64*(3), 447–458.

Safran, J. D., & Muran, J, C. (Eds.). (1998). *The therapeutic alliance in brief psychotherapy.* Washington, DC: American Psychological Association.

Safran, J. D., & Muran, J. C. (2000). *Negotiating the therapeutic alliance: A relational treatment guide.* New York: Guilford Press.

Safran, J. D., & Muran, J. (2006). Has the concept of the therapeutic alliance outlived its usefulness? *Psychotherapy: Theory, Research, Practice, Training, 43*(3), 286–291.

Skinner, B. (1982). Contrived reinforcement. *Behavior Analyst, 5*(1), 3–8.

Skinner, B. F. (1953). *Science and human behavior.* New York: Macmillan.

Skinner, B. F. (1974). *About behaviorism.* New York: Knopf.

Tsai, M., Kohlenberg, R. J., Kanter, J. W., Kohlenberg, B. S., Follette, W. C., & Callaghan, G. M. (2008). *A guide to functional analytic psychotherapy: Awareness, courage, love and behaviorism.* New York: Springer.

Tsai, M., Kohlenberg, R. J., Kanter, J. W., & Waltz, J. (2008). Therapeutic technique: The five rules. In M. Tsai, R. J. Kohlenberg, J. W. Kanter, B. S. Kohlenberg, W. C. Follette, & G. M. Callaghan, (Eds.), *A guide to functional analytic psychotherapy: Awareness, courage, love and behaviorism* (pp. 61–102). New York: Springer.

Vandenberghe, L., Coppede, A. M., & Kohlenberg, R. J. (2006). Client curiosity about the therapist's private life: Hindrance or therapeutic aid? *The Behavior Therapist, 29*(3), 41–46.

Watson, D., & Friend, R. (1969). Measurement of social-evaluative anxiety. *Journal of Consulting and Clinical Psychology, 33*, 448–457.

CHAPTER 10

■ ■ ■ ■ ■

The Therapeutic Alliance in Humanistic Psychotherapy

Jeanne C. Watson
Freda Kalogerakos

The importance of therapeutic relationship has long been central to the writings of humanistic theorists and practitioners (Barrett-Lennard, 1997; Bohart, 1991; Bozarth, 2001; Cain, 2001; Cooper, 2008; Rogers, 1951; Watson, Greenberg, & Lietaer, 1998). In his writings Rogers (1951, 1967) focused primarily on therapists' attitudes and behaviors that he saw as optimal for facilitating clients' changes in psychotherapy. The construct of the working alliance, defined as client and therapist agreement on the goals and tasks of therapy, as well as the bond or positive feelings that develop between the two participants came into focus after some humanistic practitioners became more process-directive in their work with clients. In this chapter we briefly examine how the alliance is viewed within each of these approaches before exploring the empirical literature that has emerged to guide humanistic practitioners in their interactions with clients.

For Rogers, therapy meant a genuine person-to-person experience, akin to the type described by Buber as an "I–thou relationship." Both Buber and Rogers thought that the experience of speaking truly and openly with another person could have a healing effect (Rogers, 1961, 1975). To this end, humanistic psychotherapists struggle to understand the subjective worldview of the other without judgment and to treat each person whom they encounter in therapy with deep respect and caring. They are committed to developing compassionate, authentic, and egalitarian, albeit asymmetrical—relationships that respect clients' autonomy.

Rogers (1951, 1967) posited six conditions for personality change to occur in therapy: first, that two people be in psychological contact; second, that the client be in a state of incongruence, being vulnerable or anxious; third, that the therapist be congruent; fourth, that the therapist experience unconditional regard for the client; fifth, that the therapist experience an empathic understanding of the client's internal frame of reference and endeavor to communicate this understanding to the client; and sixth, that the client perceive to at least a nominal degree the therapist's unconditional positive regard and empathic understanding (Rogers, 1967). These conditions require therapists to create warm, safe, nonjudgmental environments and to respond by showing deep understanding of clients' emotional experience. According to Rogers's view, therapists are free to set limits on behavior but not on attitudes and feelings, and they should restrain themselves from probing, blaming, interpreting, reassuring, or persuading clients (Wyatt, 2001).

Rogers (1951) viewed pathology as arising from a conflict between a person's organismic experience and internalized conditions of worth learned from early caretakers and significant others. According to this view, feelings and inner experiencing that are inconsistent with internalized conditions of worth lead to anxiety and the tendency to deny conflicting feelings. This anxiety limits the extent to which people attend to or use their organismic experiencing as a guide to living. Rogers suggested that in environments of acceptance and empathy clients would be able to moderate their conditions of worth and develop more authentic and satisfying ways of being in the world (Bozarth, 1990; Brodley, 1990; Rogers, 1951). Healthy functioning for Rogers' was characterized by openness to experience. Lietaer (1993) characterized this perspective as a way of being that is flexible and open, with an ability to hold concepts of the real and the ideal self tentatively so that they are accessible to awareness and receptive to new information and experiences and readily amenable to change whenever necessary.

THE NONDIRECTIVE APPROACH

To promote a facilitative climate Rogers emphasized a nondirective style of therapy aimed at following clients' experience and trying to mirror it in the session (Brodley, 1990). The primary objectives within a nondirective approach are to perceive the idiosyncratic meaning of clients' feelings and experiences, communicate this understanding to clients through empathic reflections, and convey warmth and acceptance of their experiences. Nondirective therapists are open and accepting as they actively listen to and strive to understand clients' feelings and personal meanings.

Unconditional Positive Regard

The first relationship condition espoused by Rogers (1967) is that therapists experience unconditional positive regard (UPR) toward their clients. This attitude signals to clients that their experience is accepted fully and valued without judgment. Bozarth (2001) sees UPR as the curative factor in client-centered therapy as therapists come to share and know their clients' experiences. UPR is the antidote to clients' conditions of worth and is particularly important for clients whose thoughts and feelings have been ignored, discounted, or harshly criticized. Empathy without UPR would be clinical, cold, and potentially destructive, just as UPR without empathy and understanding of the other might be experienced as superficial, irrelevant, and empty. However, empathy combined with warm acceptance can be a very potent source of change, leading some theorists to suggest that the two are a single condition, with each aspect balancing and enriching the other (Bozarth, 2001; Freire, 2001). In client-centered therapy UPR is essential to ensure that empathy is used benignly and in the clients' best interest, just as knowledge of the other is necessary for the transforming power of UPR to be experienced. Rogers saw UPR as an overriding need in human beings and as crucial to the development of a fully functioning self. It is through the experience of UPR that individuals are able to integrate their experiences into a concept of self (Eckert & Biermann-Ratjen, 1998; Watson & Steckley, 2001).

Empathy

The second relationship condition identified by Rogers was empathy. Rogers (1975) described empathy as a multifaceted phenomenon that involves entering into the client's world as a companion and being sensitive to the client's changing flow of felt meanings without making judgments. Drawing on Gendlin's (1981, 1996) view that within people there is a flow of experiencing to which the individual can turn as a referent in order to discover the meaning of his or her experience, Rogers saw therapists' empathy as pointing sensitively to the felt meanings that clients experience in any particular moment. Therapeutic empathy works to track the moment-to-moment unfolding of the client's experience. By pointing to the possible meanings in the flow of their experiencing, therapists help clients to focus on it, experience the meanings more fully, and move forward in their experiencing process (Rogers, 1967). Empathic responses consist of reflections of feeling, cognitions, or behaviors as well as metaphors to capture and evoke the live and poignant aspects of clients' phenomenological experience.

Empathic reflections assist with building a working alliance by, first, helping clients and therapists to negotiate a shared perspective of clients' problems—and the issues that are contributing to these problems—and to formulate a focus of treatment. Second, they help to clarify the client's internal state, including feelings and judgments about the significance of events in their lives, thereby keeping clients and therapists on the same track. Third, empathic reflections validate clients' feelings and emphasize that their internal experience is an important source of information to help them resolve problematic issues, thereby establishing clients as the experts on their experience. Fourth, by validating clients' experiences, therapists empower their clients, making them active agents in the change process and engaging them in treatment (Bohart, Elliott, Greenberg, & Watson, 2002; Vanaerschot, 1990; Watson, 2001).

Congruence

The third relationship condition that humanistic therapists strive to provide is congruence. Rogers saw it as essential that therapists be genuine in their relationships with their clients. Over time Rogers came to see this characteristic as the most important condition that therapists could offer. Being congruent requires therapists to be aware of their inner experiencing and to be able to share this awareness with their clients if they see it as helpful to the therapeutic process. Rogers was concerned that therapists not present an outward façade of one attitude while covertly experiencing another. He urged therapists to ensure that they are sincere in communicating empathy and acceptance so that there is no discrepancy between what they are communicating and what they are feeling. Lietaer (1993) refers to the inner awareness as congruence and the communication of the inner experience as transparency. This condition requires therapists to be self-aware, responsible, and real in their relationships.

Taken together, Rogers's (1951) core conditions of unconditional positive regard, empathy, and genuineness provide clients with safe and nonthreatening relationships in which they can explore their inner selves and make the intrapersonal and interpersonal changes necessary to function adaptively and healthily. Rogers's primary goal was to empower clients. He saw clients as the experts on their experience, and his belief in the growth tendency allowed him to trust that clients could effect change given the right therapeutic conditions. His objective was to remove therapists from the center of the change process. He saw them, instead, as providing a supportive function that clients could draw upon to bring about changes in their lives. He viewed therapists as handmaidens and less as the primary agents of change. Rogers's formulation of the relationship conditions can be seen to have provided therapists with the necessary and sufficient guidelines to govern their behavior with clients in order to provide healing relationships and a constructive way to avoid hostile, negative interpersonal process.

We see all four attitudes as interrelated and necessary to communicate understanding and acceptance in order to enable clients to explore their phenomenological experience in safety and overcome blocks to self-actualization. More recently some researchers have used the term "presence" to capture the relationship conditions in a holistic way (Geller & Greenberg, 2002). By "presence," these authors are referring to a way of being with clients that is focused, mindful, accepting, respectful, and nonjudgmental.

Research and the Rogerian Relationship Conditions

Numerous research studies have investigated the efficacy of the relationship conditions in promoting change. These studies continue to highlight and emphasize the importance of the Rogerian relationship conditions in facilitating change and promoting good outcome (Greenberg, Watson, Elliott, & Bohart, 2001; Norcross, 2002). After a review of the research on specific elements of the psychotherapy relationship that work, the Division 29 Task Force of the American Psychological Association stated unequivocally that empathy is a key element promoting change in psychotherapy and that positive regard and congruence are very promising elements (Norcross, 2002). Moreover a number of studies in which clients have been interviewed have found that they value speaking to someone who is warm, understanding, and involved (Lietaer, 1992; Henry & Strupp, 1994). Bent, Putnam, and Kiesler (1976) found that satisfied clients saw their therapists as warmer than did dissatisfied clients.

Further support for the relationship conditions was provided by Lietaer (1974) and Gurman (1977) in their factor analyses of empathy. They found that it included respect, unconditional positive regard, transparency, directivity, and congruence. While these studies focused on clients' self-reports of the therapeutic relationship, other studies that have looked at therapist interpersonal process using external raters highlight similar behaviors as therapeutic. Studies of client and therapist interpersonal process show that therapists in good outcome cases were supportive, affirming, openly receptive, involved, nurturing, and stimulating in their interactions with clients, whereas therapists in poor outcome cases were controlling, critical, and hostile (Henry, Schacht, & Strupp, 1990; Lorr, 1965; Najavits & Strupp, 1994; Watson, Enright, & Kalogerakos, 1998).

PROCESS-DIRECTIVE APPROACHES

The experiential approach grew out of Rogers's research program that subjected the psychotherapy process to intense study and description. Rogers (1961) and his colleagues at the University of Chicago observed in their studies of clients' process in therapy that clients with good outcomes engaged in self-exploration with little or no direction or prodding from their therapists. These clients were self-directed and explored their inner worldviews, feelings, and perceptions and posed questions about their experiencing that they would then explore in a purposeful fashion to resolve issues or create shifts in their perceptions or ways of feeling. However, poor-outcome clients did not engage in this process as readily. This led Eugene Gendlin, a colleague of Rogers, to devise the method of *focusing* in an attempt to teach clients how to engage productively in client-centered therapy (Gendlin, 1981, 1996). This technique taught clients to attend to their bodies and inner experience and to symbolize this experience through words. Subsequently, Leijssen (1990), using case study methodology, identified four steps associated with effective focusing interventions. The steps include clients' symbolization and representation of the situation, their bodily felt sense, a symbol for the bodily felt sense, and the feeling that was generated.

Following the experiential model of therapy developed by Gendlin and Rogers, Rice and Greenberg (1984) developed a research program that used task analysis to identify and analyze micro change events in a session to identify the steps that clients engaged in to resolve problematic issues in therapy. This research program found that there were certain therapist interventions that were more helpful than others in the resolution of specific types of problematic issues, for example, problematic reactions (Rice & Saperia, 1984), unfinished business, and conflict splits (Greenberg & Webster, 1982). This program of research led to the development of process–experiential psychotherapy, an emotion-focused approach to change (PE-EFT; Elliott, Watson, Goldman, & Greenberg, 2004; Greenberg, Rice, & Elliott, 1993).

Experiential approaches balance guidance with acceptance as therapists make process observations and suggestions to clients to facilitate shifts in their experiencing during the session while still providing the therapeutic conditions advocated by Rogers (1951). The primary objective for experiential therapists is to assist clients in accessing their organismic experience and to become aware of how they are blocking or distorting it from awareness or otherwise trying to control and manage their experience to conform to internalized conditions of worth or social norms and pressures. The objective is to help clients to actualize by helping them become aware of all aspects of their experience and to work out ways of expressing and balancing their needs and feelings with a system of values that they fully own and accept.

Experiential therapists distinguish between the relationship conditions and the working conditions of therapy (Rice, 1983). This distinction coincides with Bordin's (1979) conceptualization of the therapeutic alliance as consisting of an affective bond dimension as well as collaboration on the goals and tasks of therapy. The creation of a safe relational environment in experiential therapy helps to facilitate the client's exploration and processing of emotional experience. However, unlike the situation in client-centered therapy, the relationship conditions in experiential therapy also serve as a collaborative base for the accomplishment of such therapeutic tasks as two-chair work or focusing. At the molecular level, experiential therapists are highly empathically attuned to clients' moment-by-moment feelings and experiences and are focused on helping clients to feel understood and accepted. Therapists' reflections assist clients in exploring difficult issues and focus clients on facets of their experience that are most salient or poignant. At the molar level, therapists guide the process by assisting clients in symbolizing different aspects of their experiencing and expressing it, to facilitate resolution of the specific problems with which they are wrestling (Elliott et al., 2004; Greenberg et al., 1993).

PE-EFT therapists integrate the use of gestalt interventions like two-chair work with the Rogerian facilitative conditions. Greenberg et al. (1993) realized the importance of attending to clients' moment-by-moment affective experiences to guide clinical practice and develop productive working spaces to enable clients to explore their conflicts and the issues that brought them into therapy. The facilitative conditions form the bedrock of PE-EFT, with empathic reflections that convey empathic understanding as well as acceptance and positive regard for the clients' moment-by-moment experience comprising a large proportion of the work in the resolution of specific tasks involving two-chair and empty-chair work. PE-EFT therapists use their own empathic responsiveness and expressions of empathy to track their clients' experience and affect in order to assist them in identifying which specific interventions or types of responses might be appropriate at different times. Acceptance and congruence work together with empathy to establish trust and facilitate the clients' opening up to explore their experience with their therapists and resolve their blocks to self-acceptance and change.

As therapists move to suggest different ways of processing experiences, experiential therapists need to balance guidance with acceptance. In order to adhere to the Rogerian relationship conditions, experiential therapists must be highly attuned to clients' feelings of discomfort or resistance when they agree to engage in specific tasks. As therapists become more process-directive, the issue of agreement on the tasks and goals becomes more central. Watson and Geller (2005) showed that empathy mediated the impact of the working alliance on outcome in a study of depressed clients treated with PE-EFT or cognitive-behavioral psychotherapy (CBT) in a randomized clinical trial. These findings underscore the importance of therapists' empathy in negotiating and maintaining the working alliance. Therapists need to understand their clients' views of their problems as well as their goals and objectives in order to fit their responses to clients' needs and to be optimally responsive within the session.

The communication of the relationship conditions of empathy, acceptance, and congruence remains fundamental to the practice of humanistic person-centered, experiential, and emotion-focused psychotherapists, irrespective of clients' presenting issues (Bohart et al., 2002; Bozarth, 2001; Elliott et al., 2004; Vanaerschot, 1990; Watson, Greenberg, & Lietaer, 1998). Even in those humanistic approaches that have broadened the range of therapeutic interventions to include more structured interventions and guidance, like PE-EFT (Elliott et al., 2004; Greenberg et al., 1993), the Rogerian attitudes are emphasized and seen as essential elements of change. Watson and Greenberg (1994) have suggested that the implementation of specific marker-guided tasks can be conceptualized as instantiations of therapist empathy and attunement to clients' goals if they fit with clients' views of their problems and objectives. However, special care needs to be taken that interventions are not suggested and imposed such that clients are disregarded as the experts on their experience. Instead, clients must be viewed as active collaborators in the process of setting up the goals and tasks of therapy. Thus, in addition to creating an affective bond between clients and therapists, this approach highlights collaboration between clients and therapists on the goals and tasks of therapy.

RESEARCH ON FACTORS
THAT MODERATE THE ALLIANCE

There has been much research investigating factors that moderate the therapeutic alliance, including studies that have examined the participants' subjective experience and inquired about the helpful aspects of therapy, client factors that contribute to the development and maintenance of the alliance over time, and therapist factors. We review some of these studies that are especially pertinent to the development and maintenance of the alliance in humanistic psychotherapy.

Studies of Client and Therapist Subjective Experience

Studies of clients' and therapists' subjective experience during a session have found that when things are going well participants experience a sense of flow and synchrony (Geller & Greenberg, 2002; Grafanaki & McLeod, 2002; Watson & Rennie, 1994; Westerman, Tanaka, Frankel, & Khan, 1986).

These researchers report that there is a sense of collaboration with clients' showing a sense of purpose and engaging in self-exploration that yields new insights and self-understanding that leads to felt shifts. They become more aware of their needs and more able to meet them and engage in new behaviours. Both participants seem to evince little concern about the relationship when things are going well. Therapists usually describe themselves as operating intuitively and easily from this place (Bojic Ognjenovic & Watson, 2002; Geller & Greenberg, 2002; Mearns & Cooper, 2005; Rogers, 1961; Watson & Rennie, 1994).

When clients are working well, are able to turn inward and represent their inner experience, and are able to reflect on themselves and their experiences so that they pose questions and explore issues in a purposeful manner that leads to felt shifts, then humanistic therapists follow their clients' lead. At these times therapists continue to provide the optimal conditions for their clients' work by being empathic, accepting, congruent, and prizing. They are attentive to the questions clients pose about their experiences and focus their reflections accordingly.

In contrast to the sense of flow that is experienced when things are going well, studies show that therapists are aware of times when the process is highly uneven (Bojic Ognjenovic & Watson, 2002), the flow is interrupted (Watson & Rennie, 1994), or something interferes with the relationship. At these times, both participants devote more deliberate attention to their alliance and how they are interacting. When the flow is interrupted or disrupted, humanistic psychotherapists emphasize congruence and transparency to resolve difficulties in the alliance (Lietaer, 1993; Watson & Greenberg, 2000). The important role of being transparent and responding in a nondefensive way to these types of alliance difficulties has been supported by the growing research literature on resolving ruptures (Safran, Muran, & Samstag, 1994). Another useful intervention is meta-communication about the goals and tasks that are being suggested and how they may be impacting the client (Rennie, 1994; Safran et al., 1994).

Humanistic therapists have developed numerous ways to try to resolve alliance ruptures. If clients are unable to represent their inner experience or seem unaware of their feelings, experiential-humanistic psychotherapists might suggest focusing exercises to begin to teach clients how to turn inward and access their bodily felt sense and feelings and to represent these symbolically either with words or images. Alternatively, they may observe that their clients seem to be conflicted over certain courses of action or treat themselves harshly and tend to oppress or dismiss their feelings. At these times experiential therapists might suggest two-chair work to help clients become more aware of the different aspects of the conflict or how they are treating themselves. As clients become more aware of their bodies and feelings, they are able to access and represent parts of their experience in new and fresh ways. This process allows them to clearly represent the impact of how they are treating themselves and begin to develop alternative ways of being. At other times when clients seem mired in complaints or disempowered and regretful about their relationships with significant others, experiential therapists might suggest empty-chair work to try to empower clients by facilitating their expression of their feelings and needs. Working in this way, clients are able to differentiate from significant others and feel more empowered so that they are able to find alternative ways of meeting their needs in relationships. If these suggestions do not work, humanistic therapists should renew their efforts to provide accepting, empathic responses to assist their clients in symbolizing their experiences in ways that make more sense to them.

Clients' Contributions to the Alliance

Studies that have investigated the joint collaboration of clients and therapists show that a positive working alliance early in therapy is related to a good outcome in short-term therapy (Horvath & Symonds, 1991; Martin, Garske, & Davis, 2000). While these findings have been interpreted to mean that therapists who are able to establish good alliances early on in therapy can facilitate change, a review of studies on attachment and the alliance suggests that a more likely explanation is that clients who have fewer interpersonal difficulties and are more securely attached are able to form good working alliances and respond well in short-term therapy.

Numerous research studies suggest that client attachment style accounts for a large percentage (up to 33%) of the variance in client-rated working alliance. More specifically, the majority of studies have found a positive relationship between secure client attachment characteristics and working alliance ratings (Eames & Roth, 2000; Justitz, 2002; Kivlighan, Patton, & Foote, 1998; Parish & Eagle, 2003; Reis & Grenyer, 2004; Satterfield & Lyddon, 1995, 1998). That is, clients who have secure attachment styles are more likely to experience more positive working alliances with their therapists than are clients with insecure attachment styles. Results of correlation and regression analyses showed that clients who were more comfortable with closeness and intimacy in relationships, and who were more willing to trust and rely on others, formed stronger alliances with counselors. Conversely, clients who were more anxious and fearful of closeness to others, avoidant or unwilling to trust and rely on others for comfort and support, or dismissive of others experienced poorer working alliances with their counselors. These findings support those of other researchers who have found that clients with attachment difficulties have difficulty self-disclosing and being open about their experiences (Mikulincer & Nachshon, 1991; Pistole, 1993). This research suggests that clients who have been severely wounded and have come to doubt and trust their own bodily felt sense may have difficulty trusting themselves or their therapists in a short period of time.

Another client factor that can act as an impediment to building a strong therapeutic alliance is feelings of shame. An intensive analysis of six cases (three good and three poor outcomes) by Watson, Goldman, and Greenberg (2007) illuminated how feelings of shame contributed to clients' difficulties in forging strong alliances with their therapists. An examination of good and poor outcome cases showed that, while clients with both good and poor outcomes reported agreement with their therapists on the goals and tasks of therapy, they differed on the degree to which they felt liked and prized by their therapists, with poor outcome clients being less certain that their therapists liked them. These clients were also ashamed and fearful of disclosing their experiences.

These findings suggest that not only is it hard for clients who feel ashamed of their experience to share their experience with others but also often it is hard for them to acknowledge it to themselves. Clients who are ashamed have internalized harsh conditions of worth and may have difficulty working within the time constraints of a short-term treatment protocol. As Rogers suggested, these clients may benefit most from their therapists' acceptance and prizing, but these attitudes may take time to penetrate clients' intense feelings of shame. However, if therapists are patient, their acceptance and empathic responding can work together to slowly melt clients' sense of shame and give them the strength to reveal their inner experience—while believing that they and it can be prized and respected.

Another important factor in terms of clients' contributions to the development of an effective working alliance is clients' expectations (Kwan, Watson, & Stermac, 2000). Clients who come to therapy believing that it is useful and will be beneficial are more likely to forge positive, strong alliances with their therapists early on. This pattern is particularly important if short-term treatments are to be effective. Difficulties arise when clients come to therapy with expectations that are at odds with talk therapy. Some clients may come expecting advice, while others may attend even while believing that their distress is biological in origin and the cure medication. It is necessary to address these expectations early on and to explain how talk therapy can be effective and to address the interactions between biology and environment. Often these differences can be resolved and a common perspective created that enables clients to work constructively in psychotherapy.

These findings suggest that clients who are more resilient and able to cope better more likely to benefit from short-term therapy. However, many clients come to therapy precisely because they are not securely attached, as their attachment histories have contributed to their feeling distrustful of themselves and others. These clients are not resilient and have not had the opportunity to develop effective interpersonal behaviors and ways of regulating their inner experience that would allow them to live full and satisfying lives and cope with problems in day-to-day living. In these cases the relationship conditions suggested by Rogers and his colleagues may be essential to help them slowly learn to trust and regulate themselves and their inner experience, develop more effective interpersonal skills, rebuild their lives, and develop their inner resources.

Balancing Guidance with Acceptance

The working alliance is fluid and dynamic, continually evolving over the course of therapy as the two participants engage in a relationship with each other to alleviate the client's distress and realize their agreed-upon goals and objectives. In order to maintain connection and a positive therapeutic relationship, therapists need to be responsive to different things at different times. A study that examined clients' and therapists' interpersonal process using the structural analysis of social behavior found that one of the dangers of accepting and following clients is that therapists may fail to provide guidance and adequately structure clients' exploration or perceive the experiential questions that their clients are posing (Watson, Enright, & Kalogerakos, 1998). At times like this, therapists risk being laissez-faire and neglectful as they listen to their clients' concerns, grasping only the surface content of what their clients are sharing and missing their emotional meanings. To avoid neglecting their clients, experiential therapists need to be responsively attuned to their clients' experience moment to moment during the session and to guide them by offering process suggestions.

However, experiential therapists must take extra care when offering process guidance in case clients are merely following along. In his research of clients' experiences during experiential psychotherapy, Rennie (1994) has shown that therapists need to be alert to moments when their clients are deferring to them and their suggestions as opposed to staying in touch with and expressing their own needs and experiences congruently. While clients may defer to some extent in order to facilitate the work of therapy and to collaborate with their therapists, it is important that they feel free to disagree with their therapists if they are to access, trust, and express their own experience. One of the most important objectives for humanistic therapists is to help clients become aware of, symbolize, and express their inner experiencing in order to live more satisfying and fulfilling lives and solve their problems in living.

In a study to investigate ruptures in PE-EFT and CBT, McMullen and Watson (2005) found that more disagreement was expressed by clients in PE-EFT than in CBT. A closer examination of the transcripts revealed that clients in emotion-focused experiential therapy were involved in a process with their therapists to more clearly refine and differentiate what they were feeling at any given moment. Emotion-focused experiential therapists encouraged their clients to check inside to see whether their therapists' conjectures and labels adequately described how they were feeling and to correct them if necessary.

As therapists move from primarily following their clients to offering processing suggestions and observations, there is a heightened need to ensure that clients share in and agree to the tasks and goals that are being proposed. Once they become invested in achieving a particular goal or steering the clients' process in a specific direction, therapists can readily lose sight of their clients. There is a risk that therapists may become too managing and controlling, which can quickly lead to negative interpersonal process, as studies have shown that therapists can become punitive and defensive when clients reject their therapists' processing suggestions (Henry & Strupp, 1994; Watson, Greenberg, & Lietaer, 1998; Watson, 2007). Thus, experiential therapists take care not to become invested in working a specific way with their clients or in achieving specific objectives even though they think these might prove helpful to clients. Experiential therapists try not to lose trust even when they doubt their clients' capacity to know what feels right and what fits at any given time. What feels right to clients may shift over time as they come to know themselves better, gain more appreciation and awareness of their felt sense, and develop the capacity to attend, represent, and express their experience for themselves and others.

An important way that experiential therapists can maintain the balance between guidance and acceptance is to support the expression of disagreement to ensure that clients *remain the experts* regarding their inner experiencing. To ensure that their clients are not merely deferring to their professional judgment, PE-EFT therapists offer their observations and process suggestions tentatively, and clients are asked explicitly whether their therapists' observations are congruent with their experience and fit with their own goals and how they want to collaborate. Clients are encouraged to see whether their therapists' processing suggestions fit closely with their own inner experience and ways of thinking about their problems.

Another way to balance guidance and acceptance is for therapists to attend to signs of clients' resistance. A number of studies have provided clues as to how client resistance might be expressed in the session, including clients' questioning the relevance of certain tasks; being unable to engage in the task of representing various aspects of their experience; showing marked hesitation; losing track of their thoughts; and engaging in long silences, especially following therapists' requests to undertake certain exercises (Bojic Ognjenovic & Watson, 2002; Henry et al., 1990; Rennie, 1994; Safran & Muran, 1998; Watson & Rennie, 1994; Westerman et al., 1986). At other times, therapists may have the sense that what their clients are expressing is incongruent. All of these behaviors are signs that experiential therapists should stop what they are doing and inquire how their clients are experiencing the session. When therapists sense that their clients are feeling resistant, it is important for them to follow their clients more closely and be more receptive, empathic, and accepting of their clients' experience in the session. At these times therapists need to be able to listen nondefensively to their clients and try to hear what they are saying so that they can once more fall into step together.

Some clients may refuse to engage in specific tasks because they are not yet ready to assume an active role in their healing. Sometimes clients who have felt cheated of nurturance or forced to be responsible for themselves and others prematurely may not be ready to engage as quickly as might be necessary in short-term therapy. These clients need time to share their experiences, to voice their complaints and disappointments, and to feel fully supported without pressure to be different or engage in new behaviors or to take care of themselves. Experiential therapists are careful at these times not to pressure their clients but rather to trust that with time they will begin to feel stronger and assume responsibility for their own self-care.

Managing Therapists' Process

One of the problems that can interfere with the alliance and treatment overall is when therapists begin to doubt themselves or become self-critical. In a study of therapists' metacognitive processing in both good and difficult sessions, Bojic Ognjenovic and Watson (2002) found that this doubt can occur with both novice and experienced therapists. In this study, therapists reported that they felt disappointed and dispirited when their clients did not seem to make progress. Some therapists became bogged down in a spiral of self-doubt and anxiety. This experience was in contrast to that of therapists who used their recognition that things were not working to readjust what they were doing in therapy and tried to better understand their clients' objectives and what they were experiencing.

Therapists who had alternative strategies and ways of working with their clients did not feel stuck and powerless. Instead, they were able to reengage empathically and reconnect with their clients. This approach led them to reframe what was happening in the session and come up with alternative formulations that fitted better with their clients' perspectives and objectives. Therapists may need support to deal with feelings of failure and self-doubt and to avoid becoming defensive and blaming their clients for treatment failures. It can be useful to have a peer support group or another therapist to turn to during the course of therapy to facilitate reflection on the process during the course of treatment. When clients do not respond to treatment protocols, the sense of failure can be strong—along with the tendency to blame clients for being difficult, unappreciative, and too damaged to work collaboratively in therapy. Therapists can guard against blaming clients by consciously being compassionate both of their own efforts and those of their clients.

To support their clients when things are not going well requires therapists to tap into large reserves of the attitudes that remain the fundamental bases of all productive therapeutic interactions: acceptance, empathy, congruence and unconditional. When clients seem slow to change, it can be useful for therapists to remember that, by providing the optimal therapeutic conditions as prescribed by Rogers (1951), they are helping clients to learn new affect regulation skills and to develop new ways of interacting with themselves and others (Elliott et al., 2004; Watson, 2007).

REFERENCES

Barrett-Lennard, G. T. (1997). The recovery of empathy-Towards others and self. In A. Bohart & L. Greenberg (Eds.), *Empathy reconsidered: New directions in psychotherapy*. Washington, DC: American Psychological Association.

Bent, R. J., Putnam, D. G., & Kiesler, D. J. (1976). Correlates of successful and unsuccessful psychotherapy. *Journal of Consulting and Clinical Psychology*, *44*, 149–154.

Bohart, A., Elliott, R., Greenberg, L. S., & Watson, J. C. (2002). Empathy redux. In J. Norcross & M. Lambert (Eds.), *Psychotherapy relationships that work*. Oxford, UK: Oxford University Press.

Bohart, A. C. (1991). Empathy in client-centered therapy: A contrast with psychoanalysis and self psychology. *Journal of Humanistic Psychology*, *31*(1), 34–48.

Bojic Ognjenovic, O., & Watson, J. C. (2002, June). *A qualitative analysis of therapists thought processes of therapists in cognitive-behavioural and process–experiential therapy working with depressed clients*. Paper presented at the 32nd annual meeting of the International Society for Psychotherapy Research Conference, Santa Barbara, CA.

Bordin, E. S. (1979). The generalizability of the psychoanalytic concept of the working alliance. *Psychotherapy*, *16*, 252–260.

Bozarth, J. (1990). The essence of person-centered therapy. In G. Lietaer, J. Rombauts, & R. Van Balen (Eds.), *Person-centered and experiential psychotherapy in the nineties*. Leuwen, Belgium: Leuwen University Press.

Bozarth, J (2001). Unconditional positive regard. In J. Bozarth & P. Wilkens (Eds.), *Unconditional positive regard* (pp. 173–179). London: PCCS Books.

Brodley, B. (1990). Person-centered and experiential: Two different therapies. In G. Lietaer, J. Rombauts, & R. Van Balen (Eds.), *Person-centered and experiential psychotherapy in the nineties*. Leuwen, Belgium: Leuwen University Press.

Cain, D. (2001). Defining characteristics, history, and evolution of humanistic psychotherapies. In D. J. Cain & J. Seeman (Eds.), *Humanistic psychotherapies:*

Handbook of research and practice (pp. 3–54). Washington, DC: American Psychological Association.

Cooper, M. (2008). Existential psychotherapy. In J. L. Lebow (Ed.), *Twenty-first century psychotherapies: Contemporary approaches to theory and practice.* London: Wiley.

Eames, V., & Roth, A. (2000). Patient attachment orientation and the early working alliance: A study of patient and therapist reports of alliance quality and ruptures. *Psychotherapy Research, 10*(4), 421–434.

Eckert, J., & Biermann-Ratjen, E. (1998). The treatment of borderline personality disorder. In L. Greenberg, J. Watson, & G. Lietaer (Eds.), *The handbook of experiential psychotherapy* (pp. 349–366). New York: Guilford Press.

Elliott, R., Watson, J. C., Goldman, R. N., & Greenberg, L. S. (2004). *Learning emotion-focused therapy. The process–experiential approach to change.* Washington, DC: American Psychological Association.

Freire, E. (2001). Unconditional positive regard: The distinctive feature of client-centered therapy. In J. Bozarth & P. Wilkens (Eds.), *Unconditional positive regard* (pp. 145–155). London: PCCS Books.

Geller, S. M., & Greenberg, L. S. (2002). Therapeutic presence: Therapists' experience of presence in the psychotherapeutic encounter. *Person-centered and Experiential Psychotherapies, 1,* 71–86.

Gendlin, E. (1981). *Focusing.* New York: Bantam Books.

Gendlin, E. (1996). *Focusing-oriented psychotherapy: A manual of the experiential method.* New York: Guilford Press.

Grafanaki, S., & McLeod, J. (2002). Refinement and expansion of the concept of experiential congruence: A qualitative analysis of client counsellor narrative accounts of significant events in time-limited person-centered therapy. *Counselling and Psychotherapy Research, 2*(1), 20–33.

Greenberg, L. S., Rice, L. N., & Elliott, R. (1993). *Facilitating emotional change: The moment by moment process.* New York: Guilford Press.

Greenberg, L. S., Watson, J. C., Elliot, R., & Bohart, A. C. (2001). Empathy. *Psychotherapy: Theory, Research, Practice, Training, 38*(4), 380–384.

Greenberg, L. S., & Webster, M. C. (1982). Resolving decisional conflict by Gestalt two-chair dialogue: Relating process to outcome. *Journal of Counseling Psychology, 29,* 468–477.

Gurman, A. S. (1977). The patient's perception of the therapeutic relationship. In A. S. Gurman & A. M. Razin (Eds.), *Effective psychotherapy: A handbook of research.* New York: Pergammon Press.

Henry, W., Schacht, T. E., & Strupp, H. (1990). Patient and therapist introject, interpersonal process, and differential psychotherapy outcome. *Journal of Consulting and Clinical Psychology, 58,* 768–774.

Henry, W., & Strupp, H. (1994). Therapeutic alliance as interpersonal process. In A. Horvath & L. Greenberg (Eds.), *The Working Alliance: Theory, research and practice.* New York: Wiley.

Horvath, A. O., & Symonds, B. D. (1991). Relation between working alliance and outcome in psychotherapy: A meta-analysis. *Journal of Counseling Psychology, 38,* 139–149.

Justitz, S. E. (2002). The implications of adult attachment, the self-model attachment dimension, and the other-model attachment dimension on the formation of the therapeutic alliance and counseling satisfaction. *Dissertation Abstracts International Section A: Humanities and Social Sciences, 63*(6-A), 2145.

Kivlighan, D. M. J., Patton, M. J., & Foote, D. (1998). Moderating effects of client attachment on the counselor experience–working alliance relationship. *Journal of Counseling Psychology, 45*(3), 274–278.

Kwan, K., Watson, J. C., & Stermac, L. (2000, June). *An examination of the relationship between clients' social experience of psychotherapy, the working alliance and psychotherapy outcome.* Paper presented to the 31st annual meeting of the Society for Psychotherapy Research Conference, Chicago.

Leijssen, M. (1990). On focusing and the necessary conditions of therapeutic personality change. In G. Lietaer, J. Rombauts, & R. Van Balen (Eds.), *Person-centered and experiential psychotherapy in the nineties.* Leuwen, Belgium: Leuwen University Press.

Lietaer, G. (1974, June). *The relationship as experienced by clients and therapist in client-centered and psychoanalytically oriented therapy.* Paper presented at the 5th annual meeting of the Society for Psychotherapy Research, Denver.

Lietaer, G. (1992). Helpful and hindering processes in client-centered/experiential psychotherapy: A content analysis of client and therapist posttherapy perceptions. In S. Toukmanian & D. Rennie (Eds.), *Psychotherapy process research: Paradigmatic and narrative approaches* (pp. 134–162). Newbury Park, CA: Sage.

Lietaer, G. (1993). Authenticity, congruence, and transparency. In D. Brazier (Ed.), *Beyond Carl Rogers: Towards a psychotherapy for the twenty-first century* (pp. 17–47). London: Constable.

Lorr, M. (1965). Client perceptions of therapists: A study of therapeutic relation. *Journal of Consulting Psychology, 29*, 146–149.

Martin, D. J., Garske, J. P., & Davis, M. K. (2000). Relation of the therapeutic alliance with outcome and other variables: A meta-analytic review. *Journal of Consulting and Clinical Psychology, 68*(3), 438–450.

McMullen, E., & Watson, J. C. (2005). An examination of therapist and client behaviour in high and low alliance sessions in cognitive-behavioural therapy and process experiential therapy. *Psychotherapy: Theory, Research and Practice, 42*(3), 297–310.

Mearns, D., & Cooper, M. (2005). *Working at relational depth in counselling and psychotherapy.* London: Sage.

Mikulincer, M., & Nachshon, O. (1991). Attachment styles and patterns of self-disclosure. *Journal of Personality and Social Psychology, 61*(2), 321–331.

Najavits, L. M., & Strupp, H. H. (1994). Differences in the effectiveness of psychodynamic therapists: A process-outcome study. *Psychotherapy, 31*(1), 114–123.

Norcross, J. C. (2002). *Psychotherapy relationships that work: Therapists' contributions and responsiveness to patients.* New York: Oxford University Press.

Parish, M., & Eagle, M. N. (2003). Attachment to the therapist. *Psychoanalytic Psychology, 20*(2), 271–286.

Pistole, M. C. (1993). Attachment relationships: Self-disclosure and trust. *Journal of Mental Health Counseling, 15*(1), 94–106.

Reis, S., & Grenyer, B. F. S. (2004). Fearful attachment, working alliance and treatment response for individuals with major depression. *Clinical Psychology and Psychotherapy, 11*(6), 414–424.

Rennie, D. (1994). Clients' deference in psychotherapy. *Journal of Counseling Psychology, 41*, 427–437.

Rice, L. N. (1983). The relationship in client-centered therapy. In M. J. Lambert (Ed.), *Psychotherapy and patient relationships* (pp. 36–60). Homewood, IL: Dow-Jones Irwin.

Rice, L. N., & Greenberg, L. S. (Eds.). (1984). *Patterns of change: Intensive analysis of psychotherapy process.* New York: Guilford Press.

Rice, L. N., & Saperia, E. (1984). Task analysis of the resolution of problematic reactions. In L. N. Rice & L. S. Greenberg (Eds.), *Patterns of change: Intensive analysis of psychotherapy process* (pp. 29–66). New York: Guilford Press.

Rogers, C. R. (1951). *Client-centered therapy.* Boston: Houghton Mifflin.

Rogers, C. R. (1961). *On becoming a person.* Boston: Houghton Mifflin.

Rogers, C. R. (1967). The necessary and sufficient conditions of therapeutic personality change. *Journal of Consulting Psychology, 21*, 97–103.

Rogers, C. R. (1975). Empathic: An unappreciated way of being. *The Counseling Psychologist, 5*(2), 2–10.

Safran, J., & Muran, C. (1998). *The therapeutic alliance in brief psychotherapy.* New York: Guilford Press.

Safran, J. D., Muran, J. C., & Samstag, L. W. (1994). Resolving therapeutic alliance ruptures: A task analytic investigation. In A. O. Horvath & L. S. Greenberg (Eds.), *The Working Alliance: Theory, Research, and Practice* (pp. 225–255). Oxford, UK: Wiley.

Satterfield, W. A., & Lyddon, W. J. (1995). Client attachment and perceptions of the working alliance with counselor trainees. *Journal of Counseling Psychology, 42*(2), 187–189.

Satterfield, W. A., & Lyddon, W. J. (1998). Client attachment and the working alliance. *Counselling Psychology Quarterly, 11*(4), 407–415.

Vanaerschot, G. (1990). The process of empathy: Holding and letting go. In G. Lietaer, G. Rombauts, & R. Van Balen (Eds.), *Client-centered and experiential psychotherapy in the nineties* (pp. 269–294). Leuven, Belguim: Leuven University Press.

Watson, J. C. (2001). Revisioning empathy: Theory, research and practice. In D. Cain & J. Seeman (Eds.), *Handbook of research and practice in humanistic psychotherapies* (pp. 445–473). Washington, DC: American Psychological Association.

Watson, J. C. (2007). Reassessing Rogers' necessary and sufficient conditions of change. *Psychotherapy: Theory, Research, Practice, Training, 44*(3), 268–273.

Watson, J. C., Enright, C., & Kalogerakos, F. (1998). *The impact of therapist variables in facilitating change.* Paper presented to the annual meeting of the Society for Psychotherapy Research, Snowbird, Utah.

Watson, J. C., & Geller, S. (2005). An examination of the relations among empathy, unconditional acceptance, positive regard and congruence in both cognitive-behavioral and process–experiential psychotherapy. *Psychotherapy Research, 15*(1–2), 25–33.

Watson, J. C., Goldman, R., & Greenberg, L. S. (2007). *Case-studies in the experi-*

ential treatment of depression: A comparison of good and bad outcome. Washington, DC: American Psychological Association.

Watson, J. C., & Greenberg, L. S. (1994). The alliance in experiential therapy: Enacting the relationship conditions. In A. Horvath & L. Greenberg (Eds.), *The working alliance: Theory, research and practice* (pp. 153–172). New York: Wiley.

Watson, J. C., & Greenberg, L. S. (2000). Alliance ruptures and repairs in experiential therapy. *Journal of Clinical Psychology, 56*(2), 175–186.

Watson, J. C., Greenberg, L. S., & Lietaer, G. (1998). The experiential paradigm unfolding: Relationship & experiencing in therapy. In L. S. Greenberg, J. C. Watson, & G. Lietaer (Eds.), *Handbook of experiential psychotherapy* (pp. 3–27). New York: Guilford Press.

Watson, J. C., & Rennie, D. (1994). A qualitative analysis of clients' reports of their subjective experience while exploring problematic reactions in therapy. *Journal of Counseling Psychology, 41*, 500–509.

Watson, J. C., & Steckley, P. (2001). Potentiating growth: An examination of the research on unconditional positive regard. In J. Bozarth & P Wilkens (Eds.), *Unconditional Positive regard*. London: PCCS Books.

Westerman, M. A., Tanaka, J. S., Frankel, A. S., & Khan, J. (1986). The coordinating style construct: An approach to conceptualizing patient interpersonal behaviour. *Psychotherapy, 23*, 540–547.

Wyatt, G. (2001). Introduction to the series. In *Rogers' therapeutic conditions: Evolution, theory, and practice* (pp. i–vi). Ross-on-Wye, UK: PCCS Books.

CHAPTER 11

■ ■ ■ ■ ■

Therapeutic Alliances in Couple Therapy

The Web of Relationships

Adam O. Horvath
Dianne Symonds
Luis Tapia

The topic of this chapter is the alliance in couple therapy. But, unlike the case in some of the previous chapters, couple therapy is not a unique theoretical domain or practice. Therapists who work with couples use a variety of theoretical frameworks. Most of the theories used by couple therapists, however, share a common historical root that is usually labeled "systems theory."[1] In order to present a coherent picture of the literature and to identify recommendations relevant to most practitioners, we rely on the systemic framework as a "common denominator" across the various branches of couple therapy practice. It is also important to note that couple and family therapy theories and practices evolved along closely parallel lines and share much of the empirical literature; authors often refer to couple and

---

[1]To make the nomenclature more confusing, some individual therapies are also labeled "systemic," and some couples and family therapies (e.g., behavioral and Adlerian treatments) are not "systemic." Nonetheless, in practice, "systemic" is the closest approximation to a collective label for the kinds of therapies we will be talking about.

family treatments as a hyphenated single entity (Sprenkle & Blow, 2004). The distinction between couple and family therapy is based on the practical fact that couple work usually involves only two clients while family therapy often (but not always) includes additional relatives attending the sessions. As a result of this practical difference, clients seeking couple therapy present a somewhat different and narrower range of problems, typically related to some aspect of the couple's relationship difficulties[2] (Shadish & Baldwin, 2005). In the review part of the chapter we focus as narrowly as practicable on research based on couples, but in many cases the lines between couple and family therapy are blurred, and in some instances we use findings based on research on family therapy and/or studies where more than one form of treatment was implemented.

THE HISTORY OF THE ALLIANCE CONCEPT IN COUPLE THERAPY

The first thing one notes in looking through the literature on the alliance in couple therapy (CT) is the discrepancy between the large volume of rich material available that is related to individual therapy, dating back several decades, and the much smaller and more recent material on the topic in the area of couple or family therapy. Almost all of theoretical work and the lion's share of the available empirical research on the alliance relates to individual therapy. Using "alliance" as a keyword, a search of English language databases yields well over 6,000 titles, but only a minuscule fraction of these deal with multiclient treatments. Our current estimate of the available empirical data on the alliance in couple therapy is less than 50 independent data sets, including qualitative investigations, theses, dissertations, and conceptual articles based on research evidence (Horvath, 2009).

In previous reviews of the literature several authors have noted that for the first 30 years of couple and family therapy there was a bias against focusing on the relationship between therapists and clients in therapy (Coyne & Pepper, 1998; Flaskas, 2004). A close examination of the literature reveals an interesting tension: on the one side, we see a great deal of abstract theorizing about the unpredictability of outcome that results from engagement with a complex system such as families (e.g., Keeney, 1981; Selvini, Boscolo, Checcin, & Prata, 1980), and a different group voices concern about becoming entangled with clients' pathogenic interactions (e.g., Boszormenyi-Nagy & Spark, 1973; Bowen, 1978). What united these two groups was their exclusive focus on clients' relational processes with the

---

[2]Marital therapy or conjoint therapy are also used as synonyms for couple therapy.

ideal facilitator seen as relationally independent of the therapy dynamic. On the Bowenian side this construct was formalized as resisting triangulation (Kerr & Bowen, 1988), and the strategic and Milan schools recommended physically removing influential therapists from face-to-face interaction with clients by staying behind the screen as the consulting team of "experts."

On the "other side of the fence," in contrast to this kind of thinking, there were a number of equally significant early figures in couple or family therapy who prized and promoted the relatedness between therapists and clients. For example Whitaker and Bumberry (1988) argued for engagement—"dancing"—with the client to make connections between both the healthy and unconscious "crazy" aspect of therapists and clients. Virginia Satir (1967) developed a highly dramatic physical method of exploring connections and tensions between everyone in the therapy room, and made these intertwined living "sculptures" the focus of her work with couples. Minuchin used the term "joining" to describe the necessity of creating a "common cause" before therapy could start. His method of therapy was centered on using his own relationship with each client to reconfigure the existing problematic connections and hierarchies. He called this technique "unbalancing":

> [It] refers to the therapist's use of himself as a member of the therapeutic system to disequilibriate the family organization, [and] he does so by joining and supporting an individual or family subsystem at the expense of other family members. This affiliation modifies the accustomed hierarchical organization of the family introducing the possibility of new alternatives. (Minuchin, 1985)

Looking back over these two seemingly opposing historical positions, it seems evident that in the first 30 years of couple and family therapy there was a serious debate about, rather than a simple bias against, the relationship in therapy. During those years systemic therapies were in a period of vigorous theory development and diversification. In contrast, the major schools of individual treatments were more fully developed, and attention shifted from championing different theoretical orientations to locating the efficacious elements shared among different types of treatments. Interest in the alliance in couple therapy came to the fore after a period of significant reevaluation of the strong emphasis on the executive function of the therapist in systemic theories (Anderson & Goolishian, 1988). In this second "mature phase" of theorising, influenced in part by feminist critiques and narrative theories, the role of the therapist as an "expert" was replaced by a more collaborative perspective on therapy (White, 2007).

The alliance concept was introduced into the "conversation" about couple therapy by the pioneering work of Pinsof and his colleagues, who developed the first measure of alliance specifically designed for couple and family treatment, the Couple Alliance Scale (CAS; Pinsof & Catherall, 1984). The conceptualization of the alliance instantiated in this instrument blended some of the concepts of alliance from individual therapy with the role and function of the relationship in systemic therapy. In constructing the CAS, important new relational dynamics had to be added to the individual model of the alliance. It became evident that clients, in addition to having their own perception of the qualities of the alliance with the therapist, were influenced by their "guesses" of the quality and strength of the partners' relation with the therapist. This dimension, which we will refer to as "inferred" (as opposed to "direct" self-reported) alliance, adds a new vector and level of complexity to the structure of the alliance that is unique to couple and family therapy.

Pinsof (Pinsof & Catherall, 1984) also introduced the idea that in a "saturated" model of the alliance in couple therapy we need to take into account not only the various strands of alliances between each client and the therapist but, in addition, the alliance between the therapist and the "clients-as-a-couple." The client-as-a-couple is a systemic concept that has been used as a way of underscoring the idea that the couple is more than the sum of its individual parts. The couple "as such," distinct from each individual, functions as a unit and has relationships with "others" as a "we" in important and meaningful ways—legally, socially, and emotionally. This collectivity with its unique relationship qualities needs to be integrated with the individual relationships when we think of the therapeutic alliance in couple therapy (Rait, 2000).

The multiplicity of relational dynamics also raised the important issue of relational (im)balances. That is, the possibility that some of the alliances might be quantitatively stronger and/or qualitatively different than other alliances. Most theorists hypothesized that unbalanced or "split" alliances within the system would have a negative impact on therapy outcome (Glickauf-Hughes & Mehlman, 1994; Pinsof & Catherall, 1984; Pinsof, Wynne, & Hambright, 1996), but others, notably Minuchin (1951), have speculated that temporarily unbalancing the relationships among the participants, "siding" with one member or the other, might dislodge the couple's recursive negative relational cycles and thus have a positive effect on the success of therapy.

While the motivation and the interest that lead to theorizing about the relationship are historically quite different in individual and couple therapies, the interaction of the two perspectives was synergistic and generative. As a result of fitting the elements of the alliance theory to a multiperson therapy framework, existing systemic models of the therapist–client relationship gained additional "layers." For couple therapists, this process has created windows of opportunities to re-search their ideas of treating couples: it opened the opportunity to consider interactively the couple relationship within the framework of the therapist relation to the clients. This relation-within-relation model also created challenging complexities. Although the available empirical data are small in volume and the methodologies are still very much "under construction," examination of the alliance in systemic therapies has yielded some challenging questions and has offered some tantalizing leads.

RESEARCH ON ALLIANCE IN COUPLE THERAPY

Outcome and Alliance

Following on the research reports based on individual therapy, a number of investigators have examined the relation between alliance and outcome in couple and family therapy. Over all, there appears to be a reliable positive association between alliance and outcome, but the effect size of these relations is generally lower than those reported by individual treatments (Coupland & Serovich, 1999; Hight, 1998; Johnson, 1985; Robbins et al., 2008; Symonds & Horvath, 2004). There appear to be a number of possible reasons why this link between alliance and outcome is lower in multiperson treatments:

One likely cause is the complex and multidimensional nature of outcome in couple therapy: therapy success can be measured from the perspective of change in each of the individuals involved or, alternately, the change in couple functioning. From the couple's functioning perspective one can examine such outcomes as: How well are the partners getting along together? Has the quality of their relationship improved? Has the couple stayed together? While an outcome that measures the couple's functioning is most often recommended (Garfield, 2004), there are situations when separation or divorce, on reasonable terms, may be the most desirable outcome. In these situations, improvement in the functioning of each individual is a more realistic measure. Unfortunately, whether individual or couple outcome is most appropriate becomes evident only during therapy, not before, but researchers have to make a priori decisions about how outcome will be evaluated. The data we reviewed included both types of outcome and in some research studies a combination of both types of measures. This complexity itself poses a problem since a portion of improvement in couples functioning may represent a different level of progress than the same change at an individual level. Additionally, whatever approach the researcher chooses, the data come from two individuals,[3] and in order to

---

[3]In theory it would be possible to collect data generated jointly by the couple, but what if they could not agree? In any case, we did not come across such data.

link outcome to process (alliance) the individuals' responses have to be summed in some fashion.

But there are serious conceptual problems with any method of summing such data. If one partner improves X and the other regresses $-X$, does it follow that the net effect of treatment was zero? Or, if one person reports no change, but the other is a +2, can we say that the therapy outcome is a +1? To make matters more challenging, it has been shown consistently that these two kinds of outcomes (individual change and couple functioning) respond differently to treatment and are not highly correlated (Hight, 1998; Knobloch-Fedders, Pinsof, & Mann, 2007; Shadish et al., 1993). Thus, it is likely that the variability of outcome reported in studies is diminished or "smoothed out" by these averaging procedures. It follows that research reports estimating the correlation between alliance and such "homogenized" outcomes will be attenuated by the information lost in the aggregating process and will likely underestimate the true magnitude of the relation.[4] The only outcome index immune to the aggregating problem is the criterion of staying in treatment versus dropping out or premature termination. Using this measure, the couple therapy research is quite consistent with, and closely parallels, results obtained in individual therapy; poor early alliance is a reliable predictor of noncompleters or dropouts (Knobloch-Fedders et al., 2007; Robbins, Turner, Alexander, & Perez, 2003).

To avoid the dilemma of summing outcomes, researchers tend to report the relation between alliance and change for male and female clients separately. These results have been a rich source of information that will be explored in more detail below, but they do not help to gauge the overall alliance–outcome link in couple therapy. This dilemma will remain a problem until we can overcome the challenge of summing the data.

The "panoramic" view of the relation between the strength of alliance in the early phase of couple therapy and outcome is similar to that found by researchers in individual therapy. It appears that a negotiated commitment to the goals of therapy, a committed belief in, and responsiveness, to the treatment procedures, combined with positive interpersonal attachments to the therapist are important prerequisites to staying in treatment and likely facilitative of longer-term success. The strength of these relations in terms of variance accounted for in outcome is modest in magnitude, but it appears to be consistently significant across studies (Beck, Friedlander, & Escudero, 2006; Butler & Strupp, 1986; Green & Herget, 1991; Jacobson, Schmaling, & Holtzworth-Munroe, 1987; White, Edwards, & Russell, 1997).

In individual therapy research there has been a shift away from deter-

---

[4]There are more sophisticated ways of dealing with outcome, particularly using multilevel hierarchical modeling, but the fact that the two outcome sources (the two partners) are not independent tends to create problems of interpretation.

mining the overall association between alliance and outcome to investigations focusing on the specific ways that alliance contributes to change. This trend includes such studies as those that measure the impact of alliance directly (Safran & Muran, 2000) and indirectly (Castonguay et al., 2004), untangling the therapists' and clients' unique contributions (Baldwin, Wampold, & Imel, 2007) and evaluating the effectiveness of training (Hilsenroth & Cromer, 2007) as well as the role of alliance in specific types of treatment/problem combinations (Raue, Castonguay, & Goldfried, 1993). The original work demonstrating the importance of the alliance in all forms of treatment has served to focus attention on the value of developing early relationships that result in a strong therapeutic alliance. However, these more recent investigations hold greater promise for generating knowledge that can be directly applied by clinicians to help their clients more effectively. This change in research focus is also beginning to occur in multiperson treatment contexts as well (Garfield, 2004; Knobloch-Fedders et al., 2007).

Split Alliances and Whose Alliance Matters

One of the earliest and most widely held hypotheses about the alliance in couple therapy was that if the couple's alliance were split—that is, one member of the couple had a better or stronger alliance with the therapist than the other, poor outcome would result. Most but not all researchers investigating split alliances found evidence that in treatments where the couples' alliance was balanced, the outcome was better than in cases with split alliances (Glickauf-Hughes, Wells, & Chance, 1996; Hight, 1998; Knobloch-Fedders et al., 2007; Mahaffey et al., 2008; Rait, 1995; Symonds & Horvath, 2004; Wolfson, 2007). But these findings are inconsistent in a number of respects. There are both qualitative and quantitative differences in how the "split" is defined, and the magnitude of the outcome differences are varied and not always statistically reliable. There are also studies that report no differences in outcome associated with splits (e.g., Bedi & Horvath, 2004; Delany, 2007). Interestingly, even in the same data set, the question "Do split alliance predict poor outcome?" yields different answers, depending on which outcome measure is privileged and whether it is measured soon after posttherapy or followed up (e.g., Horvath, 2005).

The anomalous results raise the possibility that we are getting these diverse answers because we are not asking the question the right way. It seems likely to us that the notion of the "split" needs to be approached in a more subtle, layered fashion. For instance: Does it matter which member of the couple is better aligned with the therapist? Does it make a difference if the balance of the alliance between the participants is improving as therapy progresses? What is more important in terms of a balanced alliance—that the partners themselves report similar alliances with the therapist or that there are differences in the alliance that each partner infers in relation to the other's alliance (i.e., the client thinks his or her alliance with the therapist is lesser or greater than the partner's)?

The Effects of Gender

One way to approach this question is to look for variables that could help us identify different alliance response patterns. There are indications that gender is likely one such variable. When working with individuals, the therapist is either the same gender as the client or not. However, in couple therapy there are three people in the room. The therapist is the same gender as one partner and the opposite of the other.[5] From the moment the clients walk into the therapy room, there is a gender imbalance. How this gender imbalance plays out in therapy has been examined by a number of researchers. They have generally found that men and women respond to alliance imbalances differently. However, there is no consensus about whose alliance is more instrumental in determining the outcome of therapy. Two studies found that men's strength of the alliance was a better predictor of outcome than women's (Bourgeois, Sabourin, & Wright, 1990; Brown, 1998). In another study, Horvath and Symonds (2004) found that when men's alliances were stronger than their partner's, therapy was much more likely to be successful. Similarly, Knobloch-Fedders et al. (2007) reported that "when men's alliances with the therapist are stronger than their partners' at session 6, couples show significantly more improvement in relationship distress" (p. 255). However, Quinn, Dotson, and Jordan (1997) found that when the wife reported a stronger alliance therapy tended to be more successful.

Werner-Wilson and colleagues (1997) concluded that both therapist and client gender had significant impact on the Bond component of the alliance (female therapist and clients score higher). But, in a different study, they found that female clients were more likely to be interrupted by the therapist (Werner-Wilson, Michaels, Thomas, & Thiesen, 2003; Werner-Wilson, Price, Zimmerman, & Murphy, 1997).[6] However, Delaney (2007) found no substantial differences in outcome for either men or women when the quality of their alliances differed. In the face of these diverse findings, we have looked for other explanations to account for different outcomes.

Some of these differences may be due to the variety of ways that researchers have operationalized the imbalance between the genders. For

---

[5]This statement is true only for heterosexual couples; however, we were not able to locate data on couple therapy with nontraditional couples.

[6]In these studies individual alliance measures were used.

example, Symonds and Horvath (2004) divided the data into two groups; those couples for whom either the women's or men's alliances were stronger than their partners. Quinn et al. (1997) computed a difference score by subtracting the men's alliance scores form the women's and correlated outcome with the difference score. Some studies used alliance subscales, others total test scores.

We agree with Garfield (2004), who suggested that gender should be included as a variable in couple therapy studies since it may play a significant role in how the alliance functions. But the lack of convergence of these studies suggests caution in interpreting these early findings and call attention to the importance of a greater level of standardization of instruments and methods to determine splits, reinforcing the need for some agreement among researchers about the methods used in couple therapy research (Christensen, Baucom, Vu, & Stanton, 2005; Heatherington, Friedlander, & Greenberg, 2005).

Perhaps more clinically relevant and useful information may be found if we approach these issues from a broader perspective. For instance, instead of alliances simply being "split" (or not), we need to examine different layers of the relational balances and investigate how these interact and relate to therapy process. Rather than thinking of the balance in the alliance as a static variable (split/intact), it is more useful to consider the role of the relational dynamic as it shifts continuously over time? It also seems evident that the status of the relational equilibrium depends on which partner's perspective we are evaluating from.

Differing Perspectives on the Alliance

The most comprehensive way to look at alliance balance is to take into account the direct and inferred perspectives together. From this vantage point, one can examine the balance between the partners' direct scales (i.e., the traditional contrast between "intact" and "split" alliances), the relative strength of the client's direct scale in comparison to the inferred status of the partner, and the degree of correspondence between the partners' inferred scales (i.e., each partner's "insight" about the other's alliance).

Symonds (1999) looked at this last layer of analysis. In this study, only between 10 and 27% of the variance in one partner's score was accounted for by the other's score. This finding suggests that couples who come in for therapy are not very good judges of their partner's alliance. (Symonds found that therapists were even less accurate in gauging the clients' self rated alliance.) But, how does this level of disagreement on the alliance impact the alliance and success of therapy? Consider what might happen in therapy if the male partner's appraisal of his wife's alliance does not match her own appraisal. He is then operating under a misconception that both he and his partner agree about the utility of the therapy tasks and goals. But it is also important to recognize that he is unaware that his partner's judgment of the alliance is different! We found that the more the partners misjudged the other's comfort with and trust of the therapist (bond scale) in the beginning of therapy, the less they experienced relief in the severity of the problem that brought them into therapy (Horvath, 2009).

The consequence of clients being in a "one-up" position (i.e., his or her alliance with the therapist is better than the partner's), equal, or "one-down" state was also examined. The best outcome was associated with clients whose alliance was balanced (within 1 standard deviation). In those cases where the alliance was unbalanced, both males and females made more *individual gains* at the end of treatment if their rating of their own alliance (direct) was higher than their judgment of their partner's alliance (inferred scale) (Horvath, 2005). Interestingly, when this question was examined by using data from the same group of clients but the outcome was based on couple-level gains, no statistically reliable differences were reported among the three groups (Bedi & Horvath, 2004). These results make sense if one considers the two possible "good outcomes" in couple therapy; either the partner's relationship becomes healthier, or the partners choose to disengage but function better as individuals. Clearly the "balanced" situation is best for either outcome, but we have speculated that when the partners were working out ways to be independent, there were more competition or anger issues to work through during the early phase, and thus feeling more connected to the therapist than their partner was facilitative to the process.

Alliance over Time

Perhaps the important issue in couple therapy is not whether the couple's alliance is "balanced" at a particular point in time but rather whether the alliance is moving toward equilibrium as therapy progresses. After all, the majority of couples who seek therapy are likely to disagree on relational matters and, at the start, often try to gain the support of the therapist (Kerr & Sholevar, 2003). As noted by Rampage, Gurman, and Jacobson (2002), "Each partner may feel concern that the therapist is more interested in what the other partner has to say, or believes that the other partner's position is more valid" (p. 536). Such "jockeying for approval" likely creates tensions and imbalances, particularly during the early phase of treatment. Perhaps the therapist's ability to move the couple closer to a balanced alliance position is a more important indicator of better outcome and thus a more relevant index of the role of the alliance in couple therapy? In one investigation couples were divided into three groups: those whose self-rated alliance became more divergent, those whose alliance remained the same, and those whose self-rated alliance with the therapist became more balanced over time. If the male and female partners' quality-of-marriage scores were averaged, there were no significant differences among the three groups. However, when the male and female scores were examined separately, statistically reliable differences emerged. For both males and females, having no change in alliance strength was associated with poor outcome. In the group that moved toward closer agreement with their partners, the male clients felt better about the marriage. However, females felt the marriage was better at the end of treatment if their judgment of the therapeutic alliance became more independent of their partner's (Horvath, 2005). We hypothesized that the no-change group represented a lack of therapeutic movement. The difference between male and female patterns may be attributable to the fact that in these data (as in most other reports) females initiated therapy and started off with stronger alliances than their partners. The male partners' increase in alliance was responsible for the "improving" group. It makes sense that these men also experienced benefit from the therapy. It may be the case that once therapy progressed females unburdened themselves of the responsibility of "holding things together" in therapy.

Alliance in Later Stages of Couple Therapy

Much of what is known about the alliance is gleaned from research focusing on the early phases of treatment. Symonds (1999) explored the relation of alliance measured after the first session to measurements obtained in mid-treatment of a time-limited brief couple therapy treatment. The results indicated that for both male and female clients these alliance scores were correlated in the moderate range ($r \leq .5$). However, the Bond subscales were most highly correlated for both partners (i.e., clients stuck close to their initial judgments), and females' alliance ratings changed somewhat more than males. Interestingly, the correlation between couple-level outcome and alliance increased only slightly over time. Horvath (2002) investigated these patterns by using data in which both clients rated the same aspect of alliance (us-as-a-couple with the therapist). He found that a large proportion ($> 50\%$) of the total variance in outcome accounted for by alliance was associated with the first Session alliance scores, but the first and third session scores "predicted" *different* aspects of couple-level outcome). This pattern is consistent with the possibility that the bond (i.e., interpersonal) aspect of the alliance that develops early and remains quite stable and the task and goal aspects of the alliance relate to *different types* of therapy achievements.

Therapist Effect

A few investigations have explored therapist qualities or actions that could impact the development or maintenance of the alliance in couple therapy.

These findings are somewhat inconsistent. The commonsense wisdom in the couple literature suggests that the quality of the therapist (as contrasted to the kind of therapy) is a determining influence in the successful development of the alliance (Sexton, 2007). Interestingly, the available empirical research has not yet fully justified this claim. One study found that more experienced therapists developed better alliances and had fewer negative episodes than predoctoral practicum students (Raytek, McCrady, Epstein, & Hirsch, 1999). But another investigator found no relation between alliance level and training, instead, the age of the therapist was the better predictor of alliance levels (Wilkens, 1999).

Client Factors

The clients' early history of relationships (i.e., significant family of origin issues; Garfield, 2004) and type of psychopathology, for example, paranoia (Height, 1998) have been documented to impact the quality of the alliance in small-scale studies but these findings have not been confirmed by subsequent investigators.

Therapy Effects

In individual treatments the type of therapy does not appear to influence the relation between alliance and outcome (Horvath & Bedi, 2002; Horvath & Symonds, 1991; Martin, Garske, & Davis, 2000). There are no empirical data addressing this question in systemic therapies, but there have been suggestions that more collaborative approaches to couple therapy would produce stronger alliances (Sprenkle & Blow, 2004). However, one study concluded that providing advice and a more confrontational style might be conducive to better alliances. The same group of researchers also found that therapists with a feminist orientation developed better alliances with male but not with female clients (Werner-Wilson et al., 2003; Werner-Wilson, Zimmerman, Daniels, & Bowling, 1999).

Conclusions

What can we conclude from the available research on alliance in couple therapy? The evidence with respect to the importance of the development of an alliance—preferably early in treatment—is clear: the quality of collaborative alliance with the therapist is positively linked to outcome. Beyond this level of analysis, the research evidence speaks in "many voices." This state of affairs is likely due to a combination of methodological inconsistencies in the field and the complex web-like nature of the relationships in couple therapy.

From a methodological perspective, it is important to note that researchers have taken a variety of approaches to instrumentally define the alliance in couple therapy. The particular measure chosen by the researcher, in effect, uniquely defines what the alliance is and is not. The range of instruments and consequent instrumental definitions currently used in the couple literature includes some instruments that are based on an explicit theoretical framework (e.g., Bordin's definition in Catheral & Pinsof, 1984; CTAS scales and the WAI-Co in Symonds & Horvath, 2004). Other measures, for example de Roten and colleagues, locate the alliance in coordinated nonverbal interactions (de Roten, Fivaz-Depeursinge, Stern, Darwish, & Corboz-Warnery, 2000; Friedlander et al., 2006). Friedlander and her group (2006) the other hand, include such variables as Safety in addition to the more traditional elements associated with the alliance framework.

Another important methodological difference among researchers is that some assessment procedures assess only dyadic relations within couple therapy (i.e., the relation between the therapist and each of the two clients individually) while other instruments provide additional information about the therapist's alliance with the couple system from each participant's perspective. In addition, some instruments measure all of these different alliance dimensions, both from the direct and the inferred perspectives. Yet other researchers use instruments made for assessing alliance in individual therapy and administer these measures to each participant in therapy (Raytek et al., 1999; Robbins et al., 2003; Werner-Wilson et al., 2003) or use assessment devices made for the occasion (Werner-Wilson et al., 1999).

On one hand, the eclectic ways the concept of the alliance has been interpreted and measured in the research community has had the positive effect of broadening our conceptual horizon of this aspect of the relationship in therapy. A rich set of variables have been identified that may influence, or are important constitutive elements of, the process and outcome of treatment. On the other hand, extrapolating the alliance from the core concept of collaboration and broadly equating it with many elements beyond the "classical" conception of the alliance creates some confusion and difficulty when we try to move from research to clinical practice (Horvath, in press). If clinical practice is to benefit from the research findings, we need to have some clarity of what the alliance is and is not. Without some consensus about the boundaries of this concept, we cannot discover what the alliance is "made of." As a consequence, we don't know what kinds of therapist practices may help to strengthen it, nor are we able to fully understand how we can use it to achieve particular goals in therapy.

The second important issue is the fact that adding one more person to the therapy environment does not simply add one more (bidirectional) relationship to the mix. In addition to the second client's relation to the therapist, there is the relationship between the clients-as-a-couple and the therapist; there are the following factors: the relation and possible tension, between each client's alliance with the therapist and his or her allegiance to the partner; the influence of each client's estimate of the quality of the partners' alliance in relation to his or her own. There is also a new dimension in the relational matrix, a same-gender and a different-gender therapist–client relationship; the issue that there are likely power and motivational differences between the clients; and last but not least, the impact of the fact that the clients bring their own troubled relationship into the therapy room, both as a target for change and as a dynamic that is played out in "real time" in the therapy discourse. We therefore see the alliance in systemic therapies in general, and in couple therapy in particular, as an emerging quality of collaboration in relation to the necessary accomplishments (such as goals and tasks) of therapy. This arises from and is built upon a web of interacting relational dynamics, the main elements or "nodes" of which are listed above.

STEPS TO BUILDING
THE ALLIANCE IN COUPLE THERAPY

To explore the important challenges in developing an alliance in a couple therapy context, we start by examining segments of transcripts taken from the same first session of a time-limited couple therapy. While each couple presents unique challenges and opportunities in building an alliance, we feel that this transcript provides us with an opportunity to have an *in situ* view of some of the common features of the beginning of the alliance-building process.

The participants in this first session are the therapist (T) and clients Kale (K, male), and Bess (B, female).

Couple #10 Time 00:00–03:30 (approximate)

1 T: now the only information I have about you is that um you have seen [name of the therapist] sometime in the (past)

2 K: for ten sessions

3 T: ten sessions

4 B: uh huh ... about six

5 T: so there's been a therapist before me

6 K: right

7 T: so it's somewhere between six and ten, right

8 K: yeah around there, I guess [... date]

9 T: okay, and that was um some time ago

10 T: okay ... well [in] this [service] you may have been given a little bit of information about it ... I just want to take some time during this first session just talk a bit about ... uh the housekeeping items; give you the opportunity to ask *any* questions you want of me ... set some guidelines ... get to know a little bit about who you are ... those kinds of things ...

11 K: so are you're gonna be the person we're gonna be dealing with for the next little while here?

12 T: yup, and you're gonna be the people that I'm gonna be dealing with for the next little while ...

13 K: okay

14 T: I take lots of notes during the session. The notes I take are guided by the problems and solutions that you bring in here and like the language you use (*cough*) excuse me ... So what I would do is I would write down information that you give me ...

15 K: uh-huh

16 T: you can see those notes at anytime at all ... We're here to sort of get an understanding about what's going on, we're not making a diagnosis ... I think that's about it ... I just want to make sure I covered everything

17 T: oh there was one other item; the fact of the matter is that in this room there are two men and one woman and uh ... I try to be sensitive to that as much as possible

18 T: I don't know what it's like to be a woman in a relationship. I don't know what its like to grow up as a girl in the family, I just have my own experiences as a boy ...

19 T: how sensitive I can be to that I suppose its up to you to judge ... if I'm missing things about what it means to be a woman in the relationship ... and equally if I'm missing things about what it is to be a man in a relationship that are important um ... I sure hope that you would find a way to express that to me ... and I think it would be different if there was a woman here right um, so that's just an ... the issue about gender that I just wanted to bring up.

20 T: now do you have any questions you'd like to ask of me?

21 K: not particularly

22 T: and you've been in counselling before so you have an experience about what you're like and telling (people) what its like for you … as I said we only have six sessions so its probably a pretty good idea to be kinda specific about what we want to do in this time …

In the opening exchanges (1–22) the therapist is making some specific moves to develop a collaborative relationship: Right at the beginning, he makes explicit references to his intention to work together with the clients: For example, in exchange 10 he starts by inviting the clients to ask questions of him. Following this, in the exchange 11–12, he creates a verbal metaphor to frame the kind of reciprocity (i.e., two-sidedness of the therapeutic contract) he is seeking to establish. Although not explicitly stated "as such," the close symmetry in content and shape of his response to Kale's comment models his intention to seek a mutually interactive rather than "therapist as expert" relational context in the therapy. In exchanges 13–15 he reinforces this idea by being explicit about what his role is (#14), and he uses "you" three times in this sequence to indicate that he is responding to and guided by the clients' needs and language. In the next statement (#16), the therapist is indicating a willingness to share his notes. The clear implication of positioning himself as someone who does not make exclusive judgments and claims no special privileges for his notes is that the rights and responsibilities of therapy will be matters of negotiation and agreement. A further relational consequence is the implied invitation for the clients to be reciprocally transparent and open to negotiating active roles in the therapy process.

In exchanges #17–19 the therapist broaches the issue of gender imbalance that is endemic to every couple therapy situation. He (and we) do not yet know if this is a concern for the client, but if this *is* a matter of some concern to the female client, the therapist indicates that he is willing to have his "inexperience" supplemented by the client's. We think that a frank discussion of the therapist's limits and boundaries has the potential to legitimize the open discussion of issues concerning the differences between himself and the female client. Also, by extension, it opens the door for each client to discuss other inequalities affecting the couple in and outside the therapy situation.

It is interesting to note that in exchange #19 the therapist first recognizes the female client's unique position, and later in the same monologue he brings to the fore the less obvious matter that there may be experiences of the male client that are also outside his (therapist's) horizon. This sequence illustrates that there are relational moves that can only be accomplished in "sequence," and the choice of the ordering—that is, whose concern is recognized first—is likely to have subtle but important consequences. From the perspective of attending to the relational balances in therapy, not only between himself and each client but also between the partners, the order in which he recognizes the unique needs of each is not arbitrary; as the session unfolds, we will see that paying attention to the female partner's position first makes logical sense.

The last therapist statement in the sequence (#22) lays the groundwork for three relationally relevant issues. First, it orients the clients toward the task of developing consensual goals. Second, it recognizes their expertise; using the phrase "you've been in counseling before" and the word "specific" makes it likely that if the clients have different expectations these will emerge to be worked on. Finally, using the collective "we" in the sentence defines the task as a shared responsibility by everyone in the room.

Summary Reflections on the Opening Sequences

Beginning with the first sentence the therapist utters, he or she is building a relational structure for the treatment. He has an opportunity to define this structure primarily through the way he positions himself in relation to the clients, the process of therapy, and the problem the couple identifies. The excerpt shows the importance of the kind of language we use in positioning the therapist's self-in-action. We not only identify who we are as therapists but also indicate the level of collaboration, the kind of alliance we seek, by the topics we show interest in, the issues we are sensitive to, and the choices we make in paying attention to each client. Even without knowing the degree to which this therapist succeeded in developing a strong alliance, it is clear that the clients got a strong message of the kind of therapeutic collaboration he was seeking.

At a different conceptual level, we see in this first 3½ minutes of conversation a short but interesting illustration of the complementarity of relationship and intervention captured by the alliance concept. If we were to analyze this segment narrowly in terms of the therapist's intervention, legitimizing discussion of, and creating space for, the issue of male–female differences would be recognized as a useful *technique* in couple therapy; that is, these issues are likely relevant to the problems the couple is trying to resolve. Viewed from the relationship perspective, the therapist is demonstrating empathy with the female client's position and genuineness by making himself available to better understand and appreciate her experience. The alliance perspective integrates this duality and captures the synergy of these elements. The resultant democratic framework positions the therapist and the clients to work interactively and collaboratively to achieve their common goals for the therapy.

Time 07:00–07:30 (approximate)[7]

23 T: okay now um if … I was just curious about … how you see yourself in terms of your own … people have a difficult time … all [clients] have difficulty [answering] this question maybe you won't … how you see yourself in terms of your own particular qualities and skills and competencies um … I ask that question 'cause sometimes c-couples come into counselling what the focus is … is always on the problem and I'm just wondering I want to take you away from that for a moment … and we will get to that eventually. I I'm just curious about um … uhh how you see yourself in terms of your—as I said—qualities and skills and uh … competencies

24 B: I think I'm a very compassionate caring person

25 T: mhmm

After segment one, in response to item #22, there was some brief but unfocused discussion of the conflicts and difficulties the clients (particularly Bess) have experienced in their relationship since their last therapy about 6 years ago. At about the 7-minute mark, the therapist offers a comment in exchange 23 that is a right-angle turn from the preceding conversation. We think that the kind of sensitivity that is reflected in 23-24 is important in terms of the alliance-building process: These remarks reflect the therapist's awareness that the clients, so early in treatment, are in the process of generating a narrative description of themselves that paints them in quite dark, negative tones. We anticipate that, if this process were to continue, the clients would construe themselves in a weak "one-down" position that would invite the therapist to take the complementary position of competence and strength. In a strong positive alliance, the clients are active, energetic partners committed to take their share of responsibilities in the therapy process. In this context, the invitation by the therapist to talk about their "skills and competencies" accomplishes a double objective: it rebalances the clients' self-narrative to encompass strengths as well as difficulties and, at a more subtle level, allows Bess to present herself as the kind of person who is deserving to be liked and respected by the therapist. Thus, both a better relational balance and the interpersonal alliance are enhanced by this interaction.

---

[7]The exchange numbers are continuous between segments of transcript for ease of reference, but these segments themselves are not proximal—see the time notations.

Time: 38:10–44:00

26 T: so what I hear you saying is that um ... that uh ... given certain circumstances or certain conditions that ... this relationship can be made better and better ... yeah

27 B: yeah I think so

28 T: okay so ... is what you worked on when you were in the relationship with ... in therapy with [previous therapist ... (is) the same issue that you guys would like to work on here

29 B: I think they're quite a bit similar

30 T: okay; would you [B] like to share, in the time we have left, a little bit about what concerns you have, and then we will come back to you [K] about and talk a little bit about what your concerns are and what you'd like to work on in the five sessions or so

31 B: when we had our session with ... one of things that came up is my family ... and I re-K [husband]... thinks this plays a major role in our relationship that it hinders him a bit, or whatever, and I really don't believe that ...

32 T: I see

33 B: I. I mean, I do see a lot of my family and stuff but it never comes before us but [K] gets one weekend a month off. I get Sunday Mondays off and K only gets Sunday Mondays off, one weekend a month so when he's off ...

34 T: K let me get these days right again ... 'cause this is important so [you g-] ...

35 B: [I get] Sunday Mondays off ... [4 exchanges to clarify the dates]

36 T: okay every third weekend Saturday to Tuesday off

37 B: yeah ... so when K's working and I'm off I do spend time with my family, go to my sister's for dinner go to my mom's for dinner whatever

38 T: is it is that a problem

39 B: I don't think it is

40 T: is it a problem for K

41 B: it think it is for him

42 T: that when K's working ... that your over at your family's house having dinner ...

43 B: and spending time with [them]

44 T: [and] spending time there with your *son*

45 K: yeah

46 T: that's a problem with K

47 B: yeah (!!) ... I think it is

48 T: okay ... so um okay so the time that you ... I want to be clear about this ... the time that you spend with your family is a problem for K

49 B: I think it is

50 T: okay what's the problem for you

51 B: problem with my family

52 T: no what's the problem for you [B] what we're talking about here is ...

53 B: [what] do I see as the problem

54 T: yeah th ...

55 B: that K might see or whatever

56 T: well ... the problem that you're talking about is the problem that K has with your family

57 B: yeah.

58 T: what's the problem that you experience ... why are you here

59 B: oh ... um ... I think we need to learn to communicate better

60 T: mhmm

61 B: hmm ... to work on some issues that have been around for quite awhile ... sometimes I don't feel like I'm an equal in this relationship K tends to make a lot of the decisions and will kinda, okay, well ... what we'll do but then he'll change his mind and then expect me to know we don't talk about ... like, for example one time I remember car insurance and we were talking about you know we're gonna pay for a year and then the day K paid for it, he says but I only paid for six months ... I'm like well we had talked about this, and this is what we had decided, but you changed your mind ... like I really feel that he's ... at times doesn't consider me in lots things? Lots of choices that ... decision

62 T: okay so you don't feel like an equal partners -u-partner [in your relationship]

63 B: not always

64 T: and you'd like to feel that way

65 B: yeah

66 T: uh ... what would you like ... you would like to be able to discuss
     issues with K and come to a mutual agreement with [him]

In this segment the therapist is attempting to identify the goals each
client has in coming to therapy. He is immediately faced with the task of
disentangling the couple's confusing and paradoxical ways of relating. But
along with this responsibility comes an opportunity to challenge the old
interactional schema and instead set the framework for a more direct and
healthier way of relating.

The female partner begins by speaking for the husband and, in doing
so, making "their problem" her idea of *his problem*: her preoccupation
with her own family, a concern that she disqualifies in the same breath
(exchange 31). We have seen hints earlier (and it becomes fully evident
later in this segment (i.e., exchange 63) that she, in fact, feels that her
voice is often lost in the relationship. Apparently the couple has developed
a pattern where she takes the role of the "spokesperson" complemented
by his (Kale's) role as the silent, withdrawn "audience." It seems likely
that the more she talks, the less she feels heard. The therapist responds by
respectfully restructuring the conversation; asking Bess to speak in "her
own voice" naming her own issues. In exchanges 62–65 her goals for the
therapy are completely redefined, and the therapist is able then to introduce the concept of identifying therapy goals that reflect a mutual agreement between the partners (#66). Thus we see in this segment, on one
level, the beginning of the development of mutual goals, and, at the same
time, the clients' problematic relation is being enacted and responded to in
a therapeutically appropriate action. We believe that this example, again,
illustrates the close interaction between developing the relational—alliance—and therapy interventions.

Summary of Opening Moves

Research on the relation of alliance to outcome strongly supports the idea
that developing a "good enough" alliance early in therapy is especially
important (Horvath & Luborsky, 1993). Our analysis of the session above
illustrated several of the significant elements we believe are important in
developing a couple therapy alliance. We believe that the following points
are particularly relevant for therapists trying to develop the alliance in couple therapy:

• The key elements from which a positive alliance is created need to
be fostered from the very first contact with the client. The degree to which
clients are expected to be actively involved in, and contribute to, the work
of therapy has to be made clear as "first business."

• The most efficient way this "setting of the stage" can be accomplished is through the careful positioning of the therapist in relation to each client and the therapy itself. The degree to which the clients' ideas are solicited, how the process of therapy is explained and negotiated, and the ways in which the goals of therapy are established indicate "in action" the core features of the therapy relationship.

• The role of the therapist and the substance of the therapy, in the first instance, is determined by the therapist's positioning of self. We believe that the therapist's most potent tool in developing a collaborative alliance is his or her actions rather than mere explanations. As the curtain comes up on the therapy stage, the therapist is, in a sense, the prime mover. Depending on where he places himself in relation to the couple, who he turns to and in what order, whether he speaks his lines loudly and assertively or softly and hesitantly in brief sentences or extended monologues—sets the pace and tone of the unfolding drama. The other actors are likely to adjust the pace and substance of their contributions to the therapist's lead.

• The couple's relationship pattern is enacted and becomes interwoven into all aspects of the therapy relationship. It involves not only the clients but the therapist as well. We believe that this "relationship within the relationship" is neither avoidable nor should one *seek* to avoid it[8]; the therapist ought not to try to absent herself from this relational "triangle." It is by recognizing how the clients interact with each other that the therapist gains the greatest opportunity to place herself in a relational position that promotes better interaction (collaboration) not only in the therapy room (alliance), but by extension develops new relational options for the clients.

WORKING WITH THE ALLIANCE

Bordin, in his last published work, differentiated between the development of the alliance during the opening stages and "working with" the alliance during the middle and later stages of therapy. He suggested that management of the strains and stresses in the alliance is one of the central challenges and, indeed, the means to deal with the client's self-defeating relational patterns (Bordin, 1994). In couple therapy these relational patterns are enacted and can be observed at two interactive levels: the clients' interaction with each other and in their alliance with the therapist. In the "working phase" of treatment, if the therapist has developed a solid alliance with the client and is familiar with the partners' interactional patterns, he or she is in a position to recognize the negative transactions the clients are habitually engaged in. This

---

[8]For a contrasting view, see Bowen (1978) or Kerr and Sholevar (2003).

creates an opportunity to create a relational context that supports a different and healthier pattern. The following excerpt illustrates this process.

The clients are Pat (P) and Donald (D), the segment is preceded by their habitual conversation in which Pat is complaining about being ignored and sabotaged by Donald, and he responds by explaining how she is "always wrong."

1 P: But he just can't hear me. He doesn't listen! He doesn't care what I say or do! I am trying hard to teach [son] to be responsible. That he has to learn to earn his privileges! I tell him one thing, I tell him you have to do your chores, or this, to get the money, and then he [D] just goes ahead and gives him 50 bucks.

2 D: but you do ... <overlap>

3 P: I don't count. He just gives in to him. He doesn't care what I say!

4 D: Well, I mean, I mean he wanted to get those shoes. [Son] was going to get those shoes. So, I mean, he's going to get those shoes. How does he going to get the money? I'd rather pay for it because ... because how is he going to earn that kinda money? At least I know where he got the money from. <pause> Eventually he'll figure it out ... .

5 T: What I hear is ... what I hear is ... there are two parents trying to ... I mean one climbs into the ring and is ready to duke it out with this boy. Mom is are ready to fight to teach him how to be a *right*! Because she wants to protect him. She wants him to be ready for life. And then I see, I see D, ... dad, and he is also trying to be a good parent and protect this boy. He doesn't want him to get his money in the wrong way ... do something bad and ... getting into, like, like trouble. <pause> <pause>

5a T: And I guess it is kind of frustrating. Kind of scary when you worry about, about how things will turn out and ... so when you are so worried, as a parent. I mean, *as a parent* ... you are so *worried* that you kind of get uncoordinated. I see you both work *so hard* that it looks to *you* that you were not listening to each other. But to me, it looks like you are trying to help each other being good parents and look after this boy. And protect each other from worrying as well ...

6 P: but, but how come he doesn't, doesn't support me?

7 T: It looks to me that you are both trying to support the other ..., the other parent. But you are so nervous, so anxious about it, that each of you try to do it in your own way, the way *you* think would be best. But then ... when things don't quite work out with [Son], there is a big confusion that happens: Your son is confused,

because he's getting different kind of loving messages; and you are confused because you misunderstand what the other person is coming from, who's being protected. Anyway, it looks like this to me. But I am just a ... bystander.

8 P: well I didn't think ... I know he is worried, I know he *is* worried that [Son] is falling in with the wrong crowd. He always tried to protect him. I know that ... it's just that I feel so alone and scared ...

9 D: I am *scared,* <softly> and for you too ...

The therapist uses the strength of his alliance with the clients to redirect the evaluation of this recursive pattern from a perspective of competition (who is right) to one of collaboration on a common goal (exchange 5), albeit "uncoordinated" (exchange 5a). He identifies what unites the couple (7) and proposes an external context (confusion) that removes the negative intention (1, exchange 3). In exchange 7 we see most clearly the opportunity provided by having built a strong alliance: the therapist can step away from the deductive modality ("just a bystander") and trust that the clients have "absorbed" the framework he put out as an alternative to their usual perspective on each other. The common theme of "scared" comes from the clients themselves.

Two slightly different alternatives to the therapists' use of the couple's in-session maladaptive interactions were articulated by Minuchin (1985). He labeled the first "enactment":

> refers to the construction of an interpersonal scenario in the session in which a dysfunctional transaction among the family members is played out. Its significance for therapy resides in the fact that the transaction is not described in the past and in another context, but it occurs in the context of the session in the present and in relation to the therapist. By facilitating this transaction, the therapist is in the position of observing the family members' verbal and non-verbal ways of signalling to each other the ranges of tolerable transactions. The therapist can then intervene in the process, prolonging the time of the transaction) introducing other family members) indicating alternative transactions) and in general introducing experimental probes that will give him and the family information about the nature of the problem, the flexibility of the family solutions, and the possibility of alternative therapeutic framework. The therapist can have the family enact changed transactional patterns in the therapy session which then serve as a model for alternative interactions outside of therapy.

He labeled the other "unbalancing":

Unbalancing refers to the therapist's use of himself as a member of the therapeutic system to dis-equilibriate the family organization, he does so by joining and supporting an individual or family subsystem at the expense of other family members. This affiliation modifies the accustomed hierarchical organization of the family introducing the possibility of new alternatives.

Although Minuchin did not use "alliance language," it appears to us that both of these interventions speak to the ways in which the therapist can directly engage with the problematic transactions evident in therapy. Minuchin argued that these interventions "provide ... [the clients] with a different world view for experiencing themselves and each other. The therapist presents the conflictive and stereotyped reality of the family as a reality that has alternative interpretations. This new reality also has alternative solutions (Minuchin, 1985).

CONCLUSIONS

We began this chapter with a journey though the history of the alliance in couple therapy, explored some of the available research, and peeked briefly into the therapy room to observe a therapist setting the stage and working with the alliance. The research on the alliance highlights the complexity of the relationships in couple therapy—a "web of alliances," we called it. The available evidence indicates that being able to develop a collaborative relationship, a clear consensus on the goals and objectives that meet the needs of both clients, and an enthusiastic endorsement of the therapist as a trustworthy, reliable, and dedicated individual makes it more likely that clients will stay in therapy and very likely improves the prospects of a good therapy outcome.

We have seen that the management of relational balances (split alliances, gender imbalances, misunderstanding of the other's relational position) represents both a challenge and an opportunity for the couple therapist. It appears that these imbalances/splits can occur at a number of different levels, involve different aspects of the relationship, and have a variety of sources. But we argued that temporary alliance misalignments are endemic to couple therapy and can actually be productive, providing opportunities to reengage the couple with each other (and the therapist) in novel ways, moving beyond old dysfunctional patterns.

We also noted some important gaps. In our review of the literature we could not find any research on the alliance based on same-sex couples. This lacunae is unfortunate. Although a growing number of articles are being published on couple therapy for gay, transsexual, and lesbian clients, so far as we know, the alliance has not been specifically examined in these contexts. We believe that the general conclusions we drew are likely valid for therapists working with nonheterosexual clients, but there may be aspects of the development and maintenance of the alliance that require different approaches or emphases for these clients (Green, Mitchell, Gurman, & Jacobson, 2002).

We found that, although the relationship in general and the alliance in particular has been almost unanimously identified as an "essential component" in psychotherapy, there is little empirical data on therapist qualities that contribute to the alliance in couple therapy. This work is pressing; recent research in individual therapy has highlighted the importance of the therapists' contributions (Baldwin et al., 2007). More research on "mid-phase" alliance is another important future research opportunity, as is investigation of how specific client problems, symptom severity, and couple characteristics affect the development of the alliance.

We believe that the alliance has a uniquely central role in couple therapy. In couple therapy—perhaps more than in any other kind of treatment—the relationship is "the heart of the matter," it is both the focus and the process of therapy. Clients most often seek couple treatment because of relational issues between them, and they enact these relational difficulties in the therapy room as part of the therapy conversation. In building a sturdy therapeutic alliance, we, as therapists, have to engage with the echoes of the dysfunctional relational patterns of our clients, and we are challenged to avoid replicating these same habits. At the same time, we have an opportunity to generate the kind of alliance that demonstrates *in situ* the possibilities of a different, more productive, engagement.

REFERENCES

Anderson, H., & Goolishian, H. A. (1988). Human systems as linguistic systems: Preliminary and evolving ideas about the implications for clinical theory. *Family Process*, 27(4), 371–393.

Baldwin, S. A., Wampold, B. E., & Imel, Z. E. (2007). Untangling the alliance–outcome correlation: Exploring the relative importance of therapist and patient variability in the alliance. *Journal of Consulting and Clinical Psychology*, 75(6), 842–852.

Beck, M., Friedlander, M. L., & Escudero, V. N. (2006). Three perspectives on clients' experiences of the therapeutic alliance: A discovery-oriented investigation. *Journal of Marital and Family Therapy*, 32(3), 355–368.

Bedi, R. P., & Horvath, A. O. (2004). Balanced versus biased alliance: Perceptions of own and partner's alliance and psychotherapeutic outcome in short-term couples therapy. *Journal of Couple and Relationship Therapy*, 3(4), 65–80.

Bordin, E. S. (1994). Theory and research on the therapeutic working alliance: New directions. In A. O. Horvath & L. S. Greenberg (Eds.), *The working alliance: Theory, research, and practice* (pp. 13–37). New York: Wiley.

Boszormenyi-Nagy, I., & Spark, G. M. (1973). *Invisible loyalties*. Maryland: Harper & Row.

Bourgeois, L., Sabourin, S. P., & Wright, J. (1990). Predictive validity of therapeutic alliance in group marital therapy. *Journal of Consulting and Clinical Psychology, 58*(5), 608–613.

Bowen, M. (1978). *Family therapy in clinical practice*. New York: Jason Aronson.

Brown, P. D. (1998). *The therapeutic alliance: A predictor of continuance and success in a couples treatment program for maritally violent men*. Unpublished dissertation, State University of New York at Stony Brook.

Butler, S. F., & Strupp, H. H. (1986). Specific and nonspecific factors in psychotherapy: A problematic paradigm for psychotherapy research. *Psychotherapy: Theory, Research, Practice, Training, 23*(1), 30–40.

Castonguay, L. G., Schut, A. J., Aikens, D. E., Constantino, M. J., Laurenceau, J.-P., Bologh, L., et al. (2004). Integrative cognitive therapy for depression: A preliminary investigation. *Journal of Psychotherapy Integration, 14*(1), 4–20.

Christensen, A., Baucom, D. H., Vu, C. T.-A., & Stanton, S. (2005). Methodologically sound, cost-effective research on the outcome of couple therapy. *Journal of Family Psychology, 19*(1), 6–17.

Coupland, S. K., & Serovich, J. M. (1999). Effects of couples' perceptions of genogram construction on therapeutic alliance and session impact: A growth curve analysis. *Contemporary Family Therapy: An International Journal, 21*(4), 551–572.

Coyne, J. C., & Pepper, C. M. (1998). The therapeutic alliance in brief strategic therapy. In J. D. Saffran & J. C. Muran (Eds.), *The therapeutic alliance in brief psychotherapy* (pp. 147–170). Washington, DC: American Psychological Association.

de Roten, Y., Fivaz-Depeursinge, E., Stern, D. J., Darwish, J. E., & Corboz-Warnery, A. (2000). Body and gaze formations and the communicational alliance in couple–therapist triads. *Psychotherapy Research, 10*(1), 30–46.

Flaskas, C. (2004). Thinking about the therapeutic relationship: Emerging themes in family therapy. *Australian and New Zealand Journal of Family Therapy, 25*(1), 13–20.

Friedlander, M. L., Escudero, V. N., Horvath, A. O., Heatherington, L., Cabero, A., & Martens, M. P. (2006). System for observing family therapy alliances: A tool for research and practice. *Journal of Counseling Psychology, 53*(2), 214–225.

Garfield, R. (2004). The therapeutic alliance in couples therapy: Clinical considerations. *Family Process, 43*(4), 457–465.

Glickauf-Hughes, C., & Mehlman, E. J. (1994). Therapist's spouse as absent cotherapist. *The Family Journal, 2*(4), 368–370.

Glickauf-Hughes, C., Wells, M., & Chance, S. (1996). Techniques for strengthening clients' observing ego. *Psychotherapy: Theory, Research, Practice, Training, 33*(3), 431–440.

Green, R.-J., & Herget, M. (1991). Outcomes of systemic/strategic team consultation: III. The importance of therapist warmth and active structuring. *Family Process, 30*(3), 321–336.

Green, R.-J., Mitchell, V., Gurman, A. S., & Jacobson, N. S. (2002). Gay and lesbian couples in therapy: Homophobia, relational ambiguity, and social support. In *Clinical handbook of couple therapy* (3rd ed., pp. 546–568). New York: Guilford Press.

Heatherington, L., Friedlander, M. L., & Greenberg, L. (2005). Change process research in couple and family therapy: Methodological challenges and opportunities. *Journal of Family Psychology, 19*(1), 18–27.

Hight, C. T. (1998). *The effects of the perceived therapeutic alliance on outcome in couples therapy.* ProQuest Information & Learning.

Hilsenroth, M. J., & Cromer, T. D. (2007). Clinician interventions related to alliance during the initial interview and psychological assessment. *Psychotherapy: Theory, Research, Practice, Training, 44*(2), 205–218.

Horvath, A. O. (2002, June). *The client's appraisal of the alliance: Exploration of objective and subjective processes, and their relation to treatment outcome.* Paper presented at the Society for Psychotherapy Research, Santa Barbara, CA.

Horvath, A. O. (2005, November). Clients' *relational process in brief couples therapy: Sources of the therapeutic alliance in systemic therapy.* Second European Conference on Brief Systemic Therapy. Arezzo, Italy.

Horvath, A. O. (2009, January). *Relationships that help: Linking research to practice.* Paper presented at the Society for Social Work Research.

Horvath, A. O. (in press). Alliance in common factor land: A view through the research lens. *Research in Psychotherapy: Psychopathology, Process and Outcome.*

Horvath, A. O., & Bedi, R., P. (2002). The alliance. In J. C. Norcross (Ed.), *Psychotherapy relationships that work: Therapist contributions and responsiveness to patients* (pp. 37–70). New York: Oxford University Press.

Horvath, A. O., & Luborsky, L. (1993). The role of the therapeutic alliance in psychotherapy. *Journal of Consulting and Clinical Psychology, 61,* 561–573.

Horvath, A. O., & Symonds, B. D. (1991). Relation between working alliance and outcome in psychotherapy: A meta-analysis. *Journal of Counseling Psychology, 38,* 139–149.

Jacobson, N. S., Schmaling, K. B., & Holtzworth-Munroe, A. (1987). Component analysis of behavioral marital therapy: 2-year follow-up and prediction of relapse. *Journal of Marital and Family Therapy, 13*(2), 187–195.

Johnson, S. M., & Greenberg, L. S. (1985). Emotionally focused couples therapy: An outcome study. *Journal of Marital and Family Therapy, 11*(3), 313–317.

Keeney, B. (1981). What is an epistemology of Family Therapy? *Family Process, 21,* 163–168.

Kerr, M. (2003). Multigenerational family systems theory of Bowen and its application. In G. P. Sholevar & L. D. Schwoeri (Eds.), *Textbook of family and couples therapy: Clinical applications* (pp. 103–126). Arlington, VA: American Psychiatric Publishing.

Kerr, M. E., & Bowen, M. (1988). *Family evaluation: An approach based on Bowen theory.* New York: Norton.

Knobloch-Fedders, L. M., Pinsof, W. M., & Mann, B. J. (2007). Therapeutic alliance and treatment progress in couple psychotherapy. *Journal of Marital and Family Therapy, 33*(2), 245–257.

Mahaffey, B. A., Lewis, M. S., Walz, G. R., Bleuer, J. C., & Yep, R. K. (Eds.). (2008). Therapeutic alliance directions in marriage, couple, and family counseling. In *Compelling counseling interventions: Celebrating VISTAS' fifth anniversary* (pp. 59–69). Ann Arbor, MI: American Counseling Association.

Martin, D. J., Garske, J. P., & Davis, K. M. (2000). Relation of the therapeutic alliance with outcome and other variables: A meta analytic review. *Journal of Consulting and Clinical Psychology, 68*(3), 438–450.

Minuchin, S. (1985). Workshop: Structural couples therapy. In A. O. Horvath (Ed.) (handout ed.). Unpublished, Seattle, WA.

Minuchin, S. (1985, August). *A Structural Family Therapy Workshop.* Seattle, WA:.

Pinsof, W. M., & Catherall, D. R. (1984). *The integrative psychotherapy alliance: Family couple and individual therapy scales.* Unpublished manuscript. Center for Family Studies, Northwestern University, Evanston, IL.

Pinsof, W. M., & Catherall, D. R. (1986). The integrative psychotherapy alliance: Family, couple and individual therapy scales. *Journal of Marital and Family Therapy, 12*(2), 137–151.

Pinsof, W. M., Wynne, L. C., & Hambright, A. B. (1996). The outcomes of couple and family therapy: Findings, conclusions, and recommendations. *Psychotherapy: Theory, Research, Practice, Training, 33*(2), 321–331.

Quinn, W. H., Dotson, D., & Jordan, K. (1997). Dimensions of therapeutic alliance and their associations with outcome in family therapy. *Psychotherapy Research, 7*(4), 429–438.

Rait, D. S. (1995). The therapeutic alliance in couples and family therapy: Theory in practice. *In Session: Psychotherapy in Practice, 1*(1), 59–72.

Rait, D. S. (2000). The therapeutic alliance in couples and family therapy. *Journal of Clinical Psychology, 56*(2), 211–224.

Rampage, C., Gurman, A. S., & Jacobson, N. S. (2002). Working with gender in couple therapy. In A. S. Gurman (Ed.), *Clinical handbook of couple therapy* (3rd ed., pp. 533–545). New York: Guilford Press.

Raue, P. J., Castonguay, L. G., & Goldfried, M. R. (1993). The working alliance: A comparison of two therapies. *Psychotherapy Research, 3*(3), 197–207.

Raytek, H. S., McCrady, B. S., Epstein, E. E., & Hirsch, L. S. (1999). Therapeutic alliance and the retention of couples in conjoint alcoholism treatment. *Addictive Behaviors, 24*(3), 317–330.

Robbins, M. S., Mayorga, C. C., Mitrani, V. B., Szapocznik, J., Turner, C. W., & Alexander, J. F. (2008). Adolescent and parent alliances with therapists in brief strategic family therapy with drug-using Hispanic adolescents. *Journal of Marital and Family Therapy, 34*(3), 316–328.

Robbins, M. S., Turner, C. W., Alexander, J. F., & Perez, G. A. (2003). Alliance and dropout in family therapy for adolescents with behavior problems: Individual and systemic effects. *Journal of Family Psychology, 17*(4), 534–544.

Safran, J. D., & Muran, J. C. (2000). Resolving therapeutic alliance ruptures: Diversity and integration. *Journal of Clinical Psychology, 56*(2), 233–243.

Satir, V. (1967). *Conjoint family therapy.* Palo Alto, CA.: Science & Behavior Books.

Selvini, M. P., Boscolo, L., Checcin, G., & Prata, G. (1980). Hypothesizing, circularity, neutrality. *Family Process*, *19*(1), 60–69.

Sexton, T. L. (2007). The therapist as a moderator and mediator in successful therapeutic change. *Journal of Family Therapy*, *29*(2), 104–108.

Shadish, W. R., & Baldwin, S. A. (2005). Effects of behavioral marital therapy: A meta-analysis of randomized controlled trials. *Journal of Consulting and Clinical Psychology*, *73*(1), 6–14.

Shadish, W. R., Montgomery, L. M., Wilson, P., Wilson, M. R., Bright, I., & Okwumabua, T. (1993). Effects of family and marital psychotherapies: A meta-analysis. *Journal of Consulting and Clinical Psychology*, *61*(6), 992–1002.

Sprenkle, D. H., & Blow, A. J. (2004). Common factors and our sacred models. *Journal of Marital and Family Therapy*, *30*(2), 113–129.

Symonds, B. D. (1999). *The measurement of alliance in short term couples therapy*. Unpublished Doctoral Dissertation, Simon Fraser University, Burnaby.

Symonds, B. D., & Horvath, A. O. (2004). Optimizing the alliance in couple therapy. *Family Process*, *43*(4), 443–455.

Werner-Wilson, R. J., Michaels, M. L., Thomas, S. G., & Thiesen, A. M. (2003). Influence of therapist behaviors on therapeutic alliance. *Contemporary Family Therapy*, *25*(4), 381–390.

Werner-Wilson, R. J., Price, S. J., Zimmerman, T. S., & Murphy, M. J. (1997). Client gender as a process variable in marriage and family therapy: Are women clients interrupted more than men clients? *Journal of Family Psychology*, *11*(3), 373–377.

Werner-Wilson, R. J., Zimmerman, T. S., Daniels, K., & Bowling, S. M. (1999). Is therapeutic alliance influenced by a feminist approach to therapy? *Contemporary Family Therapy: An International Journal*, *21*(4), 545–550.

Whitaker, C. A., & Bumberry, W. M. (1988). *Dancing with the family: A symbolic–experiential approach*. Philadelphia: Brunner/Mazel.

White, M. (2007). *Maps of narrative practice*. New York: Norton.

White, M. B., Edwards, S. A., & Russell, C. S. (1997). The essential elements of successful marriage and family therapy: A modified Delphi study. *American Journal of Family Therapy*, *25*(3), 213–231.

Wilkens, T. A. (1999). *Self-disclosure and working alliance related to outcome in premarital training with couples*. Ann Arbor, MI: ProQuest Information & Learning.

Wolfson, A. N. (2007). *Alliance patterns related to dropout in couples therapy*. Unpublished dissertation, Boston University.

CHAPTER 12

■　■　■　■　■

Therapeutic Alliances and Alliance Building in Family Therapy

Valentín Escudero
Laurie Heatherington
Myrna L. Friedlander

Consider the following, possibly familiar, exchange as it unfolds in a family therapist's office:

> MOM: It's important to—that we talk.
>
> DAUGHTER: This is so stupid. Why'd you bring me here? I don't even know this woman! (*huge sigh; avoiding eye contact with mother or therapist*)
>
> MOM: Well, sometimes it's—it's good to have someone that doesn't know you, so that you can talk to them.
>
> DAUGHTER: She doesn't understand—she's not even my age!
>
> THERAPIST: What makes you feel like I can't understand you?
>
> DAUGHTER: (*sigh*) Well, you're not my age, one thing—you don't know what it's like being me. I have to live every single day without having friends, and after school I have nothing to do, and I don't want to sign up for anything—that's so stupid! (*sigh*) Clubs are just a waste of my time, like *this* is right now … (*sigh*)
>
> THERAPIST: Sarah, I understand your feelings, and, um, I think I can help you.

DAUGHTER: You don't understand, you don't understand anything! You're not *me*! Stop *saying* that!

MOM: Just give it a try, Sarah.

DAUGHTER: (*sigh*) No. (*long sigh*)

MOM: We're just worried about you, you know, I'm just worried about you, sweetie.

DAUGHTER: (*sigh*) Well, then, don't be!

MOM: I'm your mom! I want you to have friends in school—I want you to be happy! You just don't seem happy.

DAUGHTER: Just because I'm not happy doesn't mean you have to bring me here to *this woman*. (*sigh*)

MOM: (*to therapist*) I give up. I just want to help, you know, this is ... the best I can do, I guess. Nothing else is working.

DAUGHTER: I understand you wanna help me, but couldn't you just come and talk to me yourself? Why do you have to bring me *here*?

MOM: We've been trying to talk.

DAUGHTER: (*sigh*) Ugh, oh my God.

MOM: Nothing's changed.

DAUGHTER: (*sigh*) Well, I don't understand what you want me to do. What do you want?

MOM: Just, talk about what's going on. (*Therapist nods.*)

DAUGHTER: I *don't* have friends, I *don't* do anything after school. (*sigh*) I just *sit* in my room is all ...

In this short exchange, daughter, mother, and therapist are engaging in a complex interpersonal "dance," one that opens—and may very well determine the success or failure of—their work together. In contrast to the therapeutic relationships discussed in the previous chapters on individual therapies, this dance takes place on multiple levels: mother and daughter are dancing with each other, daughter and therapist pair off at times, and at other times it is mother and therapist together. Throughout, the triad is an overarching element, for even as two people interact, the third is an active observer, shaping and being shaped by the ongoing process.

Indeed, the alliance in conjoint family therapy comprises a unique set of conceptual and clinical features. Obviously, the presence of more than one client in the session, especially when they are at different developmental levels, results in a higher level of complexity for creating and maintaining the alliance. However, it is also the complexity of motives and motivations for being in therapy that make establishing therapeutic alliances in family therapy challenging. In the example above, for example, the mother's motives, at least currently, are not her daughter's.

Conflicting motives and ambivalence about participating in the therapy may involve the entire family, such as when treatment is initiated under pressure from the school. Also, beyond these multiple and possibly conflicting motivations, this is not just any collection of people. They are a system with a particular history, interpersonal dynamics, and power structure that regulates decisions that can direct or indirectly affect the initiation and process of therapy and that may make some members of the family vulnerable to other members. Families often seek help when their members are in acute conflict. Granted, clients seeking individual therapy also often present with conflicts that are interpersonal, not just strictly internal. But conjoint therapy presents extra challenges for the therapeutic alliance, not the least of which is the common expectation that when there is disagreement or conflict the therapist will take sides. Moreover, what happens in conjoint therapy sessions can have real-life consequences afterward for many people, particularly if the therapist is unable to manage the conflict during the session.

Further, in individual therapy it is the client's choice alone what to reveal and when, and the client's feelings of trust and confidence in the therapist influence the timing of these revelations. In conjoint therapy people have little control over, and no protection from, what others choose to reveal, including family secrets (Friedlander, Escudero, et al., 2006; Imber-Black, 1993). If the daughter in our earlier example were to disclose that her father is having an affair with another woman, her mother could hardly avoid the impact of having to process that information. Thus, the experience of feeling safe in conjoint treatment is qualitatively different (Friedlander, 2000). Also, "split" alliances (Pinsof, 1995; Pinsof & Catherall, 1986) can occur in family therapy and in fact are commoNPLace (Heatherington & Friedlander, 1990). Moderate splits happen when some family members are neutral about the therapist and others are quite positive, but "severe" splits happen when family members' positive feelings about the therapist are counterposed with others' intense antagonism (Muñiz de la Peña, Friedlander, & Escudero, 2009). Also, negotiating an agreement about the goals and tasks in therapy can be challenging in family therapy. The therapist's explicit agreement with one client about the goals of, or even the need for, therapy may alienate another family member who has come to the session unwillingly, as a kind of "hostage" (Beck, Friedlander, & Escudero, 2006; Friedlander, Escudero, et al., 2006).

These observations, born of clinical practice, illustrate how the emotional bonds, goals, and tasks elements of the alliance become complicated in the theory and practice of family therapy. In this chapter, we review how such observations have been used to conceptualize and theorize about the alliance in family therapy, and we summarize findings about how the alliance relates to outcomes. We then go "inside" the session for a closer look at the measures used to assess the strength of family therapy alliances. Measures are a bridge between science and practice. To measure a phenomenon requires that we truly know and understand it, and measures (especially observational measures) permit the demonstration of change over time. This methodology naturally leads to the key questions: How do we get from here to there? From the first handshakes to a strong working alliance? From a threatened or ruptured alliance back to a solid one? What is the process by which the alliance develops and deepens, and how can it be fostered within the session, in training, and in supervision? The latter half of the chapter addresses these clinical applications, with special attention to some situations that family therapists find most challenging.

ALLIANCE MATTERS: EVIDENCE FROM FAMILY THERAPY RESEARCH

Evidence that the therapeutic alliance matters in family therapy outcomes is quite convincing. Much of this evidence comes from studies of family therapy for adolescents who have externalizing problems, including substance abuse. Premature termination from treatment has been predicted from observer ratings of family members' alliances in brief strategic family therapy™ (BSFT; Waldron & Turner, 2008) and from parent alliances in multidimensional family therapy (MDFT). For example, in a sample of 13 dropout and 17 completer cases of substance abusing adolescents in MDFT (Robbins et al., 2006), the therapists' alliances with both the youths and their mothers declined over the first two therapy sessions in the dropout group, whereas in the completer group the alliances either stayed the same (among youths) or increased slightly (among mothers). In another study, the parents' alliances predicted dropout, and observer ratings (though not self-report) of the youth's alliance with the therapist predicted adolescents' post-treatment substance abuse and dependency (Shelef, Diamond, Diamond, & Liddle, 2005). Interestingly, the relationship between the youth's alliance and outcomes was moderated by the strength of the parent alliance; it was significant only when the parent alliance was moderately or very high. Thus, "Whereas the strength of the parent alliance predicts whether or not the family remains in treatment, once the family engages in treatment, it may be the quality of the alliance with the adolescent which, at least in part, determines changes in the adolescent's drug-using behavior" (Shelef et al., 2005, p. 695). In another study, the parent–therapist alliance in the second or third session was significantly predictive of reduced teen substance use and parent-reported externalizing behavior posttherapy (Hogue, Dauber,

Stambaugh, Cecero, & Liddle, 2006). Teen–therapist alliances were more complex; an early weak alliance that subsequently improved was associated with better outcomes, but stronger alliances early were associated with *more* externalizing behavior problems at posttherapy and at the 6-month follow-up. Thus, it was *growth* in the alliance rather than the overall strength of the alliance that mattered. The fact that treatment of substance abusing adolescents is often mandated requires skillful clinical interventions that foster this kind of "alliance shift" (p. 127), as we discuss later in this chapter.

In therapy other than manualized treatments for families with behavior-disordered adolescents, the alliance also matters. In brief family outpatient therapy, successful outcomes as measured by therapist and family consensus on improvement and reduced problem severity were predicted by clients' engagement in the therapeutic process, emotional connection with the therapist, safety early in therapy (Session 3), and productive within-family collaboration later on (Session 6) (Escudero, Friedlander, Varela, & Abascal, 2008). Similar results have been demonstrated in treatment-as-usual family therapy in community clinics. In a sample of low-income multiproblem families, certain subcomponents of the alliance, namely, parent safety, which seemed to facilitate productive family collaboration in the initial session, predicted ratings of improvement after Session 3 (Friedlander, Lambert, & Muñiz de la Peña, 2008). The authors of the latter study noted that "when family members express a common goal, offer to compromise, and demonstrate mutual respect in the first session, therapists can encourage more risk taking and expression of painful emotions" (p. 123).

In situations of abuse and neglect, where alliance building is particularly difficult, the strength of the alliance, particularly the emotional bonds component, moderates therapy outcome. Johnson and Ketring (2006), for example, found that alliance and posttreatment reduction in symptom distress (anxiety and depression) were significantly related and that clients' perceptions of client–therapist agreement on the goals of therapy were correlated with less family violence posttreatment. Thus, time spent early in treatment negotiating mutually agreeable goals seems to be time well spent. Further, the emotional bonds component of the alliance moderated posttreatment violence; it seemed especially important for families who reported higher levels of violence to experience warmth, trust, and connection with their therapists. Likewise, intrafamily attachments and alliance together influenced the outcomes of home-based treatment conducted after protective services referrals (Johnson, Ketring, Rohacs, & Brewer, 2006; Johnson, Wright, & Ketring, 2002). Even in more structured treatments, such as psychoeducational family treatment for schizophrenia, the therapeutic alliance is critical, predicting fewer prodromal signs of relapse and less likely hospitalization over a 2-year follow-up (Smerud & Rosenfarb, 2008).

The "big picture" is thus quite clear: in family therapy, the alliance is just as important a factor in positive outcomes as it is in individual therapy. This review of outcome research, however, has been in broad strokes, begging the more critically important questions: Just what exactly constitutes a strong alliance in conjoint family therapy? How do we know one when we see it, and how can it be assessed? Good measures are the key to assessing change over time, and change over time is at the heart of the therapeutic enterprise.

INSIDE THE SESSION: ASSESSING THE ALLIANCE

There are three ways to assess the alliance empirically: ask clients, ask therapists, and observe in-session behavior. In general, research on the alliance reveals an interesting metafinding: self-reported and observer ratings of the alliance sometimes have different associations with outcomes (Horvath & Greenberg, 1986; Martin, Garske, & Davis, 2000). Next we discuss two kinds of measures and what each contributes to understanding the alliance in family therapy.

Self-Report Measures

Early researchers realized that assessing the alliance in couple and family therapy involved taking into account the fact that each family member forms a relationship with the therapist while observing how every other family member relates to the therapist (Pinsof & Catherall, 1986). Thus, in creating their Integrative Psychotherapy Alliance Scales, the first self-report instruments specifically designed to assess the working alliance in couple and family therapy, Pinsof and Catherall (1986) crossed Bordin's (1979) three content components (goals, tasks, and bonds) with three interpersonal dimensions in couple and family therapy: self with therapist, other family members with therapist, and group with therapist. That is, each of the three interpersonal dimensions in their Couple Therapy Alliance Scale (CTAS) and Family Therapy Alliance Scale (FTAS) contains items related to goals, tasks, and bonds, for example, "I trust the therapist" (self-therapist bonds) and "My partner is not in agreement with the therapist about the goals for this therapy" (other family members–goals).

A fair amount of research has been conducted with the original CTAS and FTAS. However, Pinsof's (1994, 1995) subsequent theorizing about the nature of the alliance in conjoint therapy resulted in a recently published shortened version of the two measures, the CTASr-SF and FTASr-SF (Pinsof, Zinbarg, & Knobloch-Fedders, 2008). The new versions, each with 12 items, contain a fourth interpersonal dimension, the within-family alliance. In Pinsof's (1994) conceptualization, the within-system alliance refers to both (1) the family members' alliances with one another apart from their alliances with the therapist and (2) the therapist's alliance with other treatment providers (cotherapist, team) and/or entities (agency, institution, supervisor), reflected by such items as "My partner and I are in agreement about our goals for this therapy" and "My partner and I are not pleased with the things that each of us does in this therapy."

The question of how to meaningfully combine the scores of family members figures prominently in the concerns of clinicians; it is clear, for example, that a very strong alliance with the mother and a very weak alliance with the son does not necessarily compute to an "average" alliance with the family as a whole. Rather, a more fine-grained analysis of the entire set of alliances is needed, with attention to "meta" categories that describe the relationships of alliance scores to one another, not just the absolute value and valence of each of them. Indeed, such "meta" categories, for example, "split" alliances (Pinsof & Catherall, 1986) and "unbalanced" alliances (Robbins, Turner, Alexander, & Perez, 2003), have demonstrated clinical import (Quinn, Dotson, & Jordan, 1997). Cross-generational unbalanced alliances also matter. With Hispanic families in brief strategic family therapy, unbalanced mother–adolescent alliances predicted premature termination, whereas unbalanced father–adolescent alliances did not (Robbins et al., 2008). In functional family therapy, it was unbalanced father–adolescent alliances that predicted retention while mother–adolescent unbalance was only marginally predictive (Robbins, Szapocznik, et al., 2003; Robbins, Turner, et al., 2003).

Observational Measures

Self-report measures are useful for investigating the alliance because they can provide a sense of each family member's unique inner perspective on what is taking place in therapy (Heatherington et al., 1998). Observational measures, however, are especially useful because they reflect the clinical process. That is, therapists do not typically stop and ask clients to complete self-report measures of the alliance; rather, they observe clients' verbal and nonverbal behaviors to assess the state of the alliance as the work proceeds (Friedlander, Escudero, Horvath, et al., 2006). Also, observational measures allow real-time tracking of changes over the course of a session, thus permitting the study of how alliances are related to in-session interventions and events (e.g., reframing, enactments, interpretations).

Two observational rating systems of couple and family alliance-related behavior have appeared in the literature, one that was adapted by Diamond, Liddle, Hogue, and Dakof (1999) from individual psychotherapy, the Vanderbilt Therapeutic Alliance Scale (VTAS-R), and one that was specifically created for couple and family therapy, the System for Observing Family

Therapy Alliances (SOFTA-o; Friedlander, Escudero, & Heatherington, 2006; Friedlander, Escudero, Horvath, et al., 2006).

The VTAS-R (Diamond et al., 1999) focuses on individual family members' behaviors in relation to the therapist in a conjoint treatment context. This observer scale contains 26 items that trained judges rate from 0 (*not at all*) to 5 (*a great deal*). Based on a factor analysis of ratings made from videotapes, Robbins, Turner, et al. (2003) identified six VTAS-R items that reliably estimate "a positive working alliance" for parents and adolescents across three therapy approaches. These items reflect the client's acknowledgment of the problem, straightforward relating, open exchange with the therapist, apparent identification with the therapist's approach, experience of the therapist as understanding and supportive, and collaboration to solve the adolescent's or family's problems. After observing a session (or the segment of a session) and taking notes on behaviors as they occur, raters assign a value of 0 to 5 to each family member on all 26 VTAS-R items. However, only the 6-item positive alliance scale is typically used in CFT research.

In contrast to the VTAS-R, the SOFTA-o was developed empirically from a review of the couple and family therapy literature, the clinical experience of the authors, and an intensive analysis of videotaped family therapy sessions in which clients' perceptions of the alliance (on the FTAS) were already known. Identifying and clustering client behaviors that reflected strong and weak alliances, Friedlander, Escudero, Horvath, et al. (2006; Friedlander, Escudero, & Heatherington, 2006) created a measure that trained judges use to rate four dimensions of the alliance. One dimension, Engagement in the Therapeutic Process, is similar to Bordin's (1979) goals and tasks but includes one behavioral item that is specific to CFT, "Client complies with therapist's requests for an enactment." A second dimension, Emotional Connection to the Therapist, is similar to Bordin's (1979) bond and has both verbal ("Client expresses interest in the therapist's personal life") and nonverbal behaviors ("Client avoids eye contact with the therapist").

The two other SOFTA-o dimensions reflect unique aspects of conjoint CFT. Safety within the Therapeutic System has items that reflect safety as it is experienced in all therapy modalities, such as "Client shows vulnerability (e.g., discusses painful feelings, cries)," but also includes behaviors that imply a client's sense of safety or ease with his or her partner or family members, such as "Client directly asks other family members for feedback about his/her behavior or about herself/himself as a person" and "Client reveals a secret or something that other family members didn't know." The fourth SOFTA-o dimension, Shared Sense of Purpose within the Family, is similar to Pinsof et al.'s (1994, 2008) within-system alliance. Behaviors reflecting this aspect of the alliance include, for example, "Family members offer to compromise" and "Family members validate each other's point of view."

All four dimensions of the SOFTA-o contain elements that cut across family therapy approaches (i.e., structural-strategic, behavioral, emotion-focused) and that lead to both positive and negative alliances. Negative indicators include "Family members try to align with the therapist against each other" (Shared Sense of Purpose) and "Client refuses or is reluctant to respond when directly addressed by another family member" (Safety). After viewing the entire session, rewinding the tape as needed, raters tally the positive and negative observed behaviors, consider their valence (positive or negative), frequency, intensity, and clinical relevance, and use operational definitions and specific rating guidelines to assign each partner or family member a global rating from −3 (extremely problematic) to +3 (extremely strong) on Engagement, Emotional Connection, and Safety, where 0 refers to a neutral, moderate, or unremarkable alliance. On Shared Sense of Purpose, the couple or family is rated as a unit on the same −3 to +3 scale.

There is also a version of the observational measure that assesses the therapist's behavioral contributions to the alliance (Friedlander, Escudero, et al., 2006; Friedlander, Lambert, Escudero, & Cragun, 2008). That is, whereas a client's behavior reflects his or her thoughts and feelings about the alliance, the therapist's behavior reflects attempts to strengthen the alliance, such as "Therapist expresses interest in the client(s) apart from the therapeutic discussion at hand" (Emotional Connection) and "Therapist acknowledges that therapy involves taking risks or discussing private matters" (Safety). The therapist version of the SOFTA-o also results in global ratings from −3 to +3 that reflect the therapist's positive (+3, +2, or +1), neutral (0), or problematic (−1, −2, or −3) contributions to the alliance. Negative ratings reflect therapist behavior that detracts from the alliance, such as, "Therapist defines therapeutic goals or imposes tasks or procedures without asking the client(s) for their collaboration" (Engagement) and "Therapist allows family conflict to escalate to verbal abuse, threats, or intimidation" (Safety).

To assess the relationship between observed alliance behaviors and clients' and therapists' perceptions of the alliance, the SOFTA-o developers also created two brief self-report measures, the SOFTA-s (Friedlander, Escudero, et al., 2006; Muñiz de la Peña, Friedlander, & Escudero, 2009), whose 16 items reflect perceptions of Engagement, Emotional Connection, Safety, and Shared Sense of Purpose. Client examples include "What happens in therapy can solve our problems" (Engagement) and "All of us who come for therapy sessions value the time and effort the others put in" (Shared Sense of Purpose). Therapist items mirror the client items, for example, "What happens in therapy can solve this family's problems."

The SOFTA-o and SOFTA-s were developed simultaneously in the United States and Spain. Both the English and Spanish observational measures (Sistema de la Observacíon de la Alianza Terapéutica en Intervención Familiar, or SOATIF; Escudero & Friedlander, 2003) are available free of charge (see *www.softa-soatif.net*) in a software version, the e-SOFTA. Therapists (and their supervisors) can use the e-SOFTA to identify alliance-related behaviors, make global ratings, and write qualitative comments that are time-stamped with the videos. A recent training study showed that use of the e-SOFTA can improve knowledge of the alliance and alliance recognition skills (Carpenter, Escudero, & Rivett, 2008). In fact, the SOFTA-o was developed not only for research but also to enhance training and practice, because inferring clients' thoughts and feelings about the alliance from their observable in-session behavior is what therapists do naturally. The remainder of this chapter, therefore, is devoted to applications of conceptual and empirical understandings to facilitating the alliance, concluding with a section on special challenges to alliance building with families.

FACILITATING THE ALLIANCE

Initial Strategies to Enhance Family Engagement

We have learned a great deal about facilitating the alliance from studies that are more intensive, qualitative, and process-focused. First, there is excellent applied research on how to engage multiproblem families in therapy. A group of investigators at the University of Miami (Coatsworth, Santisteban, McBride, & Szapocznik, 2001; Santisteban, et al., 1996) for example, tested specific strategies for engaging hard-to-reach drug abusing Hispanic adolescents to attend an initial session of brief strategic family therapy. These include an intervention called strategic structural systems engagement (SSSE) that involves joining the family by demonstrating concern, interest and empathy, reframing the problem, and even visiting the reluctant client's home to forge alliances and facilitate engagement before treatment begins.

Second, an early task in many family therapy approaches is to help family members (re)construct the problem itself—and hence the goals of therapy—in a way that is less blaming, less linear, and more likely to engage each member in collaborating. Constructions such as "Our problem is that she isn't aware how demanding my work is, and she thinks I don't spend more time with her simply because I don't want to" are likely to arouse resistance in the partner, as well as cross-complaining constructions like "No, our problem is that YOU do not value the time together and my effort to improve our communication," reflecting a weak shared sense of purpose. Finding a way to (re)construct the problem definition itself—"It seems that you both agree that you are losing your way of showing each other how much you need and value love and understanding"—helps the partners engage collaboratively in the work of therapy. Sluzki (1992) articulated a "blueprint" for effecting such transformations from the "old" story to a new, more systemic, one in which each member of the family can play an active positive role. Circular, reflexive, and transformative questions, for example, "How will your wife react when you ask her for support around your stressful situation at work?," as well as exploring shared values and motivations foster in partners a sense of hope and commitment to each other (Coulehan, Friedlander, & Heatherington, 1998). Although first impressions and early engagement are especially important in family therapy, the growth, maintenance, and repair of alliances throughout the treatment are equally important (Escudero et al., 2008; Friedlander, Lambert, Escudero, & Cragun, 2008; Hogue et al., 2006). Thus we now consider selected key topics in facilitating the alliance.

Strengthening Emotional Bonds with All Family Members

The person of the therapist is obviously an important factor in facilitation of the therapeutic alliance. Clients report highly valuing therapists who are warm, active, down-to-earth, informal, trustworthy, optimistic, secure, humorous, caring, and understanding (e.g., Bischoff & McBride, 1996; Kuehl, Newfield, & Joanning, 1990). A study of 83 families seen at a child guidance center (Firestone & O'Connell, 1980) showed that the therapist's reactions to the family after the first session predicted which families eventually dropped out of treatment; not surprisingly, feelings of indifference or contempt toward the family were predictive of dropout. In fact, the bond aspect of the alliance may be the most valued component by clients (Beck et al., 2006; Johnson et al., 2002), who cite being "caring" and "understanding" as the most helpful therapist characteristics (Kuehl et al., 1990). Further, when the bond is strong, clients tend to experience their sessions as smoother and easier (Heatherington & Friedlander, 1990).

Having similar life experiences or backgrounds, as well as shared values, obviously makes this work easier. But in family therapy, especially when people are at different life stages (parents, young children, teens, grandparents), such synchrony is not evenly distributed. Self-disclosure as a way to communicate shared life experience, and humor as a way to communicate similarity in values or perspectives, can effectively transmit the implicit message that the therapist sees the family members as people, not as problems (Reynes & Allen, 1987). Humor can also serve to reduce tension, increase motivation, facilitate emotional release, and help clients develop a more realistic appraisal of the magnitude of their problems (Carroll & Wyatt, 1990). Thus, humor should not be overlooked as a means of creating an emotional connection *among* family members (even if the joke is at the expense of the therapist!) as well as between the therapist and clients.

Promoting Collaboration among Family Members

Family therapists from widely different orientations share many common strategies and behaviors for creating within-family alliances (Friedlander, Ellis, Raymond, Siegel, & Milford, 1987; Friedlander, Highlen, & Lassiter, 1985). Specific strategies to promote within-family alliances include eliciting family dialogue, using enactments (Butler & Wampler, 1999; Friedlander & Diamond, in press), circular questioning, deliberately drawing in the quieter members with questions or empathy, encouraging clients to compromise or to ask each other for their perspective, and praising family members for respecting each other's point of view even when they disagree. In order to help clients see themselves as a unit, effective therapists draw attention to family members' shared values, experiences, needs, and feelings, offering them a unifying perspective on their situation (Friedlander, Escudero, et al., 2006). In a family showing, for example, a high level of conflict, a therapist remark such as "The common denominator of your attitude toward the problem is that each of you wants to openly discuss and repair the problem, all of you share a brave attitude, and no one hides or avoids the battle" acknowledges the conflict but emphasizes what they share and positively reframes the behavior.

Sensitivity to change and co-responsibility for change are crucial ingredients for the creation of alliance in conjoint family therapy (Friedlander, Escudero, et al., 2006). For a therapeutic alliance to be strong, all participants in the therapy need to be sensitive to the changes that are slowly taking place and to attribute them to their involvement in the therapeutic process—not as an individual matter but as a mutual process. Feelings of frustration and despair can easily inundate the mood of the session and bring everyone down when change is slow-going. Thus the therapist's task is to sensitize the family to small shifts in behavior or attitude that arise from therapeutic conversations and that accompany the trying-out of new behaviors. Pointing out the changes that have already taken place or are likely to occur, or proposing simple "homework" tasks whose aim is merely to sensitize the family to change, are two interventions that can be used to draw attention to small changes. A possible homework assignment is to ask each family member to make a slight positive change in routine (e.g., hairstyle, the place he or she normally sits at the table) that is absolutely unpredictable and to keep it secret from the others; then each family member is asked to figure out what the others have done—without discussing the changes until the next session. This intervention allows the therapist to compliment the clients for their motivation and willingness to try new behavior, to compromise, to talk about feelings, and so forth, even if the behavioral change is not substantial. Along the same lines, structural therapists (Minuchin & Fishman, 1981), who work with in-session enactments, recommend "punctuating" change during a session, that is, stopping a family discussion before it disintegrates to old, familiar patterns of blame, criticism, or withdrawal.

Working with Coalitions and Conflict

A topic of particular clinical importance is avoiding coalitions. Robbins et al. (2008) described how families in conflict attempt overtly and covertly to draw the therapist into coalitions. The therapist's response to these maneuvers is critical in shaping future therapist–client and client–client alliances. Evidence suggests that using teaching, confronting, and reframing interventions affect subsequent family resistance and negativity within the session (Patterson & Forgatch, 1985; Robbins, Alexander, & Turner, 2000). Therapists must take care to avoid even inadvertently validating an angry parent's negativity about a child, alienating the child, and neglecting the other parent as an agent of change. To do so risks creating "split" or "unbalanced" alliances, which are associated with early termination and poor outcomes (Flicker, Turner, Waldron, Brody, & Ozechowski, 2008; Robbins et al., 2008).

Perhaps the most challenging situation for facilitating a strong therapeutic alliance is working with conflictual families where violence is a real risk. In these situations, the creation of safety takes priority. Of course, no therapy should be undertaken without a minimum level of safety. The therapist must deflect blame and hostility, protect clients from each other, and try to create alliances with all family members involved in the conflict. Working with such families, therapists must create a "safety zone" (Friedlander, Escudero, et al., 2006) where conflict can be approached without harm. In order to do that, the therapist must be able to contain and control the conflict, converting it into something constructive. The creation of safety depends on the context of the family conflict but also in large measure on the therapist's comfort level. While it is essential for the therapist to feel secure as the therapy unfolds, this sense of security is not always easy to guarantee. The therapist's sense of personal security may be compromised for any number of reasons—poor training, lack of experience with difficult cases, or personal characteristics or biases.

Dealing with Alliance Ruptures and Therapeutic Impasses

Of course, the process does not always go smoothly in couple and family therapy, and at times the alliance is threatened or ruptured by the behavior of the therapist or—more often—of the family members interacting with one another. Three qualitative studies (Diamond & Liddle, 1999; Friedlander, Heatherington, Johnson, & Skowron, 1994; Heatherington & Friedlander, 1990) delineated necessary steps for moving through a family impasse, that is, a rupture in the alliance that kept family members from working together productively.

In individual therapy, a client's refusal to comply or cooperate with tasks posed by the therapist can both reflect a weak alliance and threaten a stable one. In family therapy, this dynamic can involve several people, for as family therapists well know, family members sometimes resist engaging with one another (and by extension with the therapist) on tasks proposed by the therapist (e.g., "Discuss the rules you wish to set for your son's curfew"). Markers of resistance include direct refusal ("This is a waste of time") indirect disengagement (continually changing the topic, sarcasm, distraction maneuvers), and passive (minimal responding, "Whatever!") (Friedlander et al., 1994).

What can a therapist do to bring the family back to sustained engaged collaboration on the work at hand? A qualitative study (Friedlander et al., 1994) distinguished the sessions in which four families moved from disengaged to sustained engagement from those of four families in which they did not. Results showed four steps:

1. Recognition by the therapist of the cognitive–emotional basis for the impasse or rupture.
2. Communication about the impasse to the family (e.g., "So, you're afraid that if you talk about what the changes were that things will get worse?"), which in some cases included coaching family members to share these thoughts and feelings with one another.
3. Acknowledgment of the other's thoughts and feelings by the family member on the receiving end.
4. New attributions about the impasse or rupture emerging (e.g., a mother comes to understand that her son's "hatred" of her new partner is really a fear of being excluded).

Also, in each of the four successful resolutions, somewhere in the process was the realization and expression of *motivations* for engaging, such as the prospect of renewed intimacy or the potential for lost attachment. These motivations are particularly powerful when they are expressed by a family member rather than the therapist. As one man told his partner, "Well, we got this far and we can go farther ... with them two [children] out there. We got to raise them." (Friedlander et al., 1994, p. 446). This example highlights the point that in a conjoint setting family members themselves can help repair ruptures and move beyond interpersonal impasses.

In a similar manner, Diamond and Liddle (1999) studied the effectiveness of a "shift intervention" (p. 6), during which therapists work to counteract hostile, nonproductive interchanges between parent and child that can destroy a family's confidence in the therapy. This intervention involves the therapist's orchestrating a resolution of the impasse by blocking and diverting negative affect and blame, while evoking and amplifying "softer," or positive, emotions—caring, curiosity, sadness—that are present in the exchange, for example, "It must be disappointing that you don't get along with your child," or "Did you know that your mother misses you?" (pp. 483–484). In an example offered by Diamond and Liddle (1999), a negative exchange between a mother and daughter about chores was challenged by the therapist ("What's getting in the way of deciding on chores?"). In response to this shift intervention, the clients began exploring the more meaningful underlying conflict—a sense of mutual rejection. The resulting conversation was a beneficial discussion of their attachment to each other and the need for forgiveness for past hurts.

The key point here is that alliance ruptures and impasses are meaningful events in therapy. "Listening with the third ear" to their meaning affords the therapist valuable opportunities to coach the family toward a resolution and, subsequently, a strengthened alliance and commitment to the therapy.

SPECIAL CHALLENGES

Alliance challenges in conjoint family therapy can arise from different sources and contexts. In some cases, they come from home lives complicated by a lack of resources: support, time, or money. Individual differences in emotional/psychological resources can also be challenging when trying to engage and ally with the family system as a whole; most notable of these is attachment difficulties (Davila & Levy, 2006; Whiffen & Johnson, 2003). Work on trust and attachment is an explicit integral component of some systemic therapy approaches and is highlighted in attachment-based therapy for depressed adolescents (Diamond, Siqueland, & Diamond, 2003) and emotion-focused therapy for couples (Greenberg & Johnson, 1988). Indeed, there is much to be learned from the ways in which these two approaches encourage family members to engage in the therapy and with one another.

Also, differing developmental levels within the family require the therapist to be versatile in how and when to approach children, teens, parents, and elders in conjoint sessions. While some strategies used in individual child therapy may be helpful (engaging the child in a discussion of his or her interests and talents), others may backfire in the presence of parents, especially early in treatment, such as engaging a child with poor attachments and a defensive parent in a discussion of their relationship. Other strategies borrowed from individual child therapy, however, can be used to connect with children without alienating parents (Taffel, 1991).

Further, the dynamics of therapist–child–parent alliance building must be considered in the context of each family's ethnic and cultural background.

This dynamic is particularly challenging when the therapist's and family's cultures differ and/or when family members differ in their cultural expectations and values. Working respectfully within the expectations and customs of the family with regard to age and gender roles, for example, is most likely to enhance the therapist's credibility, likability, and trustworthiness. A common challenge for immigrant families is tension between younger second-generation family members who are more fully bicultural and first-generation parents/elders who are much less familiar or comfortable with the host culture and with their child's participation in it. Therapists must strive not only to understand the cultural background of the family (McGoldrick, Giordano, & Garcia-Preto, 2005) but also how their own cultural identity (especially if it is closer to the identity of the younger family members) risks fostering split alliances (Friedlander, Escudero, & Heatherington, 2006).

Adolescents often present particular challenges to alliance building. How can a family therapist working with adolescents improve an alliance that starts off on the wrong foot? Diamond et al. (1999) addressed this common dilemma in an exploratory study that involved MDFT and particularly difficult cases, that is, male adolescent substance abusers and their families with an initially poor teen–therapist alliance. Five cases in which the alliance improved by Session 3 were compared with five cases in which it did not in order to explore what "worked" to improve the alliance.

Three key alliance-building strategies were present only in the improved cases: (1) paying attention to the adolescent's experience, (2) presenting oneself as an ally, and (3) helping the teen identify personally meaningful goals for therapy. Attending to the adolescent's experience, included clarifying, summarizing, and interpreting the client's feelings, thoughts, or behaviors, for example, "It sounds like you've been responsible for yourself *and* your brother" (p. 360); presenting oneself as an ally was about indicating a willingness to advocate for the client, for example, "I will help your parents hear how humiliating it is to be yelled at" (p. 360). Presenting oneself as the teen's ally, in fact, was what most clearly distinguished the cases with improved alliances.

Also, the pacing of successful relationship-building work seems to differ for adolescents versus adults. Since children and adolescents are typically not self-referred, they are more likely to enter therapy in a precontemplative state of change (DiGiuseppe, Linscott, & Jilton, 1996). In general, staying close to the adolescent's concerns and supporting self-efficacy, at least initially, are likely to be more successful strategies than pushing for the expression of vulnerable feelings.

Several treatment models include specific interventions to engage reluctant adolescents. For example, MDFT therapists (Liddle, 2002; Liddle & Schwartz, 2002) use specific adolescent engagement interventions to show teens that they can gain something worthwhile from therapy, that their feelings will be respected, that therapy can help restore relationships, and that their participation is needed for change to come about. MDFT therapists also use parental reconnection interventions to address the adolescent–parent bond, whose objective is to generate the active participation of parents by "reestablishing parental feelings of love toward, commitment to, and influence over their adolescents" (Liddle & Schwartz, 2002, p. 465). This approach takes a lot of preliminary work, first encouraging and supporting angry youths to get in touch with and then express their "softer" emotions with regard to the relationship with their parents (disappointment, longing, etc.) while preventing the parent from becoming defensive, cutting off the child's expression, and preventing a repetition of old negative escalating patterns of interaction. The parent is helped to listen and experience his or her child's vulnerability, which if successful then allows repairs in attachment. In one case, for example, the therapist asked the father, "How do you feel about what your son just said?" to which the dad replied *to his son*:

> "That was deep. It's hard to put into words what I'm feeling right now. I know in my heart that a lot of things you've gotten into were because of me ... because I wasn't there for you when I should have been ... You've done the things you felt—you got this big barrier up in front of you, and you don't want nobody to knock that barrier down, you've put up this big wall. And then you're like, 'Damn, where's my daddy at? My daddy ain't there'. I know what you're going through because I went through the same thing with my dad. ... "

And then later:

> "I can't change what I should have done, I can't change what I could have done, I can't change what I didn't do. All I can do is try to make things better for you from this point on ... The main thing is, I haven't been there to listen to you. But the only thing I can tell you, son, is I love you, and I'll be there for you." (in Liddle & Schwartz, 2002, p. 471)

Not only adolescents but also other family members, and sometimes whole families, come to therapy reluctantly or even against their will. Brief strategic family therapists (Watzlawick, Weakland, & Fisch, 1974) and solution-focused therapists (de Shazer, 1985) offer interesting descriptions of clients' initial attitudes toward therapy that may create difficulties for the developing alliance. Solution-focused theorists, for example, define three types of therapeutic relationships: the customer, the complainant, and the visitor (de Shazer, 1988). The customer relationship is optimal for the therapeutic alliance—client and therapist define the problem together and collaboratively negotiate how to address it. In a complainant or "plaintiff" (Beck et al., 2006) relationship, client and therapist agree on the nature of the problem, but the client does not see him- or herself as part of the solution, asserting instead that others need to change in order for the situation to improve. These "others" can be family members, agencies, or outsiders who are complaining about the client. A "visitor" does not really recognize a problem to work on, and it is impossible to negotiate reasonable treatment objectives with him or her. In many cases the client believes that others are mistaken ("there *is* no problem") or that other people are the ones with problems; the visitor relationship is common when clients are pressured into therapy by others within or outside of the family. Obviously, in these circumstances the therapist risks responding to the client's lack of motivation with frustration. It is tempting to make a negative attribution about the visitor's poor motivation, but such attributions can be counterproductive for the creation of a therapeutic alliance.

Friedlander, Escudero, and Heatherington (2006) described a fourth type of therapeutic relationship, one that is unfortunately common in mandated cases, the *hostage relationship*. This relationship occurs when the client not only does not perceive a problem to be addressed but also views the therapy referral as unjust. Consequently, the client shows overt resentment or even hostility toward the therapist. Further, a hostage relationship can co-occur with other kinds of relationships, when, for example, a mother acts as consumer, the father is a plaintiff, a sibling is in the role of visitor, and the identified adolescent patient is in the position of a hostage. When a plaintiff accompanies a family member who feels like a hostage, it is likely that the clients' presentation in session mirrors the conflictual relationships that sustain the presenting problem. Typically, the hostage feels blamed by the plaintiff or by other members of the family, who feel guilty or ashamed of the hostage's behavior and their inability to control it. For therapy to work under these conditions, the therapist must first create a safe space for everyone. Seeing family members individually during the first stage of treatment may be beneficial. In any case, it is important to demonstrate early on that each person's perspectives and feelings are respected, and to block family patterns that threaten the safety and emotional bond of each person with the therapist.

When a family is forced into treatment by an external agency or institution (e.g., child protective services), the family as a whole typically comes as a hostage, visitor, or plaintiff. In such cases, the therapist needs to recognize the coercive context and—difficult as it may be—avoid seeing the family's resentment or hostility as a commentary on his or her own adequacy or skill, or as an expression of the family pathology. Paradoxically, a good alliance can be hindered if the therapist immediately and exclusively focuses on the problems for which the family was referred—particularly in cases of child neglect. When, on the other hand, the therapist makes a genuine effort to understand the family's point of view and deep mistrust of professional "helpers," the therapist's empathy with the clients' feelings of invasion or betrayal will nurture the alliance. This understanding is crucial when working with cases in which children have been removed from the home or when the possibility of removal hangs over the family.

In conclusion, we note that, just as the conjoint nature of family therapy presents unique challenges to alliance building, it also affords unique opportunities. Parents who witness the therapist establishing an emotional connection with their difficult child during the intake session typically gain confidence in the treatment. Family members who sense that the therapist is listening closely and respectfully to others may become more engaged as the session progresses. An adolescent who takes risks implicitly communicates that therapy is a safe place, and younger siblings may follow suit. When an alliance rupture between a father and the therapist is repaired, the repair strengthens not only their alliance but the alliance with the family as a whole. These events are uniquely possible in the conjoint setting, where exchanges both occur among, and are witnessed by, those whose lives are intimately connected. This exquisite sense of interconnectedness is both the great potential and promise of alliance building in conjoint family therapy.

REFERENCES

Beck, M., Friedlander, M. L., & Escudero, V. (2006). Three perspectives of clients' experiences of the therapeutic alliance: A discovery-oriented investigation. *Journal of Marital and Family Therapy, 32,* 355–368.

Bischoff, R. J., & McBride, A. (1996). Client perceptions of couples and family therapy. *American Journal of Family Therapy, 24,* 117–128.

Bordin, E. S. (1979). The generalizability of the psychoanalytic concept of the working alliance. *Psychotherapy: Theory, Research, and Practice, 16,* 252–260.

Butler, M. H., & Wampler, K. S. (1999). Couple-responsible therapy process: Positive proximal outcomes. *Family Process, 28,* 27–54.

Carpenter, J., Escudero, V., & Rivett, M. (2008). Training family therapy students in conceptual and observation skills relating to the therapeutic alliance: An evaluation. *Journal of Family Therapy, 30,* 211–424.

Carroll, J., & Wyatt, G. K. (1990). Uses of humor in psychotherapy. *Psychological Reports, 66,* 795–801.

Coatsworth, J. D., Santisteban, D. A., McBride, C. K., & Szapocznik, J. (2001). Brief strategic family therapy versus community control: Engagement, retention, and an exploration of the moderating role of adolescent symptom severity. *Family Process, 40,* 313–332.

Coulehan, R., Friedlander, M. L., & Heatherington, L. (1998). Transforming narratives: A change event in constructivist family therapy. *Family Process, 37,* 17–33.

Davila, J., & Levy, K. N. (2006). Introduction to the special section on attachment theory and psychotherapy. *Journal of Consulting and Clinical Psychology, 6,* 989–993.

de Shazer, S. (1985). *Keys to solutions in brief therapy.* New York: Norton.

de Shazer, S. (1988). *Clues: Investigating solutions in brief therapy.* New York: Norton.

Diamond, G. S., & Liddle, H. A. (1999). Transforming negative parent–adolescent interactions: From impasse to dialogue. *Family Process, 38,* 5–26.

Diamond, G. S., Liddle, H. A., Hogue, A., & Dakof, G. A. (1999). Alliance-building interventions with adolescents in family therapy: A process study. *Psychotherapy: Theory, Research, Practice, Training, 36,* 355–368.

Diamond, G. S., Siqueland, L., & Diamond, G. (2003). Attachment-based family therapy for depressed adolescents: Programmatic treatment development. *Clinical Child and Family Psychology Review, 6,* 107–127.

DiGiuseppe, R., Linscott, J., & Jilton, R. (1996). Developing the therapeutic alliance in child–adolescent psychotherapy. *Applied and Preventative Psychology, 5,* 85–100.

Escudero, V., & Friedlander, M. L. (2003). El sistema de observación de la alianza terapéutica en intervención familiar (SOATIF): Desarrollo trans-cultural, fiabilidad, y aplicaciones del instrumento. *Mosaico (Journal of the Spanish Federation of Family Therapy Associations), 25,* 32–36.

Escudero, V., Friedlander, M. L., Varela, N., & Abascal, A. (2008). Observing the alliance in family therapy: Associations with participants' perceptions and therapeutic outcomes. *Journal of Family Therapy, 30,* 194–214.

Firestone, A., & O'Connell, B. (1980). Does the therapeutic relationship matter?: A follow-up study of adherence and improvement in family therapy. *Australian Journal of Family Therapy, 2,* 17–21.

Flicker, S. M., Turner, C. W., Waldron, H. B., Brody, J. L., & Ozechowski, T. J. (2008). Ethnic background, therapeutic alliance, and treatment retention in functional family therapy with adolescents who abuse substances. *Journal of Family Psychology, 22,* 167–170.

Friedlander, M. L. (2000). Observational coding of family therapy processes: State of the art. In A. P. Beck & C. M. Lewis (Eds.), *The process of group psychotherapy: Systems for analyzing change* (pp. 67–84). Washington, DC: American Psychological Association.

Friedlander, M. L., & Diamond, G. M. (in press). Couple and family therapy. In E. Altmaier & J. Hansen (Eds.), *Oxford Handbook of Counseling Psychology.*

Friedlander, M. L., Ellis, M. V., Raymond, L., Siegel, S. M., & Milford, D. (1987). Convergence and divergence in the process of interviewing families. *Psychotherapy: Theory, Research, Practice, Training, 24,* 570–583.

Friedlander, M. L., Escudero, V., & Heatherington, L. (2006). *Therapeutic alliances in couple and family therapy: An empirically-informed guide to practice.* Washington, DC: American Psychological Association.

Friedlander, M. L., Escudero, V., Horvath, A. O., Heatherington, L., Cabero, A., & Martens, M. P. (2006). System for observing family therapy alliances: A tool for research and practice. *Journal of Counseling Psychology, 53,* 214–225.

Friedlander, M. L., Heatherington, L., Johnson, B., & Skowron, E. A. (1994). "Sustaining engagement": A change event in family therapy. *Journal of Counseling Psychology, 41,* 438–448.

Friedlander, M. L., Highlen, P. S., & Lassiter, W. L. (1985). Content analytic comparison of four expert counselors' approaches to family treatment: Ackerman, Bowen, Jackson, and Whitaker. *Journal of Counseling Psychology, 32,* 171–180.

Friedlander, M. L., Lambert, J. E., Escudero, V., & Cragun C. (2008). How do therapists enhance family alliances?: Sequential analysis of therapist–client behavior in two contrasting cases. *Psychotherapy: Theory, Research, Practice, Training, 45,* 75–87.

Friedlander, M. L., Lambert, J. E., & Muñiz de la Peña, C. (2008). A step toward disentangling the alliance/improvement cycle in family therapy. *Journal of Counseling Psychology, 55,* 118–124.

Greenberg, L. S., & Johnson, S. M. (1988). Emotionally focused couples therapy. New York: Guilford Press.

Heatherington, L., & Friedlander, M. L. (1990). Applying task analysis to structural family therapy . *Journal of Family Psychology, 4,* 36–48.

Heatherington, L., Johnson, B., Burke, L. E., Friedlander, M. L., Buchanan, R. M., & Shaw, D. M. (1998). Assessing individual family members' constructions of family problems. *Family Process, 37,* 167–184.

Hogue, A., Dauber, S., Stambaugh, L. F., Cecero, J. J., & Liddle H. A. (2006). Early therapeutic alliance and treatment outcome in individual and family therapy for adolescent behavior problems. *Journal of Consulting and Clinical Psychology, 74,* 121–129.

Horvath, A. O., & Greenberg, L. S. (1986). The development of the Working Alliance Inventory. In L. S. Greenberg & W. M. Pinsof (Eds.), *The psychotherapeutic process: A research handbook* (pp. 529–556). New York: Guilford Press.

Horvath, A. O., & Symonds, B. D. (1991). Relation between the working alliance and outcome in psychotherapy: A meta-analysis. *Journal of Counseling Psychology, 38,* 139–149.

Imber-Black, E. (1993). Secrets in families and family therapy: An overview. In E. Imber-Black (Ed.), *Secrets in families and family therapy* (pp. 3–28). New York: Norton.

Johnson, L. E., & Ketring, S. A. (2006). The therapy alliance: A moderator in therapy outcome for families dealing with child abuse and neglect. *Journal of Marital and Family Therapy, 32,* 345–354.

Johnson, L. E., Ketring, S. A., Rohacs, J., & Brewer, A. L. (2006). Attachment and the therapeutic alliance. *American Journal of Family Therapy, 34,* 205–218.

Johnson, L. N., Wright, D. W., & Ketring, S. A. (2002). The therapeutic alliance in home-based family therapy: Is it predictive of outcome? *Journal of Marriage and Family Therapy, 28,* 93–102.

Kuehl, B. P., Newfield, N. A., & Joanning, H. P. (1990). A client-based description of family therapy. *Journal of Family Psychology, 3,* 310–312.

Liddle, H. A. (2002). *Multidimensional Family Therapy: A treatment manual.* Rockville, MD: Center for Substance Abuse Treatment.

Liddle, H. A., & Schwartz, S. J. (2002). Attachment and family therapy: Clinical utility of adolescent–family attachment research. *Family Process, 41,* 455–476.

Martin, D. J., Garske, J. P., & Davis, M. K. (2000). Relation of the therapeutic alliance with outcome and other variables: A meta-analytic review. *Journal of Consulting and Clinical Psychology, 68*, 438–450.

McGoldrick, M., Giordano, J., & Garcia-Preto, N. (Eds.). (2005). *Ethnicity and Family Therapy*. New York: Guilford Press.

Minuchin, S., & Fishman, C. (1981). *Techniques of family therapy*. Cambridge, MA: Harvard University Press.

Muñiz de la Peña, C., Friedlander, M. L., & Escudero, V. (2009). Frequency, severity, and evolution of split family alliances: How observable are they? *Psychotherapy Research, 19*, 133–142.

Patterson, G. R., & Forgatch, M. S. (1985). Therapist behavior as a determinant for client noncompliance. *Journal of Consulting and Clinical Psychology, 53*, 846–851.

Pinsof, W. M. (1994). An integrative systems perspective on the therapeutic alliance: Theoretical, clinical, and research implications. In A. O. Horvath & L. S. Greenberg (Eds.), *The working alliance: Theory, research, and practice* (pp. 173–195). New York: Wiley.

Pinsof, W. M. (1995). *Integrative problem-centered therapy*. New York: Basic Books.

Pinsof, W. M., & Catherall, D. R. (1986). The integrative psychotherapy alliance: Family, couple, and individual therapy scales. *Journal of Marital and Family Therapy, 12*, 137–151.

Pinsof, W. M., Zinbarg, R., & Knobloch-Fedders, L. M. (2008). Factorial and construct validity of the revised short form Integrative Psychotherapy Alliance Scales for family, couple, and individual therapy. *Family Process, 47*, 281–301.

Quinn, W. H., Dotson, D., & Jordan, K. (1997). Dimensions of the therapeutic alliance and their association with outcome in family therapy. *Psychotherapy Research, 74*, 429–438.

Reynes, R. L., & Allen, A. (1987). Humor in psychotherapy: A view. *American Journal of Psychotherapy, 41*, 260–270.

Robbins, M. S., Alexander, J. F., & Turner, C. W. (2000). Disrupting defensive family interactions in family therapy with defensive adolescents. *Journal of Family Psychology, 14*, 688–701.

Robbins, M. S., Liddle, H. A., Turner, C. W., Dakof, G. A., Alexander, J. F., & Kogan, S. M. (2006). Adolescent and parent therapeutic alliances as predictors of dropout in multidimensional family therapy. *Journal of Family Psychology, 20*, 108–116.

Robbins, M. S., Mayorga, C. C., Mitrani, V. B., Szapocznik, J., Turner, C. W., & Alexander, J. F. (2008). Adolescent and parent alliances with therapists in brief strategic family therapy with drug-using Hispanic adolescents. *Journal of Marital and Family Therapy, 34*, 316–328.

Robbins, M. S., Szapocznik, J., Santisteban, D. A., Hervis, O. E., Mitrani, V. B., & Schwartz, S. (2003). Brief strategic family therapy for Hispanic youth. In A. E. Kazdin & J. R. Weisz (Eds.), *Evidence-based psychotherapies for children and adolescents* (pp. 407–423). New York: Guilford Press.

Robbins, M. S., Turner, C. W., Alexander, J. F., & Perez, G. A. (2003). Alliance and dropout in family therapy for adolescents with behavior problems: Individual and systemic effects. *Journal of Family Psychology, 17*, 534–544.

Santisteban, D. A., Szapocznik, J., Perez-Vidal, A., Kurtines, W. M., Murray, E. J., & Laperriere, A. (1996). Efficacy of intervention for engaging youth and families into treatment and some variables that may contribute to differential effectiveness. *Journal of Family Psychology, 10*, 35–44.

Shelef, K., Diamond, G. M., Diamond, G. S., & Liddle, H. A. (2005). Adolescent and parent alliance and treatment outcome in multidimensional family therapy. *Journal of Consulting and Clinical Psychology, 73*, 689–698.

Sluzki, C. E. (1992). Transformations: A blueprint for narrative changes in therapy. *Family Process, 31*, 217–230.

Smerud, P. E., & Rosenfarb, I. S. (2008). The therapeutic alliance and family psychoeducation in the treatment of schizophrenia: An exploratory prospective change process study. *Journal of Consulting and Clinical Psychology, 76*, 505–510.

Taffel, R. (1991, July/August). How to talk with kids. *Family Therapy Networker*, 39–45, 68.

Waldron, H. B. & Turner, C. W. (2008). Evidence-based psychosocial treatments for adolescent substance abuse. *Journal of Clinical Child and Adolescent Psychology, 37*, 238–261.

Watzlawick, P., Weakland, J. H., & Fisch, R. (1974). *Change: Principles of problem formation and problem resolution.* New York: Norton.

Whiffen, V. E., & Johnson, S. M. (Eds.). (2003). *Attachment processes in couple and family therapy.* New York: Guilford Press.

CHAPTER 13

■　■　■　■　■

The Therapeutic Alliance in Group Therapy

William E. Piper
John S. Ogrodniczuk

This chapter differs from most of the other chapters in this book by not focusing on individual therapy. Instead, it focuses on the construct of the therapeutic alliance in group therapy. In the case of individual therapy, many researchers define the alliance as the collaborative working relationship between the patient and the therapist. Agreement between the patient and therapist on the patient's goals, his or her tasks, and a positive emotional bond between the patient and therapist appear to represent generic components of the alliance (Bordin, 1979). In addition, a variety of adjectives have been used to further specify the conceptual emphasis of a particular use of the term "alliance." Examples include ego alliance (Sterba, 1934), therapeutic alliance (Zetzel, 1956), working alliance (Greenson, 1967), and helping alliance (Luborsky, 1976). Unfortunately, as this set of terms suggests, there has been a lack of agreement about how to label the construct of alliance. Difficulties with multiple labels have contributed to a lack of clear definitions and the development of few reliable measures. Such difficulties and others, such as distinguishing the alliance from positive transference, has led some of the construct's strongest supporters and most active researchers to question whether the construct has outlived its usefulness (Safran & Muran, 2006).

In the case of group therapy, the situation is even more complicated. The same difficulties that exist in individual therapy concerning multiple labels, definitions, and measures exist in group therapy. However, in group therapy, two additional parties are present: the other patients and the group as a whole. Questions immediately arise as to whether the relationships between the patient and each of the two additional parties should be incorporated under an overarching alliance construct or whether each should represent a separate type of alliance.

COHESION

To further complicate the situation, one must contend with the construct of cohesion, which overlaps, to some extent, with alliance. "Cohesion" is generally defined as the attractiveness of the group to its members. Yalom (1995) conceptualizes cohesion as the "we-ness" that is felt among group members. It refers to the "togetherness" of the group and the belonging or being valued that is sensed by individual members. The construct of cohesion incorporates a complex set of relationships that exist within any therapy group, including member-to-member, member-to-therapist, and member-to-group relationships. Unfortunately, the literature contains multiple divergent definitions and measures of cohesion in the absence of any unifying theoretical or empirical basis for the construct. This relative confusion has led reviewers to conclude that there is little cohesion in the cohesion literature (Bednar & Kaul, 1978; Dion, 2000). Despite definitional and measurement difficulties, cohesion has received considerably more attention than alliance in the group therapy literature, perhaps because of its greater heuristic value to clinicians and researchers. In many ways, the construct of alliance has been eclipsed by the construct of cohesion, which has been heralded as one of the most important therapeutic factors in group therapy (Yalom & Leszcz, 2005). As Burlingame, Fuhriman, and Johnson (2002) argue, cohesion in group therapy is *the* therapeutic relationship.

Some investigators have argued that cohesion in group therapy is analogous, if not synonymous, with the construct of alliance. Clearly though, cohesion is a more complex construct, as it incorporates multiple relationships (alliances) and thus pertains to phenomena that have no parallels in individual therapy. Yet, there remains difficulty in concluding whether the member-to-therapist aspect of cohesion differs appreciably from the patient–therapist alliance. To date, there is a lack of consensus of how to define the alliance and cohesion in order to clearly differentiate these constructs.

GROUP CLIMATE

Another complicating factor in our consideration of the alliance in group therapy is the construct of group climate. MacKenzie (1983) has described the group climate as an environmental press, that is, a property or attribute of the group environment that facilitates or impedes the efforts of an individual to reach a particular goal. The group climate consists of three dimensions: engagement (reflecting cohesion and work in the group); avoidance (reflecting group members' reluctance to take responsibility for changing); and conflict (reflecting interpersonal conflict and distrust). MacKenzie (1998) has suggested that the group climate (particularly the engagement dimension) is closely related to the therapeutic alliance. However, this interpretation is unlikely to be the case, as the group climate refers more to the relationships among the group members and less to any one member's relationship with the therapist. In fact, MacKenzie's Group Climate Questionnaire (MacKenzie, 1983) makes no reference to the group member's relationship with the therapist at all. Instead, the group climate appears to be a more complex construct that attends to multiple forces of the group, such as level of work, anger and tension, and personal responsibility for affecting change.

KEEPING THINGS SIMPLE

Given this state of affairs, group therapy researchers may be more able to make progress, at least initially, by studying the simpler construct of alliance, which focuses only on the relationship between the patient and the therapist. The fact that this has not happened to any appreciable degree may be attributed to resistance to conceptualizing groups as therapist-centered, or in other words, as focusing too much on the therapist. Practitioners of interpersonal approaches to group therapy, of which there are many, often emphasize the importance of peer relationships and peer feedback (Yalom & Leszcz, 2005). Focusing on alliance rather than cohesion may be regarded as taking a too narrow view of the different types of relationships in groups. This may be a case of theory and practice constraining research. Despite the risk of narrowness, it seems reasonable to attempt to make progress with a simple model before expanding to a complex one.

CHAPTER OBJECTIVES

Given the variety of constructs that appear to overlap with the alliance, some investigators have attempted to discover more basic underlying factors through various types of correlational and factor analyses. These are reviewed in this chapter. Also included in this chapter is a review of findings from group therapy studies that investigated the relationship between the alliance and treatment outcome. As is the case in individual therapy, authors have consistently regarded a strong alliance as a desirable condition of group therapy. Healing power has been attributed to the alliance itself and to its ability to facilitate the therapeutic effects of therapist technique. Some of these studies compare the strength of the alliance versus the strength of cohesion in predicting outcome. Other studies that investigated the relationship between potential predictor variables and alliance in group therapy are reviewed as well. Additional topics covered include the search for mediating variables, patterns of alliance over time, and the importance of forming a strong alliance early in therapy. Furthermore, we describe practice guidelines for establishing a good alliance in group therapy, consider various strategies for building a strong alliance, and provide a clinical example of how a ruptured alliance can be repaired. Finally, recommendations for further research of alliance in group therapy are considered.

EVIDENCE FOR INDEPENDENT CONSTRUCTS (ALLIANCE, COHESION, AND OTHERS)

Our review of the literature revealed only one study that had the expressed purpose of directly discovering basic underlying factors (components) from a larger set that included the alliance in group therapy (Johnson, Burlingame, Olsen, Davies, & Gleave, 2005). For most studies, the nature of the alliance construct is only a secondary issue. In the Johnson et al. (2005) study, four constructs (group climate, cohesion, alliance, and empathy) across three types of relationships (member–member, member–group, and member–leader) were included in the analyses. Three multilevel structural equations were tested, using self-reports from a large sample of group participants. Unfortunately, and despite the fact that many of the correlations between pairs of the variables were substantial, none of the three equations provided a good fit with the data, not even the model hypothesized to have one factor. Given this problem, the investigators conducted an exploratory factor analysis. The analysis revealed that the group members distinguished their relationships in groups primarily by the quality of the relationships rather than who was involved. These included positive bonding, positive working, and negative relationships. Although the components were meaningful, they cannot be regarded as valid until verified by confirmatory analysis or replicated with an independent sample. Also, some of the psychometric properties of the measures, such as the internal consistency of the group climate measure, were problematic. This is a good example of a comprehensive study that required considerable time and effort but in the end, unfortunately, dealt with only a few constructs. In addition, the constructs were not reducible to a smaller number of basic factors, nor did they provide evidence that supported their hypothesized conceptual models into a structural model. For these reasons, the study did not produce compelling findings.

Indirect evidence of considerable overlap among pairs of such constructs as alliance, cohesion, and climate has additionally been provided by studies that compared the abilities of the constructs to predict therapy outcome. For example, in a predictor study carried out by Joyce, Piper, and Ogrodniczuk (2007), a patient-rated measure of the alliance was significantly related to three of five measures of cohesion. The correlation coefficients ranged from .27 to .49. In a second study that reported correlations between alliance and cohesion (van Andel, Erdman, Karsdorp, Appels, & Trijsburg, 2003), the correlations were even higher, ranging from .65 to .73, and in a third study (Marziali, Munroe-Blum, & McCleary, 1997) the correlation was .65. Considering this set of correlation coefficients, the amount of common variance shared by the two constructs ranged from 7 to 53%, which is quite substantial.

ALLIANCE AND COHESION AS PREDICTORS OF THERAPY OUTCOME

As indicated, several studies have compared the predictive strength of alliance and cohesion in relation to therapy outcome. The group of Dutch investigators cited above (van Andel et al., 2003) provided cognitive behavioral group therapy to patients who had undergone a coronary angioplasty and who were experiencing a combination of symptoms including anxiety and exhaustion. The revised Helping Alliance Questionnaire–II (Luborsky et al., 1996) was used to measure the alliance, and the Group Cohesion Questionnaire, an instrument developed by the authors, was used to measure cohesion. The latter measure captured two facets of cohesion, the bond with the group as a whole and the bond with other group members. Both of these bond variables and the alliance variable contributed significantly and independently to posttreatment blood pressure and posttreatment quality of life. In regard to the measure of cohesion, the investigators did what many others have done: they created their own measure rather than use an already established measure. The problem with this strategy is that the field has become rather cluttered with measures that have not been used in multiple investigations and of which knowledge of their psychometric properties is somewhat limited and largely uninvestigated.

The Joyce et al. (2007) study of short-term group therapies for patients experiencing complicated grief compared a patient-rated measure of alliance, a therapist-rated measure of alliance, and three measures of cohesion rated by the patient, the other patients, and the therapist on their ability to predict therapy outcome. The cohesion variables focused on the patient's commitment to the group, compatibility with other patients, and compatibility with the therapist. Patient-rated alliance was directly related to all three primary outcome variables in the study, while therapist-rated alliance was directly related to just one. In addition, only one of the cohesion variables was directly related to one of the outcome factors. Thus, the strength of the simple relationship between patient-rated alliance and outcome was substantially higher than was the case for therapist-rated alliance and outcome. Patient-rated alliance was also more strongly related to outcome than any of the cohesion variables.

In a study similar in purpose, Marziali et al. (1997) compared a patient-rated measure of alliance with a patient-rated measure of cohesion regarding their ability to predict therapy outcome in groups for borderline patients. There was evidence that each of the two variables was significantly related to outcome, but the alliance variable accounted for significantly greater outcome variance than the cohesion variable.

Using the Working Alliance Inventory (Horvath & Greenberg, 1994) and the Group Attitude Scale (Evans & Jarvis, 1986) as their measures of alliance and cohesion, respectively, Woody and Adessky (2002) studied the effects of group cognitive-behavioral therapy (GCBT) with socially phobic patients. They found that neither the alliance nor the cohesion variable was significantly related to outcome. This finding was true for both the static level and rate of change of the variables over time. There appears to be an increase in the use of GCBT techniques in group therapy. The authors correctly noted that there is also a greater willingness to consider the relationship between the patient and therapist as an influential variable affecting outcome. They also correctly observed that the findings concerning the associations between alliance, cohesion, and outcome have been mixed in GCBT.

Finally, in a study with a small sample of depressed patients who were treated with short-term group psychodynamic therapy (Lindgren, Barber, & Sandahl, 2008), the level of alliance to the group as a whole as measured by the California Psychotherapy Alliance Scales (CALPAS; Marmar & Gaston, 1988) was predictive of two of three outcome variables. However, an early increase in alliance to the group as a whole was unrelated to outcome. Cohesion was not included in this study.

Many of the studies that have focused solely on the alliance have revealed a significant correlation with outcome. Also, studies that have pitted alliance against cohesion in regard to strength of relationship to outcome have favored the alliance. There appear to be no studies that have favored cohesion.

Predictors of the Alliance in Group Therapy

In addition to studying the relationship between alliance and outcome, some investigators have been interested in discovering predictors of alliance. It is not unreasonable to assume that there may be a causal sequence in which predictors in some way bring about an increase in alliance, which in turn brings about a favorable outcome. Thus, Johnson, Penn, Bauer, Meyer, and Evans (2008) investigated predictor variables associated with two forms of treatment (GCBT and group supportive therapy) for schizophrenic patients who had treatment-resistant auditory hallucinations. The investigators found that baseline autistic preoccupation and poor social functioning were negatively associated with midtreatment group alliance. Mid-treatment group alliance was positively associated with group insight. Furthermore, a strong alliance was associated with increased attendance and compliance with treatment. The authors pointed out some implications regarding group composition. For example, patients appeared to form stronger alliances when in a group where the other patients were high in insight rather than low in insight.

Taking a similar approach, Taft, Murphy, Musser, and Remington (2004) attempted to identify predictors of working alliance in CBT groups for men who had been violent with their partners. Working alliance was measured by the Working Alliance Inventory (Horvath & Greenberg, 1989). Motivational readiness to change (Prochaska & DiClemente, 1982) was the strongest predictor of the working alliance. Psychopathic personality traits were a strong negative predictor of the alliance. Other significant correlates of alliance were low level of borderline personality traits, low level of interpersonal problems, self-referral, marriage, age, and income.

ALLIANCE AND MEDIATING EFFECTS IN GROUP THERAPY

In search of explanatory mechanisms that could make the findings involving alliance and other variables easier to understand, investigators have explored mediator relationships. They have usually used the statistical procedure developed by Baron and Kenny (1986). For example, in the previously mentioned study by Taft et al. (2004), the investigators selected alliance as the dependent variable and then investigated such variables as personality characteristics, interpersonal characteristics, readiness to change, and certain demographic variables as potential mediators of the relationship between psychopathic characteristics and alliance. The investigators found that motivational readiness to change mediated the relationship between psychopathic characteristics and the working alliance.

Taking a different perspective, Abouguendia, Joyce, Piper, and Ogrod-niczuk (2004) selected patient-rated alliance as a potential mediator between expectancy of outcome and actual therapy outcome. Patients who met criteria for complicated grief were assigned to one of 16 therapy groups. Using Baron and Kenny's (1986) procedure, their study served as a cross-validation for a study previously conducted by Joyce, Ogrodniczuk, Piper, and McCallum (2003). There were important differences in the main characteristics of the two studies. In the Joyce study (2003), the patients were psychiatric outpatients who experienced a wide range of difficulties (e.g., anxiety, depression, low self-esteem, and interpersonal problems) rather than complicated grief, and the treatment was short-term individual therapy rather than short-term group therapy. Despite these major differences, the findings of the studies were similar. For both studies, the alliance emerged as a significant mediator of the relationship between expectancy of outcome and actual reported therapy outcome.

PATTERN OF ALLIANCE IN GROUP THERAPY

While most studies of the alliance have examined it as a static construct, a number have investigated changes in the alliance over the course of therapy. Most of these studies involved individual therapy. Unfortunately, findings of the relation between patients' patterns of the alliance and outcome in individual therapy are diverse. Several studies (Joyce & Piper, 1990; Kivlighan & Shaughnessey, 1995; Piper, Boroto, Joyce, McCallum, & Azim, 1995; Suh, O'Malley, & Strupp, 1986) reported that a linear pattern of the alliance was directly related to favorable outcome. In contrast, Horvath and Marx (1990) and Patton, Kivlighan, and Multon (1997) found that a curvilinear pattern of the alliance was related to favorable outcome. There appears to be no unifying theoretical explanation for the diverse findings concerning the nature of the general pattern of the alliance nor the diverse findings concerning the relation between individuals' patterns and their outcomes in the field of individual therapy.

Following individual therapy investigations of the pattern of alliance over time and their relationships with therapy outcome, similar analyses have been conducted for a few group therapy studies. The most common pattern reflected a linear increase in alliance over time. Significant linear increases were reported by Piper, Ogrodniczuk, Lamarche, Hilscher, and Joyce (2005); Lindgren et al. (2008); Taft et al. (2004); Tasca, Balfour, Ritchie, and Bissada (2007); and Woody and Adessky (2002). However, although the overall pattern may have been significant, the size of the increase was not necessarily significantly related to favorable outcome (e.g., Woody & Adessky, 2002). Thus, in the case of group therapy, the field is not any better off, although for a different reason. There are simply not enough group therapy studies to assess whether there are consistent patterns and whether variability among the patterns is related to therapy outcome.

FORMATION OF A STRONG ALLIANCE EARLY IN TREATMENT

Beginning approximately in the late 1960s and early 1970s, a transformation began to emerge in the psychotherapy field about what could be accomplished with short-term forms of psychotherapies. Although there were dissenters, an era of optimism began to prevail that cut across different forms of therapy, for example, behavioural, dynamic, and experiential. As time went on, the vast majority of therapies were completed in 20 sessions or fewer. Many of the therapies were time-limited, which meant that both patient and therapist agreed on the length of therapy prior to its onset. Advocates of brief therapies believed that a time limit created a beneficial pressure on both parties to get busy and work hard before time ran out. The situation appeared to be even more challenging for the participants in the case of short-term group therapy, where patients competed not only with the clock but with the other patients. Despite the appearance of a greater handicap for group therapy patients, most meta-analytic reviews of the outcome literature have reported few differences in outcomes between short-term individual and group therapies (see Burlingame, MacKenzie, & Strauss, 2004).

Clinicians who regularly practice short-term group therapies have emphasized the importance of the therapist's "hitting the ground running," that is, quickly getting off to a good start. In regard to the alliance, this advice means establishing a strong alliance early in therapy. With this thought in mind, some investigators have focused on the level of alliance early in group therapy and its relationship to therapy outcome at the end of therapy. For example, Piper et al. (2005) found a significant direct relationship between patient-rated alliance measured after one-third of therapy (Session 4 of 12) and therapy outcome. Other studies that have found a direct relationship between early alliance and favorable outcome are those of Taft et al. (2004) and Lorentzen, Sexton, and Hoglend (2004). Given the fact that short-term group therapy appears to be an underutilized therapy (Piper, 2008), we can expect that its prevalence will continue to increase. Therefore, it is likely that there will be many opportunities to study its properties.

PRACTICE GUIDELINES FOR ESTABLISHING A GOOD ALLIANCE

It is well accepted that establishing a good alliance is a critical objective for the group therapist, which seems supported by findings from a variety of research studies. Yet, despite this recognition, there are few resources that explicitly describe how a therapist can go about building a good alliance with her patients in group therapy. Some authors have suggested that certain therapist qualities and behaviors are useful for building a good alliance, regardless of whether treatment is provided in an individual or group format. For example, therapists who are warm, accepting, and convey positive regard for their patients are more apt to develop good working relationships with their patients. Additionally, therapists who are open, empathic, and display genuine interest in their patients are likely to build good alliances. Recently, the American Group Psychotherapy Association (AGPA) published a set of clinical practice guidelines for group psychotherapy. Contained within these guidelines was a discussion of the establishment of a therapeutic alliance. The discussion focused specifically on why pretherapy group preparation is imperative for laying the foundation for a strong therapeutic alliance. The AGPA guidelines provide a generic outline of methods to use during preparation for group therapy. The outline offers the following recommendations:

- The number of preparation sessions and times can vary, ranging from one session lasting an hour or less to four meetings (Piper & Perrault, 1989).

- The settings in which preparation is done can vary from meeting with patients one at a time or with two or more prospective group members in an actual pregroup preparation group (Yalom & Leszcz, 2005).

- Information is usually delivered across a spectrum from passive to more active or interactive formats with behavioral, cognitive, and experiential components (Burlingame et al., 2006). Combinations of four general methods can be identified: written, verbal, audiovisual, and experiential (Piper & Perrault, 1989).

- Passive procedures usually rely on instructions, delivery of cognitive information related to a model or example, and opportunities for vicarious learning through observation (Rutan & Stone, 2001).

- Active and interactive procedures rely more heavily on behavioral rehearsal and experiential components in which members are provided a brief structured therapy-like experience, role play, or the opportunity to watch and discuss a video of group therapy (Piper & Perrault, 1989).

- Adaptations in procedures and special consideration for neophytes to group and new members joining an ongoing group are recommended (Salvendy, 1993; Yalom & Leszcz, 2005). These may include orienting the incoming member to the current issues that the group is addressing.

- Adapting the preparations to be culturally attuned to the patient may be another important consideration (La Roche & Maxie, 2003).

• A combination of active and passive methods produces the most effective results (Yalom & Leszcz, 2005).

Unfortunately, because of the necessary brevity of the AGPA guidelines, particular techniques or strategies that therapists can use during the preparation stage that could facilitate a good alliance were not discussed. Such descriptions can be found in other sources (e.g., Piper & Perrault, 1989; Ogrodniczuk, Joyce, & Piper, 2005). For example, we have described a four-session experiential pretraining intervention for group therapy (Ogrodniczuk et al., 2005). The intervention consisted of providing patients with written material several days in advance of group training sessions. The written material focused on four concepts that were believed to be of primary importance to the type of group therapy offered in a particular outpatient clinic. These concepts highlighted here-and-now events, interpersonal processes, group processes, and member–leader relations. Patients then participated in structured group exercises that were intended to provide experiences of each concept (one session per concept)—for example, experiencing what happens in therapy when the focus is on relationships between the group therapist and patients in the group. The sessions are each 1 hour long and occur twice per week over a 2-week period. Beyond the general discussion of the role of group preparation in forming a good alliance, the AGPA guidelines do not attend specifically to alliance-building strategies to use during therapy. The work of Corey and Corey (2002) may come the closest to providing therapists with clear practice guidelines on how to form good alliances in group therapy. For example, they discuss assisting members in expressing their fears and expectations and working toward the development of trust, being open with group members and being psychologically available for them, clarifying the division of responsibility, and helping members establish concrete personal goals.

STRATEGIES FOR BUILDING A STRONG ALLIANCE

Beyond general guidelines, clinicians are interested in specific strategies for building a strong alliance with their patients. Newman's (1997) manual on establishing and maintaining a therapeutic alliance offers an excellent discussion of various alliance-building strategies. Although the manual was written for individual treatment with substance abuse patients, its relevance to psychotherapy in general (including group therapy) is clear and well worth considering by any therapist. For example, Newman recommends the following strategies for establishing the alliance at the outset of therapy (Newman, 1997, p. 183):

1. Speak directly, simply, and honestly.
2. Ask about the patient's thoughts and feelings about being in therapy.

3. Focus on the patient's distress.
4. Acknowledge the patient's ambivalence.
5. Explore the purpose and goals of treatment.
6. Discuss the issue of confidentiality.
7. Avoid judgmental comments.
8. Appeal to the patient's areas of positive self-esteem.
9. Acknowledge that therapy is difficult.
10. Ask open-ended questions, then be a good listener.

For maintaining a positive alliance over the course of therapy, Newman (1997, p. 191) suggests that therapists:

1. Ask patients for feedback about every session.
2. Be attentive. Remember details about the patients from session to session.
3. Use imagery and metaphors that the patients will find personally relevant.
4. Be consistent, dependable, and available.
5. Be trustworthy, even when the patient is not.
6. Remain calm and cool in session, even if the patient is not.
7. Be confident, but be humble.
8. Set limits in a respectful manner.

Finally, Newman (1997, pp. 197–198) recommends that therapists use the following general strategies when the alliance has suffered a setback and is in need of repair:

1. Strive to understand the pain and fear behind the patient's hostility and resistance.
2. Explore the meaning and function of the patient's seemingly oppositional or self-defeating actions.
3. Assess the patient's beliefs about therapy.
4. Assess your own beliefs about the patient.
5. Collaboratively utilize unpleasant feelings in the therapeutic relationship as grist for the mill.

CLINICAL EXAMPLE OF REPAIRING A RUPTURED ALLIANCE

The topic of ruptured therapeutic alliances (i.e., alliances that have been strained in some way) and how to repair them has received increasing attention in the literature. As noted above, Newman (1997) has offered some general guidelines of how to handle a ruptured alliance. Several other excellent resources discuss this topic in detail (e.g., Safran, Muran, Samstag, &

Stevens, 2002). Below, we provide a brief clinical example of a ruptured alliance in group therapy and how it was managed by the therapist.

Group's Background

Originally, there were 10 patients in this open-ended, long-term psychotherapy group led by a male therapist. Three patients dropped out of the group during the first few months. A fourth patient dropped out after 26 months. At this time, the therapist decided to add three new patients. The addition of new patients in a therapy group often precipitates a rupture in the relationship between the therapist and one or more of the patients who have continued with therapy. The following vignette illustrates the impact of one of the new arrivals (Carla) on one of the current group member's (Ellen's) alliance with the therapist. This is the fourth session after the arrival of the new patients. Ellen, who had rarely missed sessions, was absent from the preceding two sessions.

Ellen's Background

Ellen was a 36-year-old single woman who presented to an outpatient psychiatry clinic with complaints of "loneliness and worthlessness." She had few friends, was socially isolated, and had an unfulfilling relationship. Ellen was diagnosed with dysthymic disorder and referred to long-term group psychotherapy. Throughout the course of the group, Ellen was relatively quiet, often silenced by her shame of making her needs known.

> ELLEN: Carla, I find you more threatening than Bob—just because of your personality. (*silence*)
>
> THERAPIST: What is it about Carla that threatens you? Is it because she came in and sort of tried to take over the group?
>
> ELLEN: Uh-huh. More domineering. The way that she's, um, she's dominating you, I guess. She's ... uh, she's, yeah, she's consuming a lot of your attention right now.
>
> CARLA: That's the first time I ever heard anything like that. Oh, my God, you think I'm actually dominating? I'm just—I—I'm—I'll just shut up, I'm sorry.
>
> ELLEN: She's trying too hard or something.
>
> THERAPIST: There's something scaring you, though.
>
> ELLEN: Her aggressiveness.
>
> THERAPIST: You mean she's aggressive, as in you're afraid she's going to be angry ...

ELLEN: No, no, no. Her aggressiveness for attention bothers me.

THERAPIST: It seems to me that Carla is much more expressive of her feelings than others in the group. In my impression, group members are reacting to the possibility that because she is so emotional, she's going to seduce me somehow—get all my attention and leave you sitting out there somewhere.

DORIS: You're in a dream world. (*anxious laughter in the group*) To say to all of us that you're going to seduce her into getting all her attention. I mean ...

THERAPIST: That *I'm* going to?

DORIS: Yeah. Well—that she's going to ...

ELLEN: But that has crossed my mind. Carla, you're able to open up just like that. I envy you for that.

THERAPIST: Well, to be fair, the anger that you have—that you're talking about—really belongs toward me, and you can't really deal with me. I think it's easier to take it out on Carla.

ELLEN: We feel that maybe we—or maybe I'm—just not good enough for you ... you had to bring somebody else in.

THERAPIST: Well, you must have a lot of feelings toward me about that if that's how you feel you're being treated.

ELLEN: Yeah. I wasn't good enough, you had to abandon me almost and go on with somebody else.

THERAPIST: So, Ellen, in your heart of hearts, it feels like Carla is the one that I'm more interested in now than you.

ELLEN: (*silence, tears*) Well, I felt there was a bond, and it's been taken away—that somebody newer and better has come along.

THERAPIST: Can you put that bond into words?

ELLEN: Acceptance, mutual respect. (*silence*) Almost like a friendship. (Silence.) That's pretty much it.

CARLA: Actually, I envy you.

ELLEN: In what way?

CARLA: You have control over your emotions.

ELLEN: (*silence*) It's funny—while I'm envying you, you're envying me. (*silence, tears*)

THERAPIST: What are you feeling, Ellen?

ELLEN: Sad.

THERAPIST: It might be good to say more about that.

ELLEN: I'm feeling a bit more bonded to Carla now, but sad. (*pause*) Sorry for myself. (*pause, tears*)

THERAPIST: What's the sadness?

ELLEN: (*sobs, tears*) I think I'm sad about my inadequacies—my inability to let my emotions go—to express myself. I wish I could be freer with them. It's very frustrating.

THERAPIST: Is it possible that you're also feeling angry?

ELLEN: Why do you say that?

THERAPIST: I'm wondering about your absence from the group during the past 2 weeks. Could this be an indirect way to express your feelings? In this case, your anger toward me?

ELLEN: Yeah. (*tears, silence*)

THERAPIST: In the past, you've talked about your feelings toward your father. They were often angry feelings.

ELLEN: Yes, I can relate it to my father. Along with the feeling that I had been thrown over for my brothers. (*pause, tears*) Because I wasn't a boy.

THERAPIST: Carla isn't exactly one of your brothers, but it sounds like your reaction, especially your feelings, are similar to those you've had toward your brothers.

ELLEN: (*pause*) I see what you're getting at. I got angry with you 'cause I thought you passed me over for Carla—the same way my father passed me over for my brothers.

Comments

One can view Ellen's absences and anger with the therapist as signs of a rupture occurring in the alliance. By dealing directly with the affects being experienced by Ellen, and also by Carla, the therapist was able to successfully address the rupture and restore the strength of the alliance for Ellen. An alternative way to understand the rupture in the relationship between Ellen and the therapist is in terms of the concept of transference. Both the nature and alignment of Ellen's emotional reactions to Carla and the therapist resemble the nature and alignment of Ellen's emotional reactions toward her father and brothers. Exploration of the similarities allowed Ellen to achieve insight into current and previous relationship problems. Once these were understood and resolved, Ellen was able to restore her customary pattern of high attendance and high level of work in her therapy group.

CLINICAL AND RESEARCH IMPLICATIONS

Given the lack of research on the alliance in group therapy, it is difficult to suggest clinical implications with any sense of confidence. However, if one is cautious and tentative in making suggestions, some tentative conclusions can certainly be drawn from the relatively few studies that have been conducted. There is evidence that the alliance is directly related to favorable outcome in group therapy, particularly if a patient-rated measure is used. If so, it follows that therapists should attempt to establish a strong alliance. This can begin before the group starts. Careful preparation of the patient by the therapist can create more accurate expectations of the roles of the therapist and patients, typical processes in the group, and typical areas of difficulty that patients experience and usually overcome. The therapist can reassure the patient and facilitate positive expectations about the outcome. At the same time that the patient is becoming more informed about the workings of the group, an affective bond between the patient and therapist can be forming that represents the beginning of a trusting collaborative relationship, that is, a strong alliance.

Once the group has begun, the therapist can be vigilant regarding problems that arise that threaten a strong alliance, for example, the imminent threat of dropouts. The signs of a rupture can be subtle. However, they are commonplace and can be anticipated. Therefore, the therapist can be prepared to intervene. Repair of ruptures can be achieved by means of supportive comments and/or interpretations, depending on the technical orientation of the group. Although many articles have been written about the detection and repair of ruptures in individual therapy, very few, if any, articles have been written about them in group therapy.

Another means of detecting the strength of the alliance and ruptures is through patient self-report. Most standard means of measuring the alliance are brief (one page or less). A short questionnaire can be administered routinely after each therapy session. It has been our experience that within a short period of time routine questionnaires are hardly noticed. The procedure becomes an unobtrusive task that can be used in an indirect way to alert the therapist to potentially significant problems involving their patients.

In regard to research implications, unfortunately some very basic conceptual issues remain to be clarified. Stated as questions, they include:

- How do alliance and cohesion differ?
- What is the best measure for each?
- How much are they related to each other?
- Which is more closely related to therapy outcome?
- Is alliance a subtype of cohesion?

- Are there consistent patterns of alliance or cohesion over the course of group therapy?
- Are particular patterns or deviations from patterns related to therapy outcome?
- Are there specific strategies for strengthening alliance and cohesion?

To provide reasonable answers to these questions, at least two distinct phases of research are required. In the first phase, a small number of measures of alliance and cohesion are subjected to factor analytic techniques to determine whether they can be represented by a more basic set of constructs. From the findings, the best two or three derivatives of each (alliance and cohesion) are chosen and used in subsequent studies. Researchers restrict themselves to this small set of measures for each. They do not invent or use additional constructs and measures from other researchers. If this procedure is followed, researchers are able to compare their findings and form conclusions that are not tied to or qualified by idiosyncratic measures in the way that much of previous and current research have been. As is the case for much group therapy research, a large number of groups in each study with an accompanying large sample of patients are highly desirable in order to avoid statistical problems related to insufficient data (Baldwin, Murray, & Shadish, 2005) and low-power findings attributable to small sample sizes. As emphasized repeatedly in this chapter, to date the most significant impediment to understanding the nature of the alliance in group therapy is the lack of systematic research.

REFERENCES

Abouguendia, M., Joyce, A. S., Piper W. E., & Ogrodniczuk, J. S. (2004). Alliance as a mediator of expectancy effects in short-term group psychotherapy. *Group Dynamics: Theory, Research, and Practice, 8,* 3–12.

Baldwin, S. A., Murray, D. M., & Shadish, W. R. (2005). Empirically supported treatments or Type I Errors? Problems with the analysis of data from group-administered treatments. *Journal of Consulting and Clinical Psychology, 73,* 924–935.

Baron, R. M., & Kenny, D. A. (1986). The moderator–mediator variable distinction in social psychological research: Conceptual, strategic, and statistical considerations. *Journal of Personality and Social Psychology, 51,* 1173–1182.

Bednar, R., & Kaul, T. J. (1978). Experiential group research: Current perspectives. In S. L. Garfield & A. E. Bergin (Eds.), *Handbook of psychotherapy and behavior change: An empirical analysis* (pp. 769–815). New York: Wiley.

Bordin, E. S. (1979). The generalizability of the psychoanalytic concept of the working alliance. *Psychotherapy: Theory, Research, and Practice, 16,* 252–260.

Burlingame, G. M., Fuhriman, A., & Johnson, J. E. (2002). Cohesion in group psychotherapy. In J. C. Norcross (Ed.), *Psychotherapy relationships that work: Therapist contributions and responsiveness to patients* (pp. 71–88). New York: Oxford University Press.

Burlingame, G. M., MacKenzie, D., & Strauss, B. (2004). Small group treatment: Evidence for effectiveness and mechanisms of change. In A. E. Bergin & S. L. Garfield (Eds.), *Handbook of psychotherapy and behavioral change* (5th ed., pp. 647–696). New York: Wiley.

Burlingame, G. M., Seaman, S., Johnson, J. E., Whipple, J., Richardson, E., Rees, F., et al. (2006). Sensitivity to change of the Brief Psychiatric Rating Scale—Extended (BPRS-E): An item and subscale analysis. *Psychological Services, 3,* 77–87.

Corey, M. S., & Corey, G. (2002). *Groups: Process and practice* (6th ed.). Pacific Grove: CA: Brooks/Cole.

Dion, K. (2000). Group cohesion: From "field of forces" to multidimensional construct. *Group Dynamics: Theory, Research, and Practice, 4,* 7–26.

Evans, N. J., & Jarvis, P. A. (1986). The group attitude scale: A measure of attraction to group. *Small Group Behavior, 17,* 203–216.

Greenson, R. R. (1967). The working alliance and the transference neuroses. *Psychoanalytic Quarterly, 34,* 155–181.

Horvath, A. O., & Greenberg, L. S. (1989). Development and validation of the working alliance inventory. *Journal of Counseling Psychology, 36,* 223–233.

Horvath, A. O., & Greenberg, L. S. (1994). *The working alliance: Theory, research, and practice.* Oxford, UK: Wiley.

Horvath, A. O., & Marx, R. W. (1990). The development and decay of the working alliance during time-limited counseling. *Canadian Journal of Counselling, 24,* 240–259.

Johnson, D. P., Penn, D. L., Bauer, D. J., Meyer, P., & Evans, E. (2008). Predictors of the therapeutic alliance in group therapy for individuals with treatment-resistant auditory hallucinations. *British Journal of Clinical Psychology, 47,* 171–183.

Johnson, J. E., Burlingame, G. M., Olsen, J. A., Davies, D. R., & Gleave, R. L. (2005). Group climate, cohesion, alliance, and empathy in group psychotherapy: Multilevel structural equation models. *Journal of Counseling Psychology, 52,* 310–321.

Joyce, A. S., Ogrodniczuk, J. S., Piper, W. E., & McCallum, M. (2003). The alliance as mediator of expectancy effects in short-term individual therapy. *Journal of Consulting and Clinical Psychology, 71,* 672–679.

Joyce, A. S., & Piper, W. E. (1990). An examination of Mann's model of time-limited individual psychotherapy. *Canadian Journal of Psychiatry, 35,* 41–49.

Joyce, A. S., Piper, W. E., & Ogrodniczuk, J. S. (2007). Therapeutic alliance and cohesion variables as predictors of outcome in short-term group psychotherapy. *International Journal of Group Psychotherapy, 57,* 269–296.

Kivlighan, D. M., & Shaughnessey, P. (1995). Analysis of the development of the working alliance using hierarchical linear modeling. *Journal of Counseling Psychology, 42,* 338–349.

La Roche, M. J., & Maxie, A. (2003). Ten considerations in addressing cultural differences in psychotherapy. *Professional Psychology: Research and Practice,* *34,* 180–186.

Lindgren, A., Barber, J. P., & Sandahl, C. (2008). Alliance to the group-as-a-whole as a predictor of outcome in psychodynamic group therapy. *International Journal of Group Psychotherapy, 58,* 163–184.

Lorentzen, S., Sexton, H. C., & Hoglend, P. (2004). Therapeutic alliance, cohesion and outcome in a long-term analytic group: A preliminary study. *Nordic Journal of Psychiatry, 58,* 33–40.

Luborsky, L. (1976). Helping alliances in psychotherapy. In J. Cleghorn (Ed.), *Successful psychotherapy* (pp. 92–116). New York: Brunner/Mazel.

Luborsky, L., Barber, J. P., Siqueland, L., Johnson, S., Najavits, L. M., Frank, A., et al. (1996). The revised Helping Alliance Questionnaire (HAq-II). *Journal of Psychotherapy Practice and Research, 5,* 260–271.

MacKenzie, K. R. (1983). The clinical application of a group climate measure. In R. R. Dies & K. R. MacKenzie (Eds.), *Advances in group psychotherapy: Integrating research and practice* (pp. 159–170). Madison, CT: International Universities Press.

MacKenzie, K. R. (1998). The alliance in time-limited group psychotherapy. In J. D. Safran & C. Muran (Eds.), *The therapeutic alliance in brief psychotherapy* (pp. 193–215). Washington, DC: American Psychological Association.

Marmar, C. R., & Gaston, L. (1988). *Manual for the California Psychotherapy Alliance Scales.* Unpublished manuscript. Department of Psychiatry, McGill University, Montreal, Quebec.

Marziali, E., Munroe-Blum, H., & McCleary, L. (1997). The contribution of group cohesion and group alliance to the outcome of group psychotherapy. *International Journal of Group Psychotherapy, 47,* 475–497.

Newman, C. F. (1997). Establishing and maintaining a therapeutic alliance with substance abuse patients: A cognitive therapy approach. In L. S. Onken, J. D. Blaine, & J. J. Boren (Eds.), *Beyond the therapeutic alliance: Keeping the drug-dependent individual in treatment* (pp. 181–206). Rockville, MD: National Institute on Drug Abuse.

Ogrodniczuk, J. S., Joyce, A. S., & Piper, W. E. (2005). Strategies for reducing patient-initiated premature termination of psychotherapy. *Harvard Review of Psychiatry, 13,* 57–70.

Patton, M. J., Kivlighan, D. M., & Multon, K. D. (1997). The Missouri Psychoanalytic Counseling Research Project: Relation of changes in counseling process to client outcomes. *Journal of Counseling Psychology, 44,* 189–208.

Piper, W. E. (2008). Underutilization of short-term group therapy: Enigmatic or understandable? *Psychotherapy Research, 18,* 127–138.

Piper, W. E., Boroto, D. R., Joyce, A. S., McCallum, M., & Azim, H. F. A. (1995). Pattern of alliance and outcome in short-term individual psychotherapy. *Psychotherapy: Theory, Research, Practice, Training, 4,* 639–647.

Piper, W. E., Ogrodniczuk, J. S., Lamarche, C., Hilscher, T., & Joyce, A. S. (2005). Level of alliance, pattern of alliance, and outcome in short-term group therapy. *International Journal of Group Psychotherapy, 55,* 527–550.

Piper, W. E., & Perrault, E. L. (1989). Pretherapy preparation for group members. *International Journal of Group Psychotherapy, 39,* 17–34.

Prochaska, J. O., & DiClemente, C. C. (1982). Transtheoretical therapy: Toward a more integrative model of change. *Psychotherapy: Theory, Research, and Practice, 19*, 276–288.

Rutan, J. S., & Stone, W. N. (1002). *Psychodynamic group psychotherapy* (3 rd ed.). New York: Guilford Press.

Safran, J. D., Muran, J. C., Samstag, L. W., & Stevens, C. (2002). Repairing alliance ruptures. In J. C. Norcross (Ed.), *Psychotherapy relationships that work*. New York: Oxford University.

Salvendy, J. T. (1993). Control and power in supervision. *International Journal of Group Psychotherapy, 43*, 363–376.

Sterba, R. F. (1934). The fate of the ego in analytic therapy. *International Journal of Psychoanalysis, 115*, 117–126.

Suh, C. S., O'Malley, S. S., & Strupp, H. H. (1986). The Vanderbilt Process Measures: The Psychotherapy Process Scale (VPPS) and the Negative Indicators Scale (VNIS). In L. S. Greenberg & W. M. Pinsoff (Eds.), *The psychotherapeutic process: A research handbook* (pp. 285–324). New York: Guilford Press.

Taft, C. T., Murphy, C. M., Musser, P. H., & Remington, N. A. (2004). Personality, interpersonal, and motivational predictors of the working alliance in group cognitive-behavioral therapy for partner violent men. *Journal of Consulting and Clinical Psychology, 72*, 349–354.

Tasca, G. A., Balfour, L., Ritchie, K., & Bissada, H. (2007). The relationship between attachment scales and group therapy alliance growth differs by treatment type for women with binge-eating disorder. *Group Dynamics: Theory, Research, and Practice, 11*, 1–14.

van Andel, P., Erdman, R. A. M., Karsdorp, P. A., Appels, A., & Trijsburg, R. W. (2003). Group cohesion and working alliance: Prediction of treatment outcome in cardiac patients receiving cognitive behavioral group psychotherapy. *Psychotherapy and Psychosomatics, 72*, 141–149.

Woody, S. R., & Adessky, R. S. (2002). Therapeutic alliance, group cohesion, and homework compliance during cognitive-behavioral group treatment of social phobia. *Behavior Therapy, 33*, 5–27.

Yalom, I. (1995). *The theory and practice of group psychotherapy* (4th ed.). New York: Basic Books.

Yalom, I. E., & Leszcz, M. (2005). *The theory and practice of group psychotherapy* (5th ed.). New York: Basic Books.

Zetzel, E. R. (1956). Current concepts of transference. *International Journal of Psychoanalysis, 37*, 369–376.

PART III
▪ ▪ ▪ ▪ ▪
TRAINING PROGRAMS ON THE THERAPEUTIC ALLIANCE

CHAPTER 14

■　■　■　■　■

Developing Skills in Managing Negative Process

Jeffrey L. Binder
William P. Henry

THE BEGINNING OF A JOURNEY OF
SERENDIPITOUS DISCOVERIES: THE ANALOGUE STUDIES

The Vanderbilt Psychotherapy Research Team began with the solitary work of Hans H. Strupp, one of the pioneers in the field of psychotherapy research. His philosophy of investigation allowed for the researcher to be surprised by what he found. While his studies always had guiding hypotheses, his research methods—incorporating multiple measurement perspectives and qualitative data whenever possible—encouraged the generation of data that could produce serendipitous findings as well as relatively more intriguing and clinically relevant questions rather than simply clarifying answers. By allowing their data to guide the directions their curiosity took, he and his colleagues were able to focus most productively on the evolving dynamics of patient–therapist relationships. The Vanderbilt Psychotherapy Research Team's discoveries about largely overlooked difficulties encountered by therapists in managing the therapist–patient relationship led to proposals for radical changes in training therapists for managing therapeutic relationships and, particularly, the establishment and maintenance of the therapeutic alliance.

The work of Hans H. Strupp began at George Washington University during the 1950s and culminated with the studies conducted at the Vanderbilt University Center for Psychotherapy Research between the 1970s and 1990s. From the beginning of his work, Strupp was interested in more than the technical operations that characterized a therapist, which was one of the predominant research questions at the time. He was more intrigued with how the personal characteristics of the therapist affect his or her performance. Strupp believed that therapeutic techniques were not applied *in vacuo*. Accordingly, his doctoral dissertation at George Washington University was a study of how the theoretical orientation, training, professional experience, and other background variables affected the ways in which therapists thought about and responded to patients. He designed an analogue study in which over 200 therapists (psychiatrists and psychologists) watched a filmed interview of a real patient. During pauses in the film, they recorded their hypothetical interventions, and afterward the therapists recorded their diagnostic impressions, case formulations, and thoughts about how the therapeutic relationship would unfold. Finally, they recorded extensive autobiographic information.

The patient on the film was a male who became increasingly demanding with the interviewer. Contrary to Strupp's expectations, this provocative patient evoked widespread negative reactions from the audience of therapists. Even more surprising, the most negative reactions were elicited from the relatively more experienced therapists. The therapists' attitudes (positive or negative) tended to crystallize within a few minutes and were not subject to later change during the course of watching the film. Strupp discovered that the tone of the therapists' personal reactions appeared to influence their diagnostic and prognostic impressions as well as the treatment strategy they recommended and their hypothetical responses to the patient at film pauses during the interview. In sum, while therapists who responded negatively to the patient were aware of how they felt, they appeared not to be aware of how their personal reactions influenced their diagnostic opinions, technical recommendations, and hypothetical technical operations. Strupp was surprised at how many of the respondents reacted to the patient's hostility and demandingness with reciprocal hostility (Strupp, 1958). The findings from his dissertation study as well as his subsequent continued study of therapeutic processes solidified Strupp's belief that the therapist's contribution to the treatment process is both personal and technical. The therapist's genuine caring for and commitment to his or her patient enables the former to create the kind of interpersonal relationship in which technical interventions can have a positive impact, leading to constructive personality change (Strupp, 1960). Conversely, the absence of a positive interpersonal relationship—what we now call a strong therapeutic alliance—is associated with conditions in which the constructive impact of any technical procedure would be greatly reduced or nullified.

THE SERENDIPITOUS REDISCOVERY: VANDERBILT I

During the 1960s, the important findings about the influence of therapists' conscious personal reactions to patients' actions were overshadowed by larger research questions. Strupp had taken a position in the psychiatry department at the University of North Carolina at Chapel Hill and embarked on a collaboration with Allen Bergin to assess the feasibility of large-scale psychotherapy process and outcome studies, in order to expand the empirical base of the field. At the time, the prevalent view among clinicians was that technical operations stressed by a particular therapeutic approach or school were the necessary ingredients responsible for therapeutic change. Yet, no solid evidence had been produced that any technique per se or form of therapy was demonstrably superior to others. This state of affairs lent credence to the position of clinicians, like Jerome Frank, who posited that interpersonal relationship factors common to all forms of therapy were necessary and sufficient for therapeutic change. These opposing views created a central question for psychotherapy researchers: To what extent are therapeutic effects the result of specific techniques (such as suggestions, clarifications, and interpretations), as opposed to nonspecific factors inherent in any benign human relationship that raise the patient's positive expectations and hope?

This question captured Strupp's attention, but he did not investigate it until after taking a position in 1967 as Distinguished Professor of Psychology at Vanderbilt University and establishing the Vanderbilt Center for Psychotherapy Research. In order to study the relative contribution to treatment outcome of techniques versus relationship factors, Strupp and his students constructed an ingenious research design. He compared the time-limited therapies conducted by a group of college professors untrained in psychotherapy (but reputed to form warm and supportive relationships with undergraduates) with the therapies conducted by a group of professional, experienced therapists who (through recommendations by peers and supervisors or by their standing in the academic community) were reputed to be highly competent therapists. The researchers assumed that both groups would be composed of people capable of forming positive interpersonal relationships with the college student patients. Therefore, the main hypothesis was that the therapists' combination of good interpersonal skills and technical skills would produce better therapeutic processes and outcomes than the college professors, who relied solely on interpersonal skills.

The unexpected main findings were that, while both treatment groups did better than control groups, on the average patients of the college professors improved as much on the quantitative measures as did the patients of the professional therapists, and these comparable results were maintained at 1-year follow-up (Strupp & Hadley, 1979). Although the main effects drew the attention of the field (and the study gained a certain notoriety), subsequent analyses proved to have more lasting significance. The researchers found considerable variability among the individual patient–therapist dyads, with some patients experiencing considerable therapeutic benefit while others remained unchanged and a few showed deterioration. As a group, the professional therapists produced differentially better therapeutic results than the college professors, but only with patients who were highly motivated for therapy and evidenced low resistance to the therapist's interventions. On the other hand, while the college professors tended to obtain moderately positive outcomes with all of their patients, the professional therapists tended to obtain poor results with hostile, mistrustful, negativistic patients.

In a series of research-informed case studies, Strupp (1980a, 1980b, 1980c, 1980d) documented how the professional therapists evidenced little capacity for adapting their interpersonal stances to patient needs. While some nonanalytic and analytic therapists related in rather warm and engaging ways, other therapists, especially some of the analytic therapists, appeared to take a stance of "abstinence" and "therapeutic neutrality," which translated into a certain remoteness and aloofness. Of even greater importance for the outcome of the treatments, the therapists were unable to adapt their therapeutic approaches or techniques in an attempt to address the relationship difficulties posed by their difficult patients. Instead, they often responded to patient hostility with counterhostility or emotional disengagement.

Although his attention temporarily had been drawn to larger research issues, Strupp rediscovered the state of affairs that had surprised him in the 1950s, namely, the vulnerability of even highly experienced psychotherapists to being drawn into unproductive, hostile interactions with negativistic, mistrustful patients. In other words, Strupp again serendipitously discovered the great difficulty that therapists encounter in effectively managing what are now called therapeutic alliance "ruptures." The enormity of this difficulty was captured by the fact that analyses of the therapeutic dyads failed to identify a single instance in which a difficult patient's hostility and negativism were successfully confronted or resolved. A subsequent review of relevant clinical and empirical literatures at the time supported the proposition that therapists' negative reactions to difficult patients are far more common and far more intractable than had been generally recognized (Binder & Strupp, 1997). The extent of this difficulty and its enormous impact on therapeutic process were empirically demonstrated in a set of seminal studies conducted by Henry and his colleagues on patient–therapist dyads in the Vanderbilt I study (Henry, Schacht, & Strupp, 1986) and the later Vanderbilt II study (Henry, Schacht, & Strupp, 1990).

In the first of these studies, Henry et al. (1986) used the SASB (Structural Analysis of Social Behavior) process coding system (Benjamin, 1993) to reexamine the same eight Vanderbilt I case studies reported earlier by Strupp (1980a, 1980b, 1980c, 1980d). Henry et al.'s (1986) results confirmed Strupp's earlier observations regarding therapist hostility but did so in greater detail, and several surprising related findings emerged as well. The therapists engaged in quite different interpersonal behaviors with their good and poor outcome cases despite using similar surface techniques. Furthermore, the interpersonal processes linked with poor outcome cases were remarkably similar across therapists of diverse theoretical orientations. Patients in good outcome cases showed significantly more interpersonal processes indicative of open disclosure and affiliative expression, while the same therapists with their low outcome cases evidenced considerably more hostile control (e.g., blaming, subtly belittling the patient). Instances of "negative interpersonal complementarity" were significantly greater in the poor outcome cases while "positive complementarity" was higher in the good outcome dyads. Finally, "complex communications" (i.e., ones that simultaneously convey contradictory interpersonal processes such as acceptance and rejection) were almost exclusively a phenomena seen in poor outcome cases. Henry et al. (1990) supported these initial findings using a larger sample of 14 dyads, again split into good and poor outcome groups, and using cases drawn from the subsequent Vanderbilt II study (involving therapists who were not involved in Vanderbilt I).

NEGATIVE COMPLEMENTARITY: THE LEITMOTIF OF THE VANDERBILT STUDIES

Based on their analysis of the quantitative findings from the Vanderbilt I study as well as their extensive review of therapy session recordings from that study, Strupp and his colleagues concluded that the pursuit of evidence for the differential therapeutic benefits of relationship versus technical factors was a fruitless quest. Instead, he reconceptualized relationship and technical factors as inextricably interrelated. The therapeutic use of the patient–therapist relationship began to be viewed as a technique in and of itself, and the development and maintenance of a therapeutic alliance was seen as requiring a high level of technical skills. Strupp believed that these skills were not sufficiently recognized or appreciated in the ways psychoanalytic therapy was written about and taught at that time, as evidenced in the pervasive difficulties that the Vanderbilt I therapists encountered in managing negative transference and countertransference. This state of affairs was especially true in the area of short-term psychodynamic therapy. Since Strupp favored a psychodynamic approach, this was the type of treatment he wanted to study. The treatment, however, had to be short-term for practical reasons (e.g., limiting data to manageable amounts, research funding schedules).

The pioneering short-term dynamic psychotherapies that were developed during the 1960s and 1970s were characterized by a strategy of identifying a core unconscious conflict as a therapeutic focus and then interpreting the link between evidence of that focal conflict in the "transference" and supposed childhood origins of the conflict. Strupp and his research team hypothesized that if they developed a form of time-limited psychodynamic therapy that stressed the identification and management of "here-and-now" transference–countertransference patterns and that could be used to train experienced therapists, they could demonstrate that the problem of treating difficult patients could be overcome. Strupp and Jeffrey L. Binder, in particular, had been influenced by the writings of Merton Gill (1982), who had used object relations and interpersonal theories to reconceptualize transference and countertransference as inextricably intertwined actions in which a patient inevitably enacts within the therapeutic relationship a core maladaptive interpersonal pattern that evokes a reaction from the therapist that represents a role within the maladaptive interpersonal pattern. From the perspective of the therapeutic alliance, Gill's conception of transference and countertransference, as well as his corollary technical strategy, focused on the identification and resolution of therapeutic alliance ruptures.

Strupp and Binder (1984) applied object relations and interpersonal concepts and principles, as well as Gill's view of therapeutic process and technical strategies, to a planned time-limited format. They called the model time-limited dynamic psychotherapy (TLDP). The research team was convinced that this model of short-term treatment would be especially effective with the hostile, negativistic, mistrustful patients with whom even highly experienced therapists had been so ineffective in the Vanderbilt I studies. By the time Strupp and his research team were ready to design another study, it was necessary to use treatment manuals for any psychotherapy study to be supported by National Institute of Mental Health funds. The team was caught up in the enthusiasm for treatment manuals that had swept the psychotherapy research community and believed, like many other researchers, that such manuals would "revolutionize" therapy training. Accordingly, the team presumed that the use of state-of-the-art training methods (described in detail below), based on a TLDP manual, would be highly effective in training therapists to implement TLDP.

The Vanderbilt II study was designed to test the hypothesis that, compared to treatment as usual (as practiced by experienced psychiatrists and psychologists), a manual-guided training program that taught TLDP would result in the participating therapists' obtaining therapeutic outcomes superior to their treatment as usual, especially with relatively more difficult patients. The project received National Institute of Mental Health approval and funding in the early 1980s. The study was designed for the therapists to act as their own controls through the use of repeated data measurements obtained before and after the experimental component.

The study was conducted in three phases. In the first phase, 16 therapists each conducted two planned short-term therapies of up to 25 sessions using their usual treatment approach. This phase lasted until all of the treatments were completed or nearly so. The second phase consisted of a year-long training program (which will be described below). The third phase began after the completion of the training program and consisted of each therapist conducting two treatments using TLDP for up to 25 sessions. Patients were recruited from the Vanderbilt University Department of Psychiatry Outpatient Clinic as well as from a newspaper advertisement offering subsidized psychotherapy. The patients were screened by the research team, and those who met the study criteria were assigned to the participating therapists, who saw the patients in their private practice offices. The only exception to this arrangement was the videotaping of Sessions 3 and 16 in the Vanderbilt Center for Psychotherapy Research offices. All patients suffered from symptoms of anxiety and/or depression and had relationship problems. All had DSM-III Axis I diagnoses, and most had Axis II diagnoses. As part of the study design, in phases 1 and 3, respectively, each therapist was assigned a relatively good prognosis patient and a relatively poor prognosis patient, as evaluated by independent raters on a scale measuring "capacity for dynamic psychotherapy" (Thackrey, Butler, & Strupp, 1985). It was expected after TLDP training the therapists would evidence differentially more success with their poor prognosis patients as compared with pretraining outcomes.

The participating therapists were licensed clinical psychologists and psychiatrists who had reputations for competence and ethical practice in the local professional communities. The final group was composed of eight psychologists and eight psychiatrists with a combined mean postgraduate experience of 5.3 years. There were 10 men and 6 women. The research team's primary source of recommendations was senior faculty members from the Vanderbilt University departments of psychology and psychiatry, who had trained many of the clinicians that they recommended. Although Nashville, Tennessee is a midsized city with a substantial number of practicing psychotherapists and three major clinical training programs, Strupp and his team were concerned about being able to recruit and retain sufficient study participants. The team was particularly concerned about the risk of therapist attrition over the year-long training component. The practitioners' major incentives for participating in the project were the opportunity to discuss cases with Strupp and his team as well as their peers and to learn a new short-term treatment model. While these appeared to be strong incentives,

Strupp and his team were concerned that the time demands of the therapists' practices would jeopardize continuing involvement in the training program. This nervousness likely influenced the therapist selection strategy, which involved reliance solely on the recommendation of senior faculty members with no further evaluation of the therapists' actual performance skills (e.g., reviewing recordings of therapy sessions). It is even more likely that the team's apprehension about losing any of the participating therapists during the course of a rather long study contributed to a certain gingerly treatment of the therapists in the training groups. This factor probably played a larger role in Strupp's training groups, because he especially was concerned about possible attrition. Whether or not this concern about therapist attrition contributed to reducing any potential training effect remains a matter of speculation.

The Vanderbilt II Therapist "TLDP" Training Program

The training component of the study used methods that represented (and still do) prevalent models of graduate clinical education. The number of contact hours in the training (an average of 100) was equivalent to about two to three graduate semester courses. The therapists were divided into four training groups of four therapists each, with Hans Strupp and Jeffrey Binder (the authors of the treatment manual and senior clinicians on the research team) each leading two groups. The two primary criteria for choosing group memberships were (1) to balance the number of psychologists and psychiatrists in each training group and (2) to accommodate the therapists' varying schedules. The training lasted approximately 12 months and consisted of approximately 50 weekly 2-hour seminar and supervision sessions, which were audiotaped. The didactic component of each session involved the group leaders presenting TLDP principles and techniques that corresponded to sections of the manual that the therapists were asked to read. This part of the training session was routinely followed by clinical examples drawn from transcripts and audio- or videotapes of the seminar participants and the leaders/supervisors (Strupp, Binder, and postdoctoral members of the research team were conducting videorecorded therapies that were used as training materials). During the training period, each therapist conducted a therapy and received supervision in his or her training group. Audio- and videotaped recordings of the cases were discussed in detail by the group leaders and members to highlight TLDP principles and techniques. Records were not kept of attendance and punctuality; however, our recollections are that both were fairly good throughout the training program.

During the year-long training period, no attempt was made to evaluate its impact. In other words, unlike the typical manual-guided treatment research study conducted at that time, in which participating therapists were trained up to a predetermined level of technical adherence before commencing the treatment to be evaluated, Vanderbilt II was designed for the unique purpose of evaluating the processes and impact of the training itself. Consequently, all process and outcome assessments were conducted *after* the training phase

The participating therapists received their formal clinical training during a period when teaching psychotherapy skills was an important part of both clinical psychology and psychiatry training programs and the majority of psychiatry programs were psychoanalytically oriented. Consequently, the participating psychiatrists typically practiced what they considered to be psychoanalytically oriented therapy (although their personal styles produced treatments that varied widely in appearance), and the participating clinical psychologists practiced a variety of psychodynamic, client-centered, and eclectic treatment approaches. In sum, while the therapists varied widely in their individual styles, their basic principles and methods of doing therapy overlapped substantially. Consequently, these therapists and the project trainers more or less explicitly agreed that a secondary training goal would be to heighten the therapists' sensibilities to the basic therapy knowledge and skills they already possessed. The primary training goal was to add to their existing therapeutic knowledge and skills a short-term approach to conducting a specific form of psychodynamic-interpersonal therapy. Knowledge largely new to these therapists consisted of concepts and principles from interpersonal and object relations theories of personality and psychopathology and contemporary ideas about the roles of transference and countertransference in therapeutic process as well as strategies for exploring and interpreting transference. Skills with which some of the therapists may have been familiar but which none of them had used consistently included (1) case formulation based on a salient recurrent maladaptive interpersonal pattern; (2) consistently exploring the identified maladaptive pattern within and across sessions; (3) stressing exploration of the maladaptive pattern as a transference–countertransference enactment; (4) self-monitoring and limiting one's own participation in the maladaptive pattern; and (5) exploring the influence of the maladaptive pattern on how the patient experiences and reacts to termination.

The training program stressed (1) the refinement of generic therapy technical skills that all parties presumed were already possessed by the therapists and (2) the acquisition of new technical skills associated with TLDP. The generic skills were represented in the items composing one of two subscales of the adherence measure constructed to assess the impact of the training program on the therapists' conduct of their posttraining treatments (Butler, Henry, & Strupp, 1995). These items emphasized attentive listening, encouraging a detailed and focused line of inquiry into the patient's subjective experiences, and collaborative work. TLDP-specific items focused on exploring the patient's experience of and reactions to the patient–therapist relationship and the person of the therapist as well as identifying and tracking a salient and maladaptive interpersonal theme, especially as it was enacted in the patient–therapist relationship.

Results of the "TLDP" Therapist Training Program

After training, the ratings of therapists' behavior showed a considerable increase in technical adherence to TLDP but no noteworthy increase in general interviewing skill (Henry, Strupp, Butler, Schacht, & Binder, 1993). This impact on therapist performance, however, was temporary and disappeared after about 16 sessions. A completely unexpected and problematic finding appeared in the ratings of the quality of the patient–therapist relationships. After training, the therapists appeared more hostile toward their patients, as reflected in more "complex" communications (as rated on the SASB coding system). This increase in hostility was attributable to increased verbal activity by the therapists rather than an increase in the proportion of hostile communications. Another indication of posttraining deterioration in the quality of the therapist–patient relationships was the ratings of the therapists' attitudes toward their patients. They were judged to be significantly less optimistic, less supportive, spent less time exploring patients' feelings, and were more authoritarian. The therapists also tended to show less overt approval of their patients and were more defensive (Henry et al., 1993). In other words, the TLDP training appeared to have contributed to at least a temporary deterioration in the ability of the therapists to establish a positive therapeutic alliance.

CONCLUSIONS FROM THE VANDERBILT II STUDY

The posttraining (phase 3) findings led Strupp and his research team to the unavoidable conclusion that they had significantly overestimated the impact that the training program would have on enhancing the therapists' skills. In particular, they had to face the fact that the training program appeared to have in some respects caused at least a temporary deterioration in the therapists' abilities to manage negative therapeutic process, which was precisely the component of therapist performance they had expected to most favorably affect.

The Vanderbilt II study was designed around 1980, and almost 30 years of subsequent psychotherapy process/outcome research, as well as clinical experience, contributed to hindsight concerning two basic assumptions that were the conceptual foundation of Vanderbilt II and that turned out probably to be erroneous.

The first assumption was that even in short-term psychodynamic therapy more or less significant difficulties in the patient–therapist relationship would always occur and these difficulties would be in the form of transference–countertransference enactments that reflected whatever salient interpersonal theme should be the focus of treatment. In other words, using the common definition of therapeutic alliance rupture as a transference–countertransference enactment, TLDP was based on the principle that most therapy sessions would have a therapeutically significant alliance rupture. A corollary assumption was that the most effective therapist strategy for managing alliance ruptures would be consistent interpretation of the transference. Years of subsequent clinical experience has led at least some of us from the Vanderbilt II research team to conclude that in short-term psychodynamic therapy indications in the clinical material of transference (that is, significant therapeutic alliance ruptures), and particularly of transference representing the thematic therapeutic focus, are sparse unless the patient has a severe personality disorder (Binder, 2004). Consistent with this clinical impression is solid evidence accumulated over the past decade that in short-term psychodynamic therapy a technical strategy based on high "doses" (it is convention to define "high doses" as more than four interventions per session) of transference interpretations tend to be negatively correlated with treatment outcome and that even lower doses of transference interpretations are effective only with some patients. Furthermore, short-term psychodynamic therapy patients with relatively high levels of interpersonal relating (who, therefore, are less prone to contributing to therapeutic alliance ruptures) tend to have good treatment outcomes regardless of whether transference interpretations are ever made (Hoglend et al., 2006; Hoglend et al., 2008). The serendipitous Vanderbilt II findings are, in fact, consistent with this research on transference-focused versus nontransference-focused short-term psychodynamic therapies. In Vanderbilt II, treatment outcomes were more or less equivalent before and after training, even though posttraining there was a significant technical shift toward more actively attempting to interpret transference.

Adherence to prescribed techniques, however, is only one of a set of skills that makes up therapy competence (Schaffer, 1983). Two researchers (Edward Bein and Timothy Anderson) who were not members of the team during the years in which the study took place later evaluated the Vanderbilt II therapists' performances and concluded that 14 of the 16 therapists had not demonstrated in their posttraining cases that they had achieved competence in conducting TLDP (Bein et al., 2000). When the Vanderbilt II therapists attempted to implement TLDP-specific techniques, they would sometimes ask about the therapeutic relationship "out of the blue," make hasty transference interpretations without a context of clinical material that would make the comments meaningful to the patient, persist in focusing on the patient–therapist relationship even when the patient did not appear to understand the purpose, and appear unsure of how to follow up with transference interpretations.

Bein et al. (2000) argued that in the posttraining cases outcomes were not enhanced because the training program had been inadequate, resulting in therapists providing inadequate versions of TLDP. While training problems may have contributed to the results of Vanderbilt II (we will address the issue of training below), we believe that another significant reason the therapists strained and stumbled in their attempts to incorporate systematic transference analysis into their technical repertoire is because a sizable percentage of patients in short-term psychodynamic therapy do not manifest transference of sufficient intensity to have a noticeable impact on the therapeutic relationship. Consequently, in these treatments, therapeutic alliance ruptures are not evident, and corresponding transference material is not available for interpretation. If the therapist tries to focus on finding and interpreting transference enactments, he or she runs the risk of confusing the patient and appearing to strain at trying to create something out of nothing.

When designing the Vanderbilt II study, the second assumption made by the research team was that the therapy training methods typically employed by graduate programs in psychology and psychiatry, as well as recommended in manual-guided research programs, were reasonably effective. We believe this assumption is widely held by psychotherapy researchers and teachers. It has far-reaching consequences, because it reduces the incentive to study the effectiveness of current therapy training methods, develop new methods, and compare these new methods with the ways in which therapists are currently trained. Indicative of how research on training methods has been neglected is the absence since 1986 of a chapter on this topic in Bergin and Garfield's classic *Handbook of Psychotherapy and Behavioral Change* (Lambert, 2004). Without a solid foundation of empirical findings, the belief that our typical psychotherapy training methods are effective is no more than a "myth" (Bickman, 1999). Certainly, the Vanderbilt II study, which to our knowledge is the only major study that has focused primarily on the impact of training, did not provide encouraging evidence.

As the research team began to look at the data, we became increasingly impressed with the complex interactions between therapist personality characteristics, training methods, and training content. The senior clinicians on the team realized that we had no coherent pedagogic theory to guide our training efforts because no such theory existed at the time— and, to our knowledge still doesn't. Psychotherapy teachers rely far too much on stretching clinical theories and concepts to provide a conceptual framework for therapy training, as exemplified by the relative neglect in discussions of the contribution to therapeutic alliance ruptures of therapist technical errors in comparison to the emphasis placed on therapist countertransference. An example of how training therapists involves figuratively "flying by the seat of your pants" is the difference in training styles between Hans Strupp and Jeffrey Binder. Strupp had a relatively nondirective style and focused primarily on general issues and patient dynamics, while Binder had a relatively more directive and detail-oriented style and focused primarily on the rationale behind therapists' actions. These differences in training styles were the unwitting products of the trainers' respective personalities and of their prior experiences as trainers and as trainees. Any personal theories of psychotherapy training that they had developed over the years were limited to having only a tacit influence on their training strategies.

Systematic review of recordings of a representative sampling of the training sessions revealed the differences in Strupp's and Binder's training styles were significantly associated with at least temporary enhancement of one fundamental therapeutic skill, namely, adherence to prescribed techniques. The therapists in Binder's training groups accounted for most of the use of TLDP-specific techniques after training (Henry, Schacht, Strupp, Butler, & Binder, 1993). Another variable that contributed to the therapists' receptiveness to the technical portion of the TLDP training was their self-treatment as measured by the SASB Intrex (the self-report version of the Structural Analysis of Social Behavior coding system; Benjamin, 1993). Approximately one-third of the therapists yielded Intrex ratings that indicated "hostile self-control/self-criticism." For reasons that are still unexplained, these therapists tended to show greater adherence to TLDP techniques after training.

Unfortunately, even the therapists in Binder's training groups tended to revert back to their usual ways of conducting therapy by the 16th session. Perhaps the therapists were not exposed to the training for a sufficient period of time to fully incorporate the new techniques into their established technique repertoire. We suspect that a major reason is that we overgeneralized the application of a transference-focused technical strategy. In any event, we believe that a more structured approach focused on the trainee's affective reactions and thought processes leading to action is a promising pedagogic strategy at least for facilitating a therapist trainee's acquisition and use of prescribed techniques. Accordingly, we recommend that trainers/ supervisors should:

1. Designate specific learning tasks for each training/supervision session (e.g., identifying and addressing subtle indications of the patient's avoidance of a relevant issue).
2. When reviewing a recorded treatment session, focus on specific

patient–therapist interactions that appear to reflect more general interpersonal patterns that characterize the session and/or the therapy.
3. Use recorded therapeutic interactions to illustrate important theoretical concepts and principles.
4. Focus on the trainee's performance rather than patient dynamics, posing questions about the trainee's affective reactions and thought processes and how these influence his or her understanding of and interactions with the patient, the trainee's understanding of the immediate therapeutic process, and the rationale for the trainee's actions.
5. Give the trainee precise feedback about his or her actions that acknowledges good performance and that constructively critiques problematic or deficient performance (Binder, 2004).

We believe that the findings from the Vanderbilt II study with the most far-reaching consequences for psychotherapy training were the lack of evidence that the therapists improved their ability to identify and manage interactions that reflected patient dissatisfaction, mistrust, emotional disengagement, or outright hostility. In other words, the project focused on improving therapist skills in identifying and managing therapist alliance strains and ruptures, and it was somewhat successful in getting the therapists to use techniques that we thought would achieve this goal; but, ultimately the therapists demonstrated no increase in skills at managing alliance ruptures.

Our experiences in the training sessions provided clear indications that Strupp and Binder successfully sensitized the therapists to the occurrence of negative processes in the interactions with their patients. The therapists learned to articulately discuss the concepts of transference and countertransference, and they demonstrated increasing skill in identifying clinical illustrations of these phenomena when watching video recordings of their peers and of themselves conducting therapy. The therapists' skills at actually managing negative therapeutic interactions, however, appeared to be mostly limited to retrospective critiques of video recordings. The gap between their increased appreciation and conceptual understanding of negative therapeutic process and their ability to actually manage it in the moment ironically appeared to have left the therapists, after training, increasingly suspicious and wary of their patients. Consequently, not only had the therapists not acquired the technical skills to effectively manage therapeutic alliance ruptures; but also, after training, their increased appreciation of the possibility of alliance ruptures appeared to have reduced the sorts of positive sentiments toward their patients that are the bedrock of the affective bond component of a good therapeutic alliance.

THE SEARCH FOR IMPROVED METHODS
OF PSYCHOTHERAPY TRAINING

The research team members responded to the discouraging findings as another instance of the Vanderbilt team's proclivity for making serendipitous discoveries. To try to understand the nature and causes of the deficiencies that we discovered in our therapist training, we first consulted a colleague at Vanderbilt University, John Bransford, who is a cognitive scientist well known in the area of instructional psychology. He introduced us to the issue of "inert knowledge," that is, conceptual knowledge (e.g., knowledge about therapy techniques and principles for using them) that is divorced from ingrained guidelines for spontaneously accessing this knowledge in real-world situations where its application would be highly useful. For example, a therapist trainee whose knowledge of psychotherapy has been acquired solely through coursework and viewing recordings of other people conducting therapy may have a large fund of "declarative" knowledge (i.e., conceptual knowledge) but relatively little if any "procedural" knowledge (i.e., the spontaneous application of relevant knowledge under actual clinical circumstances). In order to overcome the problem of "inert" knowledge, Bransford and his colleagues developed a learning environment called "anchored instruction," in which students learn basic facts, concepts, and principles in environments that more or less simulate real-world circumstances where the knowledge acquired would be practically useful (Bransford, Franks, Vye, & Sherwood, 1989). We realized that the typical psychotherapy training curriculum in which the trainee abruptly transitions from coursework to seeing actual patients promotes the maintenance of "inert" knowledge about psychotherapy and, consequently, is a very inefficient method for facilitating the acquisition of therapy skills (Binder, 1993).

We discovered the areas of the cognitive sciences concerned with studying the nature and development of complex performance skills and studying methods for effectively teaching these skills across various performance domains (e.g., Ericsson, Charness, Feltovich, & Hoffman, 2006). We became particularly interested in evidence for the role of "deliberate practice" in the attainment of expertise in any complex performance domain (Ericsson, Drampe, & Tesch-Romer, 1993). Deliberate practice consists of three components: (1) performance of well-defined tasks at an appropriate level of difficulty; (2) immediate and informative feedback; and (3) opportunities for repetition and correction of performance errors. Trainees in many complex performance domains clearly engage in deliberate practice, with music and athletics being perhaps the most clear-cut examples. Other domains, however, such as laboratory research and to an increasing extent medicine also are incorporating the principles of deliberate practice. Trainees in these domains practice the components of complex performances in simulated real-world settings before having to actually perform similar tasks in real life. A novice musician would not take courses in music theory and then go directly to performing on stage. Yet, the predominant format of psychotherapy training requires the trainee to go directly from coursework to seeing real patients. No matter how talented the supervisor, the supervision of real patients only minimally approximates the requirements of "deliberate practice" (Binder, 1993, 1999).

As we learned more about the nature of expertise in complex performances like psychotherapy, we realized that we had not successfully facilitated the therapists' acquisition or refinement of two fundamental generic skills: interpersonal pattern recognition and self-monitoring of ongoing performance. These skills appear to be especially important for effectively managing therapeutic alliance ruptures. Our training methods (perhaps including the length of the training program) had not improved the therapists' ability to "reflect-in-action," (Schön, 1983) that is, in the course of therapeutic interactions to stand back and identify any negative processes and to monitor one's own responses to them. Similarly, as we learned more about methods for training complex performance skills, we began to envision a new and improved format for psychotherapy training.

This format would address the issue of inert knowledge by using computer-generated virtual reality environments to create simulations of any desired therapeutic situation (e.g., different forms of therapeutic alliance confrontation or withdrawal ruptures). Interactive computer technologies would be used to link the trainee and a supervisor/coach with the virtual reality environment. The software for this technology would consist of video-recorded vignettes of real therapy interactions that can be artificially elaborated by using avatars (i.e., lifelike simulations of people based on digital recordings of real people). A specific clinical situation would have a root vignette along with several alternative consequent narrative sequences. These alternatives would illustrate the consequences of productive or unproductive interventions by the trainee. The choice of which alternative narrative would be the most likely consequence of the trainee's intervention would be decided by a supervisor/coach, who would activate that narrative for the trainee to experience. If the consequent narrative illustrated an unproductive intervention, the trainee would receive feedback from the supervisor, and they would discuss it. Then, the trainee would have the opportunity to repeat the situation in the root vignette and again intervene. This iterative process would continue until the trainee demonstrated enhanced understanding of and skill in managing the particular clinical situation.

While the components of psychotherapy theories could be introduced in didactic formats, they could be practically understood by applying them in this simulated clinical environment. These practice environments could be laboratory components of psychotherapy courses in formal training programs as well as laboratory components of manual-guided research projects that include a training program. Students (or research project therapists) could demonstrate a certain proficiency with the therapy skills to be acquired before they tried them out with real patients.

We must confess that these suggestions for improving the training of therapists, including training in the skills necessary for managing therapeutic alliance ruptures, are limited to untested speculation. There have been earlier proposals to pilot and test this technology with psychotherapy training (Beutler & Harwood, 2004; Binder, 1993, 1999), but to our knowledge these proposals have not yet been acted on. Doing so would be a natural next step for the Vanderbilt Research Team. Unfortunately, our original leader, Hans Strupp, is no longer with us, and the team disbanded years ago. Individual members of the team (such as Jeffrey Binder, William Henry, and Timothy Anderson) plan to explore some of these proposals. However, we urge other researchers who may have the resources to mount full-scale development efforts to seriously investigate the psychotherapy training potential associated with relevant theories from the cognitive sciences and with the virtual reality technology available to implement proposed new training formats.

REFERENCES

Bein, E., Anderson, T., Strupp, H. H., Schacht, T. E., Biner, J. L., & Butler, S. F. (2000). The effects of training in time-limited dynamic psychotherapy: Changes in therapeutic outcome. *Psychotherapy Research, 10*, 119–132.

Benjamin, L. S. (1993). *Interpersonal diagnosis and treatment of personality disorders*. New York: Guilford Press.

Beutler, L. E., & Harwood, T. M. (2004). Virtual reality in psychotherapy training. *Journal of Clinical Psychology, 60*, 317–330..

Bickman, L. (1999). Practice makes perfect and other myths about mental health services. *American Psychologist, 54*, 965–978.

Binder, J. L. (1993). Is it time to improve psychotherapy training? *Clinical Psychology Review, 13*, 301–318.

Binder, J. L. (1999). Issues in teaching and learning time-limited dynamic psychotherapy. *Clinical Psychology Review, 19*, 705–719.

Binder, J. L. (2004). *Key competencies in brief dynamic psychotherapy. Clinical practice beyond the manual.* New York: Guilford Press.

Binder, J. L., & Strupp, H. H. (1997). "Negative process": A recurrently discovered and underestimated facet of therapeutic process and outcome in the individual psychotherapy of adults. *Clinical Psychology: Science and Practice, 4*, 121–139.

Bransford, J. D., Franks, J. J., Vye, N. J., & Sherwood, R. D. (1989). New approaches to instruction: Because wisdom can't be told. In S. Vosniadou & A. Ortony

(Eds.), *Similarity and analogical reasoning* (pp. 470–497). New York: Cambridge University Press.

Butler, S. F., Henry, W. P., & Strupp, H. H. (1995). Measuring adherence in time-limited dynamic psychotherapy. *Psychotherapy, 32,* 629–638.

Ericsson, K. A., Charness, N., Feltovich, P. J., & Hoffman, R. R. (Eds.). (2006). *The Cambridge handbook of expertise and expert performance.* New York: Cambridge University Press.

Ericsson, K. A., Drampe, R. T., & Tesch-Romer, C. (1993). The role of deliberate practice in the acquisition of expert performance. *Psychological Review, 100,* 363–406.

Gill, M. M. (1982). *The analysis of transference I: Theory and technique.* New York: International Universities Press.

Henry, W. P., Schacht, T. E., & Strupp, H. H. (1986). Structural analysis of social behavior: Application to a study of interpersonal process in differential psychotherapeutic outcome. *Journal of Consulting and Clinical Psychology, 54,* 27–31.

Henry, W. P., Schacht, T. E., & Strupp, H. H. (1990). Patient and therapist introject, interpersonal process, and differential psychotherapy outcome. *Journal of Consulting and Clinical Psychology, 58,* 768–774.

Henry, W. P., Schacht, T. E., Strupp, H. H., Butler, S. F., & Binder, J. L. (1993). Effects of training in time-limited dynamic psychotherapy: Mediators of therapists' responses to training. *Journal of Consulting and Clinical Psychology, 61,* 441–447.

Henry, W. P., Strupp, H. H., Butler, S. F., Schacht, T. E., & Binder, J. L. (1993). Effects of training in time-limited dynamic psychotherapy: Changes in therapist behavior. *Journal of Consulting and Clinical Psychology, 61,* 434–440.

Hoglend, P., Amlo, S., Marble, A., Bøgwald, K. P., Sørbye, Ø., & Sjaastad, M. C. (2006). Analysis of the patient–therapist relationship in dynamic psychotherapy: An experimental study of transference interpretations. *American Journal of Psychiatry, 163,* 1739–1746.

Hoglend, P., Bøgwald, K. P., Amlo, A., Marble, A., Ulberg, R., & Sjaastad, M. C. (2008). Transference interpretations in dynamic psychotherapy: Do they really yield sustained effects? *American Journal of Psychiatry, 165,* 763–771.

Lambert, M. J. (Ed.). *Bergin and Garfield's handbook of psychotherapy and behavior change* (5th ed.). New York: Wiley.

Schaffer, N. D. (1983). Methodological issues of measuring the skillfulness of therapeutic technique. *Psychotherapy, 20,* 486–493.

Schön, D. A. (1983). *The reflective practitioner.* New York: Basic Books.

Strupp, H. H. (1958). The psychotherapist's contribution to the treatment process. *Behavioral Science, 3,* 34–67.

Strupp, H. H. (1960). Nature of psychotherapist's contribution to treatment process: Some research results and speculations. *Archives of General Psychiatry, 3,* 219–231.

Strupp, H. H. (1980a). Success and failure in time-limited psychotherapy: A systematic comparison of two cases (Comparison 1). *Archives of General Psychiatry, 37,* 595–603.

Strupp, H. H. (1980b). Success and failure in time-limited psychotherapy: A systematic comparison of two cases (Comparison 2). *Archives of General Psychiatry*, *37*, 708–716.

Strupp, H. H. (1980c). Success and failure in time-limited psychotherapy: With special reference to the performance of a lay counselor (Comparison 3). *Archives of General Psychiatry*, *37*, 831–841.

Strupp, H. H. (1980d). Success and failure in time-limited psychotherapy: A systematic comparison of two cases (Comparison 4). *Archives of General Psychiatry*, *37*, 947–954.

Strupp, H. H., & Binder, J. L. (1984). *Psychotherapy in a new key. A guide to time-limited dynamic psychotherapy*. New York: Basic Books.

Strupp, H. H., & Hadley, S. W. (1979). Specific versus nonspecific factors in psychotherapy: A controlled study of outcome. *Archives of General Psychiatry*, *36*, 1125–1136.

Thackrey, M., Butler, S. F., & Strupp, H. H. (1985, June). *Measurement of patient capacity for dynamic press*. Paper presented at the annual meeting of the Society for Psychotherapy Research, Evanston, IL.

CHAPTER 15

■ ■ ■ ■ ■

Training in Alliance-Fostering Techniques

Paul Crits-Christoph
Katherine Crits-Christoph
Mary Beth Connolly Gibbons

BACKGROUND AND RATIONALE
FOR ALLIANCE-FOSTERING PSYCHOTHERAPY

In 1994 our research group at the University of Pennsylvania was contemplating ways to examine empirically the role of the patient–therapist alliance in psychotherapy. Meta-analytic studies (Horvath & Symonds, 1991, and later Martin, Garske, & Davis, 2000) had documented consistent correlations between the quality of the alliance and psychotherapy outcome across a diverse range of psychotherapies. Such correlations, of course, do not prove causality. A number of "third variables" might be responsible for the correlational links between the alliance and outcome. For example, patients who improve over the course of the initial one or two psychotherapy sessions would likely both rate their therapeutic relationship more positively and achieve relatively better treatment outcomes (Barber, Connolly Gibbons, Crits-Christoph, Gladis, & Siqueland, 2000). In addition, several studies had indicated that patient pretreatment variables predict the quality of the alliance (e.g., Connolly et al., 2003; Mallinckrodt, Coble, & Gantt, 1995; Muran, Segal, Samstag, & Crawford, 1994; Piper et al., 1991). To the extent that the alliance is a function of what the patient brings to therapy, not what happens in therapy, the alliance concept would have little relevance to the conduct of psychotherapy or the training of psychotherapists other than to warn therapists that poor alliances happen with some patients.

Based on the logic above, we reasoned that what was needed were studies that documented whether or not the alliance can be influenced by therapist behaviors. If certain therapist interventions could produce relatively better alliances, then the alliance concept would be highly relevant to the teaching of psychotherapy and models of psychotherapy. Our initial thoughts about how to test this empirically led to a proposal to compare one treatment condition in which therapists (randomly assigned) have been trained to enhance the alliance to another treatment condition in which therapists were not trained to enhance the alliance. Feedback from grant reviewers raised the question of whether it would make more sense to ask a preliminary question: Can therapists be successfully trained to enhance the alliance? If therapists could not be trained to improve their alliances, then an experimental test of high alliance versus typical alliance would not be possible. Based on this feedback, we redesigned the study as a training study to see if we could improve average therapists' alliances.

In order to conduct such a study, a treatment manual was a necessity, and accordingly we created our alliance-fostering psychotherapy manual in preparation for the study. The treatment manual was a collaboration between researchers familiar with the alliance literature and a senior clinician/supervisor who had extensive experience in training therapists in psychotherapy studies. Potential alliance-enhancing techniques were drawn from both the clinical and research literature, but with a primary emphasis on the research literature. In particular, we drew therapy elements from a variety of existing psychotherapies, including an emphasis on such concepts as empathy and positive regard from client-centered therapy (Rogers, 1957) and motivational enhancement therapy (MET) (Miller & Rollnick, 1991). The supportive principles described by Luborsky (1984) were a central part of the approach.

To guide the overall concept of the alliance-fostering manual, we relied on the definition of the alliance articulated by Bordin (1979). This definition consists of three alliance components: agreement on tasks, agreement on goals, and therapeutic bond. An existing comprehensive review of the research literature on aspects of the therapeutic bond that predict outcome (Orlinsky, Grawe, & Parks, 1994) was a useful resource for extracting techniques related to the bond component. To establish agreement on tasks and goals during the course of psychotherapy the concept of collaborative stance was helpful, but we believed that further clinical strategies were needed to evaluate and enhance this aspect of the alliance (as described in the next section).

While the alliance has been found to be relevant to treatment outcome across a wide range of disorders, in designing our study of alliance-fostering psychotherapy it was important to focus on one particular disorder. The rationale for focusing on one clinical disorder was twofold: (1) by limiting variability in the alliance that might be due to disorder (e.g., certain personality disorders like borderline personality disorder might be expected to have chaotic and sometimes highly negative alliances), the likelihood of achieving a training effect on the alliance would be greater (this is particularly true for small sample size pilot studies where one or two cases might influence the overall results); and (2) results of the study could more easily be compared to studies in the literature.

We chose major depressive disorder (MDD) as the focus for our alliance-fostering therapy. MDD was chosen because many of the studies in the literature linking alliance to outcome targeted MDD patients. Thus, by choosing MDD, we could be more confident that enhancing the alliance would produce better outcomes. A second reason that we chose MDD was that this disorder has high prevalence and therefore any study results would have greater generalizability to typical clinical practice.

In creating a treatment manual that has the clinical goal of enhancing the alliance, it was also important to make the treatment approach credible. Our concern was that, if psychotherapists only focused directly on the alliance, patients would not experience the treatment as relevant to their specific problems and goals. The history of the development of other psychotherapy approaches informed our decision on this issue. For example, the techniques of client-centered therapy—a therapy that overlaps considerably with our alliance-fostering approach—were originally outlined by Rogers (1951) as primarily consisting of empathy, unconditional positive regard, and genuineness. However, subsequent conceptualizations of client-centered therapy expanded beyond Rogers's original model to include other techniques that focus on specific therapy tasks and client goals (Rice, 1984). Similarly, MET is a treatment model that borrows alliance-enhancing techniques from client-centered therapy (e.g., empathy, positive regard) but adds further techniques that go beyond just the establishment of rapport with the patient (e.g., an increase in the client's awareness of a discrepancy between where his or her life is currently vs. where he or she wants it to be in the future, eliciting client discussion about positive change).

To address this concern, we formulated our alliance-fostering approach as a group of techniques that could be "grafted" onto a variety of diverse psychotherapies. For our planned study, we made the decision to "graft" the alliance-fostering techniques onto a version of Luborsky's (1984), an interpersonally oriented psychodynamic therapy (supportive–expressive therapy). This combination was a natural "fit," given that, as mentioned, the alliance-fostering techniques were drawn in part from supportive–expressive therapy. Moreover, we had previously conducted a study that documented a strong relationship between the central technique of supportive–expressive therapy—interpretation of repetitive maladaptive interpersonal themes— and the development of the alliance over the course of psychotherapy (Crits-Christoph, Barber, & Kurcias, 1993). Thus, we had an empirical basis for including interpretation of relationship themes within our treatment manual for alliance-fostering therapy. Furthermore, our clinical trainers were highly experienced in training therapists in supportive–expressive therapy, and therefore we expected the integration of the two sets of techniques to be seamless from a conceptual and practical viewpoint.

SUMMARY OF THE TREATMENT MODEL

The alliance-fostering treatment was specified as a 16-session brief therapy. Sessions were held once per week and lasted for 50 minutes. The basic orientation of the treatment approach generally followed an interpersonal– psychodynamic stance, although with a relatively active therapeutic style characteristic of brief interpersonal and psychodynamic therapies. However, the beginning of the manual (P. Crits-Christoph & K. Crits-Christoph, 1998) makes clear to the reader (e.g., therapist in training) that the manual is an integrative model that goes beyond traditional brief psychodynamic and interpersonal models to include some active techniques for fostering the alliance.

As mentioned, the treatment was designed as a therapy for major depressive disorder. Thus, an early section of the manual orients the therapist-in-training to basic information about major depressive disorder. This section is followed by another providing a rationale for why greater attention to fostering the alliance may be able to achieve enhanced outcomes in the treatment of major depressive disorder.

Beyond these introductory sections, our alliance-fostering treatment manual is organized around general principles for fostering the alliance that are illustrated with examples. The general principles are presented in terms of the three main components of the alliance as articulated by Bordin (1979): agreement on goals, agreement on tasks, and the therapeutic bond.

Agreement on Goals and Tasks

The primary techniques designed to maximize agreement on goals are (1) establishing explicit goals and (2) regularly reviewing the goals in subsequent sessions. Establishing goals is done as described in many brief therapies, particularly by Luborsky (1984). Regularly reviewing the goals occurs at the beginning of each session (after goals are established, generally in Session 1 or 2). A suggested therapist approach to reviewing goals is given in the following example:

> "Last time we came up with some goals. These were [name them]. I want to review these with you to see if anything has changed. Sometimes people change their perspective on their goals, or therapy or other events in life lead to new goals or reprioritizing goals. Do you still feel these should be your goals?"

In regard to agreement on the tasks of therapy, alliance-fostering psychotherapy uses an initial socialization process, conducted during the first one or two sessions, to orient the patient to the general tasks of treatment. While this approach provides a relatively high likelihood that there is initial agreement on the tasks of therapy, therapists are instructed to review tasks regularly (approximately every other session) and assess whether there is still agreement with the patient about such tasks. This review can be initiated by asking a general question to see what is on the patient's mind about the tasks of therapy:

> "How have you been feeling about the work that we are doing?"

If the therapist has a sense that there might be an emerging lack of agreement on tasks, the following suggested comment is cited in the manual:

> "At the beginning of therapy, we talked about different aspects of therapy and how it goes. What are your thoughts at this point about what is most useful about therapy for you? Do you think we should modify therapy at this point to meet your needs?"

The therapist's aim is to have a clear sense of what the patient finds helpful and not helpful in the therapy. Some discussion about these issues is likely warranted if any disagreements are evident. After eliciting and understanding the patient's views of therapeutic tasks, the therapist makes a statement like the following:

> "So, it looks like we agree, then, that the best way for us to proceed is. ... "

This type of wording communicates that there is mutual agreement and that the therapist will proceed with treatment in a way that is accords with the patient's views.

Therapeutic Bond

For the patient–therapist bond element of the alliance, we relied upon the list of techniques provided by Orlinsky et al. (1994) that were thought to enhance the bond. These techniques include personal role involvement, interactive coordination, communicative contact, and mutual affirmation. In our manual, we address personal role involvement by first evaluating the patient's motivation for change and then, if needed, using techniques to enhance motivation drawn from the stages of change model (Prochaska & DiClemente, 1984). The initial focus in therapy for patients who are unaware that there is a problem that needs to be changed is to review the costs of depression to the patient empathically, to increase the motivation for treatment. As treatment progresses, therapists must closely monitor patient involvement in the process of treatment in terms of their attentiveness and activity level.

Two approaches are used to help establish a collaborative climate for therapy ("interactive coordination"). One approach involves the general empathic stance of the therapist, with empathy being demonstrated by the therapist's communicating that he or she understands the patient's experiences, feelings, and behavior. Thus, in this approach simple reflective clarifications are used with relatively high frequency. Empathy is also communicated by accurately addressing the patient's core conflictual relationship theme (discussed at greater length). A second way of establishing a collaborative climate is by frequently using the word "we" (or other words suggestive of working together as a team) during sessions or collaborating on a role play with the patient to establish a "we" bond. An example of a statement that communicates this type of teamwork is "Let's work together and figure out where to go next—what are your thoughts?" Generally, the therapist in alliance-fostering therapy is encouraged to use the words "we," "us" or "let's" several times in every session. For example, the therapist can introduce new topics or agenda items using the team concept thusly:

> "I thought we might spend some time reviewing your progress on your goals."

When important issues come up in sessions, the therapist can use the team concept as one way to explore the issue in greater depth, for example:

> "You said you've been getting angry at your spouse. Why don't we look at that more closely."

Another important aspect of enhancing the bond, as described by Orlinsky et al. (1994), is simply maintaining communicative contact. In alliance-fostering therapy this type of bonding is facilitated by using a conversational style (i.e., a back-and-forth discussion, but avoiding being "chatty" and unfocused), making repeated acknowledgments that the patient is being "heard," and frequently using reflective clarifications. Often, however, communicative contact might be ruptured during a session, at times evidenced by verbal or nonverbal distancing by the patient. In these situations, the therapist works to have the patient express his or her underlying feelings, such as anger or anxiety, and the interpersonal issues connected to them in an empathic and accepting climate—so that the patient no longer feels the need to distance him- or herself. Another common issue is that a patient may appear connected but may not really be bringing up relevant material. In these situations, the therapist simply asks the patient how the therapist can help the patient raise more emotionally meaningful issues.

A final approach to enhancing the bond is mutual affirmation, which is defined as a sense of caring, respect, acceptance, warmth, and positive regard. The manual for alliance-fostering psychotherapy instructs the therapist to enhance mutual affirmation through such nonverbal signs or signals as smiling, leaning forward, with facial expressions exhibiting interest and respect, as well as the tone of one's voice and the verbal content specifically noting positive attributes and changes.

Addressing Core Conflictual Relationship Themes

As already noted, for our own purposes, we largely "grafted" the foregoing alliance-fostering techniques onto supportive–expressive psychotherapy (Luborsky, 1984). Drawing upon the central technical strategy of supportive–expressive psychotherapy, the alliance-fostering therapy manual includes a section on learning how to formulate and address Core Conflictual Relationship Theme (CCRT) patterns (Luborsky & Crits-Christoph, 1998). The CCRT is a method for formulating interpersonal issues in terms of the patient's main wishes or needs expressed toward others, the responses of others toward the patient, and the subsequent responses of the patient. Details on how to formulate and interpret CCRT patterns were taken from Luborsky's (1984) manual.

There were three reasons why interpretation of CCRT patterns was a useful addition to the alliance-fostering therapy manual. To begin with, a core aspect of the alliance-fostering approach is therapist empathy, and patients typically experience accurate CCRT interpretations as empathic, supportive statements. In fact, accurate CCRT interpretations have been demonstrated to lead to increases in the alliance over time (Crits-Christoph et al., 1993). A second reason for including CCRT interpretations in the alliance-fostering manual was the felt need to have more of an agenda than merely focusing solely on the alliance. The other alliance-building techniques (enhancing the bond, reviewing goals, and reviewing the tasks of therapy), in themselves, are not likely to be compelling as a "therapy" for many patients. A related final reason to include CCRT interpretations was that they provided the opportunity to focus on patients' depressive symptoms directly, as these symptoms (e.g., depressed mood, helplessness, guilt) are often addressed as part of the "response of self" component of the CCRT.

With the inclusion of CCRT-related techniques, the alliance-fostering manual is somewhat similar to other interpersonal–psychodynamic treatment models, especially the supportive–expressive model. Despite the similarities, the alliance-fostering manual differs from Luborsky's (1984) traditional supportive–expressive psychotherapy in both style and emphasis. In terms of style, alliance-fostering therapy is "warmer" and more active than traditional supportive–expressive therapy. In terms of emphasis, the addition of several new elements (frequent review of goals and tasks, efforts to increase the bond, managing of alliance ruptures) inevitably means that there is relatively less time that can be devoted to pure expressive (interpretative) work by the therapist, as compared to the case with traditional supportive–expressive therapy.

Sequence of Techniques over the Course of Treatment

The techniques used in alliance-fostering therapy were designed to unfold over the course of therapy in the following typical sequence. Sessions 1 and 2 are devoted to socialization to therapy, reviewing of treatment expectations, reviewing the history of previous treatment, and the establishment of patient's goals. In most subsequent sessions, the therapist regularly evaluates agreement on goals and tasks, works toward better agreement on goals and tasks, and establishes and maintains a bond with the patient. In addition to these ongoing tasks, during Sessions 3–5, the therapist formulates and addresses an initial CCRT. During Sessions 6–16 the therapist both expands and thoroughly works through the CCRT. The final three sessions are normally devoted to address impending termination.

SUMMARY OF THE RESEARCH EVIDENCE

We have conducted one preliminary study that evaluates whether therapists can be trained to materially improve their patient alliances by using alliance-fostering psychotherapy (Crits-Christoph et al., 2006). The design of the study included a pretraining phase, a training phase, and a posttraining phase. Five early-career psychotherapists participated in the study. During each of the three study phases, each of the five therapists was randomly assigned three patients (in total, 45 patients participated). The purpose of the pretraining phase was to determine each therapist's typical alliance level.

The training phase involved intensive supervision led by an experienced supportive–expressive clinician–trainer. This training phase was designed to teach the techniques of alliance-fostering therapy. The purpose of the posttraining study phase was to see whether therapists could successfully implement the alliance-fostering techniques on their own, without close supervision.

Our primary hypothesis was that training in alliance-fostering therapy would produce increases in the average alliance for a therapist caseload. The alliance was measured with two patient-report scales administered at the end of each treatment session: the California Psychotherapy Alliance Scale—Patient Version (CALPAS; Gaston, 1991) and the Helping Alliance Questionnaire (HAQ-II; Luborsky et. al., 1996). Additional patient measures were also examined as secondary outcomes. The study was designed as a pilot feasibility study; there was low statistical power for testing the significance of differences between therapist alliance scores before versus after training.

Patients recruited for the study were adults with a primary diagnosis of major depressive disorder. Excluded was anyone with current or past history of schizophrenic disorders, bipolar disorders, Cluster A Axis II personality disorders (schizoid, schizotypal, or paranoid), or a diagnosis during the past 12 months of alcohol or substance dependence, obsessive–compulsive disorder, eating disorder, or borderline personality disorder. Patients were recruited through the outpatient psychiatric referral system at the Department of Psychiatry at the University of Pennsylvania and through newspaper advertisements.

The therapists for the study were three women and two men, all of whom were relatively inexperienced PhD or PsyD psychologists (1–3 years of postdegree experience) who were currently working as clinicians in the community. We selected relatively inexperienced therapists because we were concerned that experienced therapists would have developed their own ways of achieving high alliances and therefore would have little room to improve their alliances. Two of the therapists were primarily cognitive-behavioral in orientation, two were psychodynamically oriented, and one was primarily trained in family systems therapy.

Given the small sample of therapists, the statistical analysis failed to reveal any significant effects by study phase (pretraining, training, posttraining) on alliance scores. However, examination of effect sizes (Cohen's d) revealed that alliance increased over the course of the study phases. Comparing the pretraining average alliance scores to the posttraining average alliance scores yielded an effect size of 0.48 for the CALPAS and 0.77 for the HAQ-II, indicating moderate to large improvement in the alliance following training in alliance-fostering therapy.

The examination of changes for specific therapists revealed substantial variability in the effects of training. Focusing on the CALPAS Working Capacity scale, we found that Therapist 2 improved from pre to during training by approximately 1.5 standard deviations, Therapist 5 improved 1.3 standard deviations from pre- to posttraining, and Therapist 1 improved from pre- to during training by approximately two-thirds of a standard deviation (SD). In contrast to these marked improvements, Therapist 4 decreased from pretraining to during training (by about two-thirds of a standard deviation) and continued to decrease during the posttraining phase. Therapist 3 decreased substantially (by about 1.5 standard deviation) from pretraining to during training; posttraining the therapist recovered to a level about one-half of a standard deviation above pretraining levels. From these numbers, we can cautiously infer that some therapists readily respond to training and their alliances improve, and that some therapists struggle with the new techniques but then master them and eventually have better alliances. However, one therapist was not able to make use of the training to enhance patient alliances. In fact, for this therapist training appeared to have a negative impact, possibly because the general therapy orientation was highly discrepant from that therapist's own style and previous training (which was in cognitive-behavioral psychotherapy).

We also had therapists complete an adherence checklist at the end of every session during the training and posttraining phases to evaluate how often each of the alliance-fostering techniques was used. These data show that the average number of techniques (out of 12) used during the typical session during the training phase was 7.81 (SD = 1.25), while the average number of techniques used per session in the posttraining phase was 7.26 (1.53). Certain techniques were more commonly used. "Reviewed patient goals for treatment to facilitate agreement on goals" was used in 68% of the sessions; "made an attempt to bond with the patient through mutual affect" was used in 79% of sessions; "discussed what we have done, or are going to do, in therapy to facilitate agreement on the tasks of therapy" was used in 68% of sessions. Less common techniques were "made an attempt to connect to the patient in regard to the patient's interests" (18% of sessions), "noticed and explored verbal distancing" (19%), and "noticed and explored non-verbal distancing" (11%).

We also conducted analyses to see if adherence was related to improved alliance scores. These analyses revealed that, during the training phase of the study, adherence in a given session was significantly correlated with alliance scores at the subsequent session. However, alliance at the current session was unrelated to adherence at the subsequent session. These results are supportive of the view that the alliance-fostering techniques actually impacted on subsequent patient-reported alliances.

The ultimate goal of alliance-fostering therapy is to improve patient outcomes. In our study, there were no statistically significant differences between the study phases in regard to outcome (as mentioned, however, the statistical power for significance testing was very limited). Examination of effect sizes revealed a small to moderate effect (Cohen's $d = 0.41$) on the Beck Depression Inventory (Beck, Steer, & Garbin, 1988) from pretraining to during and posttraining on termination scores, and a small to moderate effect ($d = 0.39$) comparing the posttraining phase to the pretraining phase at follow-up. Of note was a large effect ($d = 0.76$) in regard to improvement in patient quality of life comparing the training phase to the pretraining phase. Quality of life was measured with the Quality of Life Inventory (Frisch, Cornell, Villanueva, & Retzlaff, 1992).

DESCRIPTION OF THE TRAINING MODEL

Before conducting the study described in the preceding section, we had no empirical basis for knowing how to structure a clinical training program for enhancing therapists' alliances by using our alliance-fostering therapy manual. The training model we implemented, therefore, was simply based on the typical set of therapist training procedures that we, and others, had used in conducting psychotherapy efficacy studies. Training consisted of two major components, an initial training workshop and training cases with supervision.

The training workshop was a 1-day event held prior to the initiation of the training phase of our study. The goals of the workshop were to review the alliance-fostering therapy manual, discuss therapists' reactions to, and concerns about, the treatment approach, and to give examples of how the techniques were implemented. The clinical supervisor led the training workshop. Immediately after the workshop, training cases were recruited and assigned to therapists.

Each therapist was provided with training cases. For each training case, the clinical supervisor listened to audiotapes of all treatment sessions. All treatment sessions were then reviewed with the therapist in one-on-one supervision sessions. The supervisor also reviewed the therapist adherence checklists prior to each supervision session. The goals of supervision were: (1) to evaluate the quality of the alliance in each session, including alliance ruptures, and review this evaluation with the therapist; (2) to ensure that the therapist was following the treatment manual and using the appropriate alliance-fostering techniques; (3) to review the therapist's ongoing CCRT formulation of a patient and make refinements as needed; and (4) to make recommendations for the next treatment session.

As mentioned, there was a posttraining phase in our pilot investigation in which therapists each treated three patients, using the alliance-fostering psychotherapy. During this phase, supervision was provided on a monthly basis. This supervision was provided because the therapists were relatively inexperienced and the patients in the study all were diagnosed with major depressive disorder (and therefore significant clinical concerns such as suicidality could emerge). The focus of this supervision was only on any significant clinical concerns and did not involve additional teaching of the alliance-fostering techniques.

The foregoing training procedures of course, were utilized in the context of a research study. If we were training therapists outside of the context of a research study, we would begin with a workshop and three training cases as a reasonable starting point. Therapists who were not adequately learning the approach could receive additional training cases. The posttraining supervision to address significant clinical concerns would not be necessary; however, some degree of ongoing consultation with a supervisor post-training would likely be useful. Some consultation could serve to provide reminders and to address unusual issues that did not arise in the context of the training cases.

In the context of our study, the clinical supervisor/trainer was a highly experienced clinician (not a researcher) with more than 15 years' experience in training therapists in manual-based (interpersonal–psychodynamic) treatments and was also a coauthor of the alliance-fostering treatment manual. While the supervisor's style was warm and respectful of the clinical skills of the therapists, supervision sessions were also somewhat didactic and focused on teaching further skills and modifying therapist behavior to conform to the approach in the alliance-fostering manual.

LESSONS LEARNED FROM TRAINING

From our experiences with the study, there were a number of "lessons learned" about training therapists to improve their alliances. As mentioned, our research study employed an adherence checklist that served not only as a research assessment but also as an element of the clinical supervision process. One lesson learned was that the use of this checklist was a very valuable addition to the supervision process. The checklist was a useful way of creating a "we" bond in the supervisor–therapist relationship—by having a separate objective standard for the therapist to target as a goal, with the supervisor providing supportive guidance toward that goal. Without this checklist to guide the use of intervention, in standard clinical supervision an exaggerated role for the supervisor as "expert" and the trainee as "student" could at times cause difficulties. The trainee's discomfort with this hierarchy could lead to arguments or to the trainee's outright rejection of the supervisory input, in order to "feel competent." Although the hierarchy is inherently part of any supervisor–trainee relationship, these types of reactions to the hierarchy are defused by structuring the supervision around a separate objective goal. In many clinical and research contexts, the existence of a treatment manual or coherent clinical theory may provide this "objective" goal for the learning process to some degree, but most clinical approaches (including the current one) have substantial clinical flexibility in the within-session implementation of clinical techniques, and therefore the "expertise" of the supervisor can dominate. As in therapy, having a successful working alliance between the supervisor and trainee is key. Mutual respect, a "we" bond, mutual affirmation, empathy, and support help maintain a productive and positive supervisor–trainee relationship.

Another lesson learned during the training of therapists for our project was the importance of including a psychotherapy socialization procedure in the first treatment session. This socialization was provided not only to educate the patient but also to allow the patient to react immediately to the expectations, tasks, and goals of therapy so that any disagreements on these issues could be discussed. Through our experience during the training phase, we came to realize that the socialization material should not simply be "read" or presented as routine instruction by the therapist. Rather, it should be presented at the appropriate time and worded so as to enhance the initial alliance with the client. For example, a good opportunity to provide socialization occurs during discussion of what the patient thought about the efficacy of past therapies and whether the patient perceives the current therapy as the same or different. If the therapist did need to refer to notes about the socialization procedures, it was useful for the therapist to say that "in order to cover everything, I might have to refer to my notes, but please feel free to interrupt me as much you want."

A further lesson learned related to the research procedures. We learned that to enhance alliance it was very important to let the patient express any concerns or frustrations with the research procedures (e.g., the extensive baseline assessments) and for the therapist to just empathize (i.e., not try to justify or defend the research as much as possible). By allowing the patient to express any concerns about the research, particularly in the first treatment session, the therapist has set the tone for the patient to express his or her negative feelings or skepticism about anything including the therapist or treatment—without being judged.

An additional important lesson learned was that the clinical techniques for alliance building always need to be titrated and modified, based on the patient's relational abilities and style. The key to enhancing the patient's level of trust with the therapist, which is part and parcel of the alliance, is the therapist's ability to ascertain the level of disclosure and exploration acceptable to the client, which is subject to change as therapy proceeds. Even an "empathetic" remark could be experienced as intrusive if given too early to a distrusting client who needed to control and closely gauge what feelings are expressed and then noticed by the therapist. Therapists who were either "too supportive" or "empathetic" without being able to assess reactions might run into as much trouble as those who treated the manual as a compendium of techniques to be implemented with no regard for the patient's relational abilities or proclivities. Some beginning therapists often err on the side of being overly "touchy-feely," but others—especially those coming from a cognitive-behavioral background—are perhaps too eager to implement as many items as possible on the adherence checklist for alliance-fostering therapy. The ability to empathize with the feelings the patient is expressing in relation to the therapeutic alliance must also be balanced with the therapist giving the patient enough space for uncomfortable feelings to be expressed. Another way to implement this delicate balance is for the therapist to allow both projections and transferential concerns to be expressed but to empathize with them in a way that fosters a positive alliance (i.e., step out of the "blank screen").

In summary, two overarching themes were apparent in our "lessons learned." One is that establishing a positive working relationship between the supervisor and trainee requires well-calibrated work that is essential to providing the platform on which further learning can be grounded. The second theme is that clinical flexibility is always needed to tailor any set of technical recommendations to the specific patient. Some might suggest that this clinical flexibility is so critical as to render psychotherapy "manuals" useless. On the contrary, our experience was that a treatment manual for fostering the alliance provides a highly useful and effective way to teach therapists to improve their alliances. Supplementing the core technical principles with additional suggestions on how to personalize the treatment for individual patients, however, is essential in extending the range of the treatment approach. By orienting therapists to the importance of fostering the therapeutic relationship *throughout* therapy, our approach likely does far more than teach a few specific "tricks" for building the alliance. The therapist is encouraged also to hone his or her skills at tuning into interpersonal issues. These enhanced skills enable therapists, with experience, to tailor the alliance-building techniques to the unique expectations, needs, and personalities of diverse patients.

REFERENCES

Barber, J. P., Connolly Gibbons, M. B., Crits-Christoph, P., Gladis, L., & Siqueland, L. (2000). Alliance predicts patients' outcome beyond in-treatment change in symptoms. *Journal of Consulting and Clinical Psychology, 68,* 1027–1032.

Beck, A. T., Steer, R. A., & Garbin, M. G. (1988). Psychometric properties of the Beck Depression Inventory: Twenty-five years later. *Clinical Psychology Review, 8,* 77–100.

Bordin, E. S. (1979). The generalizability of the psycho-analytic concept of the working alliance. *Psychotherapy: Theory, Research, and Practice, 16,* 252–260.

Connolly, M. B., Crits-Christoph, P., de la Cruz, C., Barber, J. P., Siqueland L., & Gladis, L. (2003). Pretreatment expectations, interpersonal functioning, and symptoms in the prediction of the therapeutic alliance across supportive–expressive psychotherapy and cognitive therapy. *Psychotherapy Research, 13,* 59–76.

Crits-Christoph, P., Barber, J. P., & Kurcias, J. S. (1993). The accuracy of therapists' interpretations and the development of the therapeutic alliance. *Psychotherapy Research, 3,* 25–35.

Crits-Christoph, P., Connolly Gibbons, M. B., Crits-Christoph, K., Narducci, J., Schamberger, M., & Gallop, R. (2006). Can therapists be trained to improve their alliances?: A pilot study of Alliance-Fostering Therapy. *Psychotherapy Research, 13,* 268–281.

Crits-Christoph, P., & Crits-Christoph, K. (1998). *Alliance-fostering therapy for major depressive disorder.* Unpublished manuscript, University of Pennsylvania.

Frisch, M. B., Cornell, J., Villanueva, M., & Retzlaff, P. J. (1992). Clinical validation of the Quality of Life Inventory: A measure of life satisfaction for use in treatment planning and outcome assessment. *Psychological Assessment, 4,* 92–101.

Gaston, L. (1991). Reliability and criterion-related validity of the California Psychotherapy Alliance Scales—patient version. *Psychological Assessment, 3,* 68–74.

Horvath, A. O., & Symonds, B. D. (1991). Relation between working alliance and outcome in psychotherapy: A meta-analysis. *Journal of Counseling Psychology, 38,* 139–149.

Luborsky, L. (1984). *Principles of psychoanalytic psychotherapy: A manual for supportive–expressive treatment.* New York: Basic Books.

Luborsky, L., Barber, J. P., Siqueland, L., Johnson, S., Najavits, L. M., Frank A., et al. (1996). The revised Helping Alliance Questionnaire (HAQ-II): Psychometric properties. *Journal of Psychotherapy: Practice and Research, 5,* 260–271.

Luborsky, L., & Crits-Christoph, P. (1998). *Understanding transference: The Core Conflictual Relationship Theme Method* (2nd ed.). Washington, DC: American Psychological Association.

Mallinckrodt, B., Coble, H. M., & Gantt, D. L. (1995). Working alliance, attachment memories, and social competencies of women in brief therapy. *Journal of Counseling Psychology, 42,* 79–84.

Martin, D. J., Garske, J. P., & Davis, M. K. (2000). Relation of the therapeutic alliance with outcome and other variables: A meta-analytic review. *Journal of Consulting and Clinical Psychology, 68,* 438–450.

Miller, W. R., & Rollnick, S. (1991). *Motivational interviewing: Preparing people to change addictive behavior.* New York: Guilford Press.

Muran, J. C., Segal, Z. V., Samstag, L. W., & Crawford, C. E. 1994). Patient pretreatment interpersonal problems and therapeutic alliance in short-term cognitive therapy. *Journal of Consulting and Clinical Psychology, 62,* 185–190.

Orlinsky, D. E., Grawe, K., & Parks, B. K. (1994). Process and outcome in psychotherapy: Noch einmal. In A. E. Bergin & S. L. Garfield (Eds.), *Handbook of psychotherapy and behavior change* (4th ed., pp. 270–376). Oxford, UK: Wiley.

Piper, W. E., Azim, H. F., Joyce, A. S., McCallum, M., Nixon, G. W. H., & Segal, P. S. (1991). Quality of object relations versus interpersonal functioning as predictors of therapeutic alliance and psychotherapy outcome. *Journal of Nervous and Mental Disease, 179,* 432–438.

Prochaska, J. O., & DiClemente, C. C. (1984). *The transtheoretical approach: Crossing traditional boundaries of therapy.* Malabar, FL: Krieger.

Rice, L. (1984). Client tasks in client-centered therapy. In R. F. Levant & J. M. Shlien (Eds.), *Client-centered therapy and the person-centered approach: New directions in theory, research, and practice.* Westport, CT: Praeger Publishers.

Rogers, C. R. (1957). The necessary and sufficient conditions of therapeutic personality change. *Journal of Consulting Psychology, 21,* 95–103.

CHAPTER 16

■ ■ ■ ■ ■

Developing Therapist Abilities to Negotiate Alliance Ruptures

J. Christopher Muran
Jeremy D. Safran
Catherine Eubanks-Carter

We developed our training protocol in the Beth Israel Psychotherapy Research Program (see Muran, 2002) primarily in response to a number of general findings in the research literature. First, outcome research has in sum demonstrated there is a good deal of room for improvement. Meta-analyses have suggested that 30–40% of patients fail to benefit (Lambert, 2004), and dropout rates average approximately 50% (Wierzbicki & Pekarik, 1993). Outcome research also has shown that patients with comorbid diagnoses (especially those with personality disorders or pathology) are especially challenging and resistant to treatment, resulting in more negative process, higher attrition rates, and greater treatment length (Benjamin & Karpiak, 2002; Clarkin & Levy, 2004; Westen & Morrison, 2001). This is particularly significant, given that comorbidity estimates of patients seeking treatment in our clinics and practices range from 40 to 70% (Kessler et al., 1994), with as many as 45% diagnosed with personality disorders (Zimmerman, Chelminski, & Young, 2008).

When it comes to considering how or where to improve the impact of our treatments, we have chosen to focus on therapist abilities to negotiate the therapeutic alliance because of the consistent finding in the research literature that the quality of the alliance (and the interpersonal process between patient and therapist) is a robust predictor of outcome—in fact, stronger than most technical interventions (Horvath & Bedi, 2002; Horvath & Symonds, 1991; Martin, Garske, & Davis, 2000; Wampold, 2001). What has also influenced us in choosing this focus is the finding that therapists' individual differences strongly predict alliance quality and treatment success (see, for example, Baldwin, Wampold, & Imel, 2007; Luborsky et al., 1986; Nagavits & Strupp, 1994; Wampold, 2001). In this regard, the research suggests that some therapists are consistently more helpful than others and that these same therapists are better able to facilitate the development of the therapeutic alliance.

DEFINING RUPTURES IN THE THERAPEUTIC ALLIANCE

Our understanding of the therapeutic alliance has been organized around Bordin's conceptualization (1979), which has formed the basis for much of the research demonstrating the predictive validity of the concept. Bordin redefined the alliance as mutual agreement on the tasks and goals of treatment and the affective bond between patient and therapist. His definition suggested an inextricable relationship between the technical and the relational—that every intervention has relational meaning. It also suggested a more mutual and dynamic process of ongoing negotiation, which stands in contrast to previous conceptualizations that emphasized the therapist's support or the patient's identification with the therapist and acceptance of the therapist's values for the psychotherapy process (Muran & Safran, 1998).

We have developed this notion of negotiation to suggest that the alliance concept can include a view of the psychotherapy process as involving an ongoing push and pull of various patient and therapist affective states, underlying needs, and interpersonal behaviors (Safran & Muran, 2000, 2006). This conception is in part informed by the mother–infant research on affect regulation (Tronick, 1989) and the research on interpersonal complementarity (Kiesler, 1996). Our conceptualization suggests an *intersubjective negotiation* (Benjamin, 1990; Pizer, 1998) in which patient and therapist are seen as engaged in a struggle for *mutual recognition* regarding their respective subjectivities—a struggle that involves ongoing power plays and inevitable hostilities, accommodations, and refusals to accommodate. We have conceptualized this struggle as basic to every rupture in the therapeutic alliance.

Alliance ruptures have received increasing attention over the past 25 years in the research literature, with growing evidence that they are common events (e.g., they are reported by patients in as much as 50% of sessions, they are observed by third-party raters in 70% of sessions), they predict premature termination and negative outcome, but when resolved they predict good outcomes (see Safran, Muran, Samstag, & Stevens, 2002; Eubanks-Carter, Muran, & Safran, Chapter 5, this volume). We have defined ruptures as (1) breakdowns in the negotiation of treatment tasks and goals and deterioration in the affective bond between patient and therapist; (2) markers of tension between the respective needs or desires of the patient and therapist as they continuously press against each other; and (3) indications of an enactment—a *relational matrix* of patient and therapist beliefs and action patterns, a vicious cycle involving the unwitting participation of both patient and therapist (Mitchell, 1988; Wachtel, 2007). This definition suggests that ruptures represent critical events and opportunities for awareness and change.

We have also defined ruptures in terms of two specific types of patient behaviors, communications or markers—withdrawal and confrontation. A *withdrawal* marker is a patient behavior indicating disengagement from an emotional state, from the therapist, or from some aspect of the treatment. It includes patient *movements away* from the therapist (away from the other); examples include silences, minimal responses, topic shifts, abstract talk, and storytelling; these are movements toward *autonomy and isolation*. Withdrawal also includes patient *movements toward* the therapist (away from self); examples include begrudgingly or too readily complying with a therapist, doing something with great anxiety or cynicism; these are movements marked by *compliance or appeasement*. A *confrontation* marker is most commonly a direct expression of anger or dissatisfaction by the patient about the therapist or some aspect of the treatment. It essentially involves patient *movements against* the therapist; these are movements marked by *aggression and control*; examples can also include coercions like being overly friendly or seductive.

Another way of understanding the distinction between withdrawal and confrontation draws on a theory of motivation that has received a great deal of transtheoretical attention in the psychotherapy literature since the 1980s (Blatt, 2008). Under this theory, withdrawal and confrontation markers can be understood as reflecting different ways of coping with the dialectical tension between two fundamental human motivations: *the need for agency versus the need for relatedness*. Ruptures mark a breakdown in the negotiation of these needs with another. Thus, a withdrawal rupture could be understood as the pursuit of *relatedness* at the expense of the need for *self-agency*, and a confrontation rupture the expression of *self-agency* at the expense of *relatedness*. Ruptures can be understood, then, as an opportunity to learn how to negotiate these needs with another.

A STAGE-PROCESS MODEL OF RUPTURE RESOLUTION

Our research program began as a study of rupture events and resolution processes with the specific aim of sensitizing clinicians to patterns that are likely to occur and to facilitate their abilities to intervene (Safran, Crocker, McMain, & Murray, 1990; Safran & Muran, 1996; Safran, Muran, & Samstag, 1994; see also Eubanks-Carter, Muran, & Safran, Chapter 5, this volume). We have proposed a typology of rupture resolution strategies, both direct and indirect, that approaches ruptures at a surface and a depth level (see Safran & Muran, 2000, and Figure 16.1). For example, a direct surface approach can involve simple clarification of the treatment rationale or the misunderstanding between the therapist and patient, whereas an indirect surface approach can involve simply changing a treatment task or goal when there is disagreement. Similarly, a direct depth approach would involve exploring a core relational theme, while an indirect depth approach would involve providing a new relational experience, which can also be a consequence of any of the resolution strategy types.

Our research has concentrated on the study of a direct depth strategy that explores a core relational theme, and in this regard we developed two stage-process models for the resolution of withdrawal and confrontation ruptures. Each of the models begins with the therapist attending to the rupture marker. The critical task is for the therapist to recognize the rupture and invite an exploration of it. To progress, the therapist must facilitate a disembedding from the relational matrix or unhooking from the vicious cycle. The key principle in this regard is to establish communications about the communication process, or metacommunication (Kiesler, 1988, 1996). The typical progression in the withdrawal resolution process is from increasingly

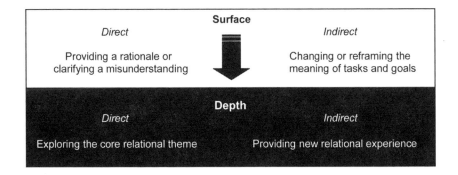

FIGURE 16.1. A typology of rupture resolution strategies. Adapted from Safran and Muran (2004). Adapted by permission. Copyright 2004 by The Guilford Press.

clearer expressions of negative sentiments to self-assertion. The typical progression in the confrontation resolution process is from expressions of anger to hurt and disappointment to vulnerability and contacting the need for nurturance. The essential task for the therapist to facilitate this movement is to empathize, to remain nondefensive, and to take responsibility where appropriate. Throughout such progressions, there are often shifts away, movements that reflect the patient's anxiety about expressions of assertion or vulnerability, which the therapist should explore.

From a series of studies (Safran & Muran, 1996), we provided confirmatory evidence for a generic model of rupture resolution, which represents the general process in the more specific resolution models described above (see Figure 16.2 for an illustration). It depicts the different pathways of intervention that therapists should pursue in response to various patient states or positions, including attending to the rupture marker, exploring the rupture experience, clarifying any mixed expressions (e.g., qualified assertions or angry expressions of hurt), exploring any avoidant movement away from communicating about the rupture, and finally recognizing the patient's expression of an underlying wish or need—whether it be the need to assert or the wish for nurturance. It is important to note that our research suggests that resolution or productive process does not require progression through all these pathways and reaching all these patient states, especially within any given session (see Safran & Muran, 1996, 2000). Instead, any exploration of a rupture or avoidance in and of itself can be experienced by patients as very meaningful.

DEVELOPING AN ALLIANCE-FOCUSED TREATMENT

Based on this research, we developed an alliance-focused treatment and training model with support from a grant awarded by the National Institute of Mental Health in the early 1990s (Muran & Safran, 2002; Safran, 2002; Safran & Muran, 2000). The alliance-focused treatment has been alternatively called *brief relational therapy* (BRT). In this grant study, we compared the treatment efficacy of BRT to two traditional time-limited treatments (a short-term dynamic psychotherapy and a cognitive-behavioral therapy approach) and found it to be at least equally effective in the treatment of patients presenting with a personality disorder, with a lower attrition rate (Muran, Safran, Samstag, & Winston, 2005). We also found preliminary evidence to suggest that BRT may be more effective with patients determined to be at risk for treatment failure based on having difficulty establishing an alliance with a previous therapist (Safran, Muran, Samstag, & Winston, 2005).

BRT is organized around several key principles: (1) it assumes a two-

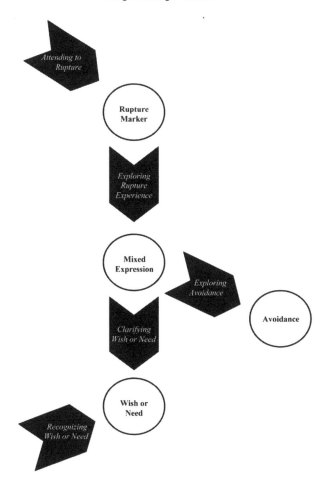

FIGURE 16.2. Therapist intervention pathways to critical patient states in the rupture resolution model.

person psychology and a social constructivist epistemology; (2) there is an intensive focus on the here and now of the therapeutic relationship; (3) there is an ongoing collaborative exploration of both patients' and therapists' contributions to the interaction; (4) it emphasizes in-depth exploration of the patients' experience in the context of unfolding interactions; (5) it makes use of therapist self-disclosure; (6) it emphasizes the subjectivity of the therapist's perceptions; and (7) it assumes that the relational meaning of interventions is critical. BRT generally involves the following protocol:

Establishing the Collaboration

The beginning of treatment in BRT is marked by defining the tasks and goals of treatment, even though this relational model remains relatively less structured or directive than other short-term dynamic models (and especially so, compared to cognitive-behavioral treatments).

Establishing the Rationale for Treatment Tasks

The process of explicitly establishing a rationale for treatment is one that is often neglected in more insight-oriented therapies. This omission fails to recognize the critical role that agreement about tasks and goals plays in creating an alliance. We typically give the patient concise reading material at the beginning of therapy and spend time early in treatment discussing how therapy works, with particular attention paid to the role of awareness and the use of the therapeutic relationship. It is critical to convey a rationale for such therapeutic tasks as becoming aware of emotional experience, exploring perceptions and beliefs, and examining what takes place in the therapeutic relationship.

Demonstrating the Task of Mindfulness

In light of the importance of establishing agreement on tasks, we also recommend the use of a mindfulness exercise to experientially demonstrate the notion of bare or nonjudgmental attention. For example, one might ask patients to close their eyes and focus on their breath and each breathing cycle, paying attention to where their mind goes and then redirecting their attention back to their breath. The purpose here is to sensitize patients to attending in an accepting manner to an emerging and ongoing process, much in the same way that they will be asked to attend to their feelings.

Clarifying Expectations Regarding Treatment Goals

When conveying the rationale at the beginning of therapy for a short-term and time-limited therapy, it is important to begin the process of trying to establish reasonable expectations about what can take place in such a framework. Our time-limited treatment is conceptualized for patients as a process of providing them a new experience, which involves primarily cultivating a new skill of attention and awareness as well as shining a beam of light on some core relational themes, such that patients can continue to grow and develop after the end of treatment.

Navigating the Treatment Course

The course of BRT involves many tasks and challenges for the therapist. Here, we outline some of the more important ones.

Oscillating between Content and Process

A major task for therapists in this model involves oscillating their attention between the *content* and *process* of communication. As communication theorists maintain, there are always report and command aspects to any communication. The report aspect of the communication is the specific content of the communication. The command aspect of the communication is the interpersonal statement or the statement about the current relationship that is being conveyed by the patient's communication. The therapist should always be monitoring both the content of *what* the patient says and the process of *how* the patient says it.

Observing the Interpersonal Field

Relatedly, the therapist should always be monitoring the current interpersonal field as it shifts over time. A cue of critical importance about the interpersonal field consists of the therapists' sense of interpersonal contact or engagement with the patient. Therapists should always be monitoring how related, connected to, or disconnected from the patient they are feeling at any given moment. Moments of disconnectedness provide the therapists with very important information about what is presently transpiring.

Exploring the Patient's Experience

In tracking patient experience, therapists should pay particular attention to not only emotionally salient experiential states in the patient but also transitions in patient experience, the seams between one self-state and another. These may reflect important underlying processes that should be explored and clarified. Often it is the case that these transitions indicate an avoidance of or a defensive operation against an experience. And often therapists find themselves losing contact with the patient as a result of this movement away. The task is to help the patient become aware of avoiding or defending against that experience, including the reasons for and ways of doing it.

Exploring Self-Experience

At the same time as tracking patient experience, therapists should track their own inner experience as well. Here it is critical to go beyond simply identifying a feeling such as sadness or anger at a more gross somatic level and to articulate the nature of one's inner experience in a more differentiated way. The process of articulating one's own inner experience involves a movement back and forth between the level of feelings grounded in bodily felt experience and a conceptual elaboration of those feelings. This parallels the task in which we invite patients to engage.

Oscillating between the Self and Other Experience

Implicit in what is being said already is that therapists are always directing their attention back and forth or alternating their attention between the patient's inner experience and therapist's own inner experience. One of the primary points of orientation for therapists is their experience of contact with the patient's inner experience. So long as therapists experience empathic contact, they are naturally inclined to establish the kind of therapeutic environment in which their patient can grow. Over the course of any session, however, it is common for therapists' experience of empathic contact to shift back and forth. Whenever the therapist experiences a lack of contact with the patient's inner experience, the key task then becomes to recognize the shift, explore it, and the let reconnection follow as a natural consequence.

The Ongoing Process of Embedding and Disembedding

The course of treatment in the best of cases invariably involves an ongoing process of embedding and disembedding from various relational matrices. Being embedded in a matrix is an inevitable part of the therapeutic process, and therapists must be able to accept the fact that they will go through extended periods of being embedded without being aware of being embedded and will also go through extended periods of feeling "stuck." Therapists should also come to understand that they are always embedded in some sort of matrix with their patient—faced with the endless task of disembedding from one and embedding into another, with no other place to go (Stern, 1997).

Approaching the Termination

The end of treatment naturally evokes certain themes. With each patient, it often poses challenges for therapists that are not unlike those they faced in working through ruptures with their patient throughout the course of treatment (though perhaps more intense). Thus, we have considered the termination process as the resolution of the *ultimate alliance rupture*.

Separation and Loss

Termination obviously involves separation and loss, and thus it can evoke sadness as well as tension between the needs for individuation and relatedness. The process of individuating is inherently guilt-producing and fraught with anxiety since it threatens relatedness. Paradoxically, however, the attainment of individuation and relatedness are dependent upon each other. As attachment researchers have observed (e.g., Bowlby, 1973), one needs a sense of security in a relationship with a significant other before engaging in the exploratory behavior necessary to facilitate individuation. Conversely, one cannot maintain a mature form of relatedness to others until one has developed a sense of oneself as an individual. This is a critical theme that the therapist and patient must negotiate as treatment nears the end.

Acceptance

In the final analysis, therapists must have tolerance for their own impotence as helpers and their own inability to solve patients' problems for them or take their pain away. It is inevitable that patients will want the impossible from their therapists. They will want them to transform their lives and take their pain away. Therapists who have difficulty accepting their own limitations and being *good enough* as helpers will respond defensively in the face of patients' impossible demands. It is thus critical for therapists to come to terms with the fact that in the end there is a limited amount that one human being can do for another.

Being Alone

As human beings we thus spend our lives negotiating the paradox of our simultaneous aloneness and togetherness. We begin our lives attempting to remain in proximity to attachment figures, and the pursuit of interpersonal relatedness continues to motivate our behavior throughout our lifetime. No matter how hard we try, however, we cannot—except for brief periods—achieve the type of union with others that permits us to escape from our aloneness. This theme can also become salient as the patient faces the end of treatment and the therapeutic relationship. The critical task for the therapist is to help the patient work through this disappointment in a constructive way.

A TRAINING MODEL ON RUPTURE RECOGNITION AND RESOLUTION

In 2006 we were awarded another grant by the National Institute of Mental Health to evaluate the additive effect of our training model on a cognitive-behavioral treatment (CBT) for personality disorders. In this study, inexperienced therapists trained to conduct CBT on a challenging patient population were introduced at different intervals to additional training specifically designed to improve their skills in recognizing and resolving alliance ruptures. The overall objective of the study was to evaluate the effect of our alliance-focused training model on the treatment process, that is, the interpersonal process between patient and therapist. The study resulted in a more detailed definition of our training model, which we describe in detail in this section.

Basic Therapist Skills

The training model concentrates on the development of the therapist's abilities to recognize ruptures and to resolve them. With regard to rupture recognition, our training targets three specific skills—*self-awareness*, *affect regulation*, and *interpersonal sensitivity*—which we see as interdependent and as critical to establishing an optimal observational stance. By *self-awareness*, we mean to developing therapists' immediate awareness and bare attention to their internal experience. Our aim here is to increase therapists' attunement to their emotions so that they may use them as a compass to understanding their interactions with their patients. By *affect regulation*, we mean to developing therapists' abilities to manage negative emotions and tolerate distress—their own as well as their patients'. In other words, we try to facilitate their abilities to resist the natural reaction to anxiety, namely, turning one's attention away from or avoiding dealing with it in some way, which amounts to not attending to or exploring a rupture. By *interpersonal sensitivity*, we mean increasing therapists' empathy to their patient's experience and their awareness of the interpersonal process they engage in with their patients. In this regard, we try to balance therapists' attention on what they or their patients say with a heightened sensitivity to how statements are communicated, the impact of expressions, and the nature of their interactions with patients.

The Technical Principle of Metacommunication

The training also attempts to teach the various rupture resolution strategies, from direct to indirect and from surface to depth, but with special attention to the technical principle of metacommunication, which we have found useful in exploring core relational themes. The principle represents an attempt to step outside of or dismembed from the relational matrix involving patient and therapist that is currently being enacted by treating it as the focus of collaborative inquiry. It is an attempt to bring immediate awareness to bear on the interactive process as it unfolds. It involves a low degree of inference and is grounded as much as possible in the therapist's immediate experience of some aspect of the therapeutic relationship. It also reflects a dialogic sensibility based on the recognition that ruptures are not only the result of a collaborative effort but also can only be understood or resolved through the collaboration of both patient and therapist (see Safran & Muran, 2000). Therapists are not seen as being in a privileged position of knowing. Rather, their understanding of the communication process is considered only partial in our model.

Metacommunication can begin with questions or observations by the therapist that focus the patient's attention on three parallel dimensions of their relationship (see Figure 16.3 for an illustration). The therapist might start by focusing the patient's attention on his or her own experience with a direct question such as "What are you feeling right now?" or with an observation about the patient's self-state: "You seem anxious to me right now. Am I reading you right?" The therapist might also direct attention to the interpersonal field by asking "What's going on here between us?" or by observing "It seems like we're in some kind of dance—does that fit with your sense?" A third approach is to bring the therapist's experience into relief by asking a question that encourages the patient to be curious about the therapist's self-state: "Do you have any thoughts about what might be going on for me right now?" Alternatively, the therapist could make a

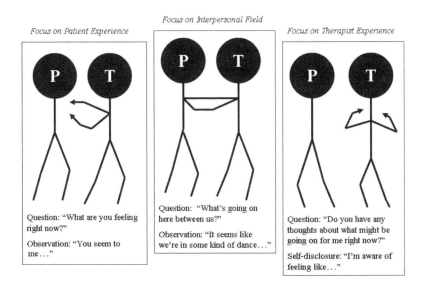

FIGURE 16.3. Metacommunication: Parallel dimensions. P, patient; T, therapist.

self-disclosure about his internal experience, such as "I'm aware of feeling defensive right now."

We have outlined a number of general and specific principles of meta-communication (see Safran & Muran, 2000), but some basic ones include the following:

Inviting a Collaborative Inquiry and Establishing a Climate of Shared Dilemma

The implicit message should always be one of inviting the patient to join the therapist in an attempt to understand their shared dilemma. Patients often feel alone and demoralized during a rupture. Therapists should try to frame a rupture as something co-created that needs to be explored collaboratively to undo. In the same vein, therapists should communicate observations in a tentative, exploratory manner that signals openness to patient input rather than conveying information with a seemingly objective attitude. In this way, instead of being yet one more in an endless succession of authority figures who do not understand the patient's struggle, the therapist allies him- or herself closely with the patient.

Keeping the Focus on the Immediate and Privileging Awareness over Change

The focus should be on the here and now—the concrete and specific—of the therapeutic relationship rather than on events in prior sessions or even earlier in the same session, and rather than on abstract intellectualized speculation. A specific immediate focus helps patients become observers of their own behavior and more aware of their own experience. Therapists should also try to convey the message to resist the urge to just make things different or better. The emphasis should be on awareness over change, with change should be understood as a byproduct of awareness, that is, with greater awareness comes change.

Recognizing That the Relationship Is Constantly Changing and Continually Gauging Relatedness

By this principle, we mean to highlight the fluidity of experience: therapists need to remember what was true a moment ago may not be true now. They should try to stay present and not get stuck in a prior moment ago, which can be very difficult when anxiety levels are high. Likewise, therapists should continually gauge relatedness to the patient and patient responsiveness to whatever they say or do. In this regard, therapists should pay close attention to their emotional experience as an important source for understanding the quality of relatedness with patients in a given moment. And they should always try to use whatever is emerging in the moment as a point of departure for further metacommunication.

Emphasizing One's Own Subjectivity and Being Open to Exploring One's Own Contribution

Therapists should emphasize the subjectivity of their perceptions. This principle plays a critical role in establishing a climate that emphasizes the subjectivity of all perceptions and helps to establish a collaborative, more egalitarian, relationship where the patient feels freer to decide how to make use of the therapist's observations. In addition, therapists should be open to exploring their own contributions to the interaction with the patient in a nondefensive manner. This process can help patients become less defensive, more able to look at their contributions, and more aware of feelings that they have but are unable to clearly articulate for fear of the therapist's response.

Expecting Initial Attempts to Lead to More Ruptures and to Be Just Beginnings in a Resolution Process

Therapists should understand that their first attempts at metacommunication are just the beginnings of a conversation to disembed from a relational matrix. They should resist the reluctance to metacommunicate and recognize that it is just one step in a resolution process rather than an ultimate intervention. Their initial attempts may lead to more ruptures and may even perpetuate an enactment, but therapists need to get *into* an enactment in order to get *out*. Even the momentary experience of hopelessness may be a necessary step toward resolution. In short, there is nothing magical or elegant in metacommunication, but it can serve as an act of freedom (Symington, 1983)—an act of breaking away from the grip of an interpersonal field (Stern, 1997).

Fundamental Training Principles

In this section, we outline some of the fundamental principles that guide our alliance-focused approach to training.

Recognizing the Relational Context

The relational context is of upmost importance in training, as in therapy. It is impossible for the supervisor to convey information to the trainee that has meaning independent of the relational context in which it is conveyed.

Supervision thus must to be tailored to the specific needs and development of the trainee. Supervisors should recognize and support trainees' needs to maintain their self-esteem and calibrate the extent to which they have more of a need for support versus new information or confrontation in any given situation. It is also critically important that supervisors continually monitor the quality of the *supervisory alliance* in a way that parallels the ongoing monitoring of the quality of the therapeutic alliance. When strains or tensions emerge, closer attention to the supervisory relationship should assume priority over other concerns.

Establishing an Experiential Focus

For many trainees, the process of establishing an experiential focus involves a partial unlearning of things that they have already been taught while doing therapy. Often the formalized training of therapists emphasizes the conceptual at the expense of the experiential. Trainees study the formulations of various psychotherapy theorists and learn to apply the ideas they are learning to their clinical experience. Although this type of knowledge is essential, it can also serve a defensive function. It can help them to manage the anxiety that inevitably arises as a result of confronting the inherent ambiguity and chaos of lived experience and lead to premature formulations that foreclose experience. It can also help them to avoid dealing with the painful and frightening conflictual feelings that inevitably emerge for both patients and therapists. In some respects, this conceptual knowledge can be useful in navigating one's anxieties and therapeutic impasses, but in certain circumstances it may serve to tighten deadlocks.

Emphasizing Self-Exploration

Although there are times when specific suggestions about ways of conceptualizing a case or intervening are useful, our approach emphasizes helping therapists to find their own unique solution to their struggle with the patient. The particular therapeutic interaction that is the focus of supervision is unique to a particular therapist–patient dyad. Therapists will thus have their own unique feelings in response to a particular patient, and the particular solution they formulate to their dilemma must emerge in the context of their own unique reactions. An important aim of training therefore is to help therapists to develop a way to dialogue with their patients about what is going on in the moment that is unique to the moment and their experience of it. Suggestions about what to say provided by supervisors or fellow trainees may look appropriate in the context of a videotape being viewed but may not be appropriate in the context of the next session. The supervisor's task is thus to help trainees develop the ability to attend closely to their own experience and use it as a basis for intervening.

Training Strategies and Tools

Our training program makes use of various strategies to develop therapist abilities and essential skills for recognizing and resolving alliance ruptures. The main training strategies we use include the following.

Manualization

In this regard, we use our book *Negotiating the Therapeutic Alliance: A Relational Treatment Guide* (Safran & Muran, 2000) as a training manual. It provides background and justification for our relational approach to practice and training. Probably the most important benefit of this book is that it presents various clinical principles and models, including our own empirically derived rupture resolution model (Figure 16.2), that can serve to help therapists organize their experience, regulate their affect, and manage their anxiety in the face of a very difficult treatment process (see Aron, 1999, for more on this point).

Process Coding

We provide a brief orientation to various research measures of psychotherapy process, such as those that focus on vocal quality, emotional involvement, and interpersonal behavior, in order to sensitize trainees to the psychotherapy process. This orientation can be very important to the development of one's clinical ear, namely, how to observe and listen to process (and not just content). Trainees may even be asked to track one of their sessions with a particular coding scheme in mind. The use of such measures (in addition to the rupture resolution model) is a good example of how research can influence practice.

Videotape Analysis

We also conduct intensive analysis of videotaped psychotherapy sessions. This type of analysis provides a view of a treatment process unfiltered by the trainees' reconstructions and an opportunity to step outside their participation and to view their interactions as a third-party observer. It facilitates an orientation to interpersonal process. There are many useful ways to use videotape, including as a prompt for accessing and defining trainees' internal experience as well as providing them with subjective feedback about the impact of the patient on others—which can be validating when it corresponds, but also illustrative of the uniqueness of interactions when it differs.

Mindfulness Training

We introduce mindfulness meditation to our trainees, which we consider a systematic strategy for developing an optimal observational stance toward internal experience. Often trainees have difficulty at first in distinguishing between their experience and their ideas about their experience, and it is useful to use structured mindfulness exercises to help them grasp this distinction and develop openness to their experience. Such exercises also help trainees sharpen their abilities to become participant–observers. We also appreciate the benefits of this training in developing affect regulation and interpersonal sensitivity. We incorporate mindfulness in supervised sessions, but we also encourage trainees to establish a personal practice of it.

Awareness Exercises

We make extensive use of awareness-oriented exercises, including the use of role plays and two-chair techniques to practice metacommunication. For example, trainees might be asked to alternate between playing their patient and then themselves around a difficult enactment observed on video, the aim being to explore their experience (especially their fears and expectations regarding the patient) and to experiment with different ways of trying metacommunication. These exercises are at the heart of the training model. They are valuable for grounding training at the experiential level and promoting self-awareness and empathy.

Training Process and Structure

Our primary mode of supervision is by group format in a 90-minute session. The group setting poses many challenges for the supervisors, given the relational orientation. It can be quite daunting for the supervisor to be sensitive to the group process and the complexity of negotiating multiple supervisory alliances while trying to maintain group cohesion. This challenge is intensified when you consider the focus on rupture events and the emphasis on self-exploration. We try to establish a culture of struggle and support. Every case poses problems for every therapist. No one is beyond this. We do privilege the presentation of difficult moments. Because of this, we expect that presenting will be especially fraught with anxiety and shame in our training sessions, and so we are careful to continually track the trainee's experience and take great pains to grant control to the trainee, allowing him or her to feel as free as possible to rein in the process at any time. We make it clear that, while self-exploration plays a central role in the training process, it is also critical for therapists to respect their own needs for privacy and their own fluctuating assessments of what feels safe to explore in front of supervisors and fellow trainees at any point in time.

Each supervisory session follows a typical structure. We usually begin with a mindfulness induction exercise. We then canvass group members to check in on their progress and to decide on which cases will be the focus of the session. Usually we focus on cases that are posing particular problems or those that have not been presented lately. When it comes to playing videotaped session segments, although we allow trainees to preface their presentation with some sort of case history (primarily to grant the trainee a sense of control), we also encourage the playing of the taped session without any introduction, based on the perspective that all the history you really need to know is captured in the patient–therapist interactions. As for the amount of the session viewed, we always err on the side of playing more rather than less. And often we invite trainees to provide narration of what they remember experiencing during the session to the best of their ability as they watch it in the group setting. As for the other trainees, we typically direct their attention toward their affective awareness rather than exhibiting their conceptual skills, which too often result in competition in the group and defensiveness in the presenter.

The initial task upon viewing the video is defining the rupture event. From this observation, we design an experiential exercise. In addition to the example described above where trainees play themselves and the patient in a two-chair exercise, we might do a role play where the presenting trainee plays the patient and the other trainees take turns trying to metacommunicate. During these exercises we try to establish a climate of experimentation and mutuality. As previously mentioned, we recognize that in the final analysis the resolution of rupture is both personal (depending on the trainee's own history and experience) and interpersonal (requiring the participation of the patient). We conclude each session by debriefing the group, gathering any final impressions, and finally we check in with the trainee who presented to see where he or she is experientially with regard to the group and then the case presented.

SOME FUTURE DIRECTIONS

Much more research needs to be conducted to evaluate our training model—in addition to our current effort to collect data on its additive effect on a CBT for personality disorders (the results of which have yet to be determined). As part of our current protocol, we are also conducting semistructured interviews with our therapists and supervisors to assess their experience of the training model, its various strategies, and its impact on the development of their clinical skills, including self-awareness, affect regulation, and interpersonal sensitivity. We have recorded supervision sessions and plan to continue to collect periodic recordings (along with postsession ratings of the group supervision process, including measures of cohesion and alliance) that will allow for more intensive analysis of our training process. There are several elements to our training model, including a variety of strategies and tools, so future efforts should attempt to evaluate what components are most essential through dismantling studies. In general, the research literature on training is relatively thin. The field has yet to approach the study of supervision with the same attention and technology that have been applied to the psychotherapy process. Although we are far from understanding the process of psychotherapy in any definitive sense, much more exacting study of the training process should represent the next frontier.

REFERENCES

Aron, L. (1999). Clinical choices and the relational matrix. *Psychoanalytic Dialogues, 9*, 1–29.

Baldwin, S. A., Wampold, B. E., & Imel, Z. E. (2007). Untangling the alliance–outcome correlation: Exploring the relative importance of therapist and patient variability in the alliance. *Journal of Consulting and Clinical Psychology, 75*, 842–852.

Benjamin, J. (1990). An outline of intersubjectivity: The development of recognition. *Psychoanalytic Psychology, 7*, 33–46.

Blatt, S. J. (2008). *Polarities of experience: Relatedness and self-definition in personality development, psychopathology, and the therapeutic process.* Washington, DC: American Psychological Association.

Bowlby, J. (1973). *Attachment and loss: Vol. 2. Separation.* New York: Basic Books.

Clarkin, J. F., & Levy, K. N. (2004). The influence of client variables in psychotherapy. In M. J. Lambert (Ed.), *Bergin and Garfield's handbook of psychotherapy and behavior change* (5th ed., pp. 194–226). New York: Wiley.

Horvath, A. O., & Bedi, R. P. (2002). The alliance. In J. C. Norcross (Ed.), *Psychotherapy relationships that work* (pp. 37–70). New York: Oxford University Press.

Horvath, A. O., & Symonds, B. D. (1991). Relation between working alliance and outcome in psychotherapy: A meta-analysis. *Journal of Counseling Psychology, 38*, 139–149.

Kessler, R. C., McGonagle, K. A., Zhao, S., Nelson, C. B., Hughes, M., Eshleman, S., et al. (1994). Lifetime and 12-month prevalence of DSM-III-R psychiatric disorders in the United States: Results from the National Comorbidity Study. *Archives of General Psychiatry, 51*, 8–19.

Kiesler, D. J. (1988). *Therapeutic metacommunication: Therapist impact disclosure as feedback in psychotherapy.* Palo Alto, CA: Consulting Psychologists Press.

Kiesler, D. J. (1996). *Contemporary interpersonal theory and research: Personality, psychopathology, and psychotherapy.* New York: Wiley.

Lambert, M. J. (2004). *Bergin and Garfield's handbook of psychotherapy and behavior change* (5th ed.). New York: Wiley.

Luborsky, L., Crits-Christoph, P., McLellan, A. T., Woody, G., Piper, W., Liberman, B., et al. (1986). Do therapists vary much in their success? Findings from four outcome studies. *American Journal of Orthopsychiatry, 56,* 501–512.

Martin, D. J., Garske, J. P., & Davis, M. K. (2000). Relation of the therapeutic alliance with outcome and other variables: A meta-analytic review. *Journal of Consulting and Clinical Psychology, 68,* 438–450.

Mitchell, S. A. (1988). *Relational concepts in psychoanalysis.* Cambridge, MA: Harvard University Press.

Muran, J. C. (2002). A relational approach to understanding change: Plurality and contextualism in a psychotherapy research program. *Psychotherapy Research, 12,* 113–138.

Muran, J. C., & Safran, J. D. (1998). Negotiating the therapeutic alliance in brief psychotherapy: An introduction. In J. D. Safran & J. C. Muran (Eds.), *The therapeutic alliance in brief psychotherapy* (pp. 3–14). Washington, DC: American Psychological Association.

Muran, J. C., & Safran, J. D. (2002). A relational approach to psychotherapy. In F. W. Kaslow & J. J. Magnavita (Eds.), *Comprehensive handbook of psychotherapy: Psychodynamic/object relations* (Vol. 1, pp. 253–281). Hoboken, NJ: Wiley.

Muran, J. C., Safran, J. D., Samstag, L. W., & Winston, A. (2005). Evaluating an alliance-focused treatment for personality disorders. *Psychotherapy: Theory, Research, Practice, Training, 42,* 532–545.

Najavits, L. M., & Strupp, H. H. (1994). Differences in the effectiveness of psychodynamic therapists: A process-outcome study. *Psychotherapy, 31,* 114–123.

Pizer, S. A. (1998). *Building bridges: The negotiation of paradox in psychoanalysis.* Hillsdale, NJ: Analytic Press.

Safran, J. D. (2002). Brief relational psychoanalytic treatment. *Psychoanalytic Dialogues, 12,* 171–195.

Safran, J. D., Crocker, P., McMain, S., & Murray, P. (1990). Therapeutic alliance rupture as a therapy event for empirical investigation. *Psychotherapy: Theory, Research, and Practice, 27,* 154–165.

Safran, J. D., & Muran, J. C. (1996). The resolution of ruptures in the therapeutic alliance. *Journal of Consulting and Clinical Psychology, 64,* 447–458.

Safran, J. D., & Muran, J. C. (2000). *Negotiating the therapeutic alliance: A relational treatment guide.* New York: Guilford Press.

Safran, J. D., & Muran, J. C. (2006). Has the concept of the therapeutic alliance outlived its usefulness? *Psychotherapy: Theory, Research, Practice, Training, 43,* 286–291.

Safran, J. D., Muran, J. C., & Samstag, L. W. (1994). Resolving therapeutic alliance ruptures: A task analytic investigation. In A. O. Horvath & L. S. Greenberg (Eds.), *The working alliance: Theory, research, and practice* (pp. 225–255). New York: Wiley.

Safran, J. D., Muran, J. C., Samstag, L. W., & Stevens, C. (2002). Repairing alliance ruptures. In J. C. Norcross (Ed.), *Psychotherapy relationships that work: Therapist contributions and responsiveness to patients* (pp. 235–254). New York: Oxford University Press.

Safran, J. D., Muran, J. C., Samstag, L. W., & Winston, A. (2005). Evaluating alliance-focused intervention for potential treatment failures: A feasibility study and descriptive analysis. *Psychotherapy: Theory, Research, Practice, Training, 42,* 512–531.

Stern, D. B. (1997). *Unformulated experience.* Hillsdale, NJ: Analytic Press.

Symington, N. (1983). The analyst's act of freedom as an agent of therapeutic change. *International Review of Psycho-Analysis, 10,* 783–792.

Tronick, E. (1989). Emotions and emotional communications in infants. *American Psychologist, 44,* 112–119.

Wachtel, P. L. (2007). Commentary: Making invisibility visible—probing the interface between race and gender. In J. C. Muran (Ed.), *Dialogues on difference: Studies of diversity in the therapeutic relationship* (pp. 132–140). Washington, DC: American Psychological Association.

Wampold, B. E. (2001). *The great psychotherapy debate: Models, methods, and findings.* Mahwah, NJ: Erlbaum.

Wierzbicki, M., & Pekarik, G. (1993). A meta-analysis of psychotherapy dropout. *Professional Psychology: Research and Practice, 24,* 190–195.

Zimmerman, M., Chelminski, I., & Young, D. (2008). The frequency of personality disorders in psychiatric patients. *Psychiatric Clinics of North America, 31,* 405–420.

CHAPTER 17

■ ■ ■ ■ ■

Coda

Recommendations for Practice and Training

Brian A. Sharpless
J. Christopher Muran
Jacques P. Barber

The doctor–patient relationship has been recognized as a central feature of good care and healing since the ancient beginnings of professional medical practice (e.g., Hippocrates' *On the Physician*, Jones, 1868) and the first descriptions of the psychotherapy process (Breuer & Freud, 1955). Today this important relationship is being discussed within the context of several wide-ranging movements related to "professionalism" and "competency" in both medicine and psychology (e.g., Cohen, 2006; Foulds et al., 2009; Kenkel & Peterson, 2009; Mead & Bower, 2000; Suchman & Matthews, 1988) and is discussed in several of the general competencies identified by the Accreditation Council for Graduate Medical Education (ACGME; 2002). There is clearly overlap among the many proposals regarding what constitutes professional and competent patient care and the therapeutic alliance literature. Therefore, the efforts undertaken in this book are highly relevant to those who practice psychotherapy across the various disciplines as well as individuals in other helping professions.

In spite of the extensive history of clinical discussion and the accumulated (and significant) research base on the therapeutic alliance (using any

number of definitions and operationalizations of the concept), we appear
to be somewhat lagging behind in the area of defining practice and training
guidelines. Thus, our intention in this chapter is to condense and formulate
tentative guidelines and regulative ideals to help both novice and experienced therapists alike navigate the sometimes murky waters of the therapeutic alliance within the psychotherapy process. To accomplish this goal, we
prioritize findings with empirical support and, where data are not available,
supplement these contributions with points of consensus linking the many
experts who contributed to this volume.

Any useful set of alliance practice and training guidelines, especially at
this stage, would need to include a list of the many factors that therapists
should remain mindful of when assessing patients (see Table 17.1). Some of
these could be considered to be "warning signs" that may predict a poorer
or stronger alliance. From the outset, however, we would strongly caution
readers that any overly simplistic or nonreflective attention to the patient
and therapist variables enumerated below is risky. These personal elements
are obviously quite context-dependent, and it would be unwise to reify any
guidelines and have them run the risk of becoming self-fulfilling prophecies—
or, worse, blind a therapist to other relevant patient information and behaviors. On the other hand, an attunement to variables that possess demonstrated empirical value may serve to moderate alliance fluctuations and in
some cases enable therapists to avoid being surprised unduly, or caught
unawares, by disruptions. Should one or more of the negative variables be
present, we would recommend paying even closer than usual attention to
the alliance, as these may provide useful clues that permit one to circumvent
premature termination of therapy.

PATIENT AND THERAPIST VARIABLES
RELEVANT FOR THE ALLIANCE

One factor contributing to the complexity of conducting good psychotherapy is the fact that it essentially consists of the interaction of two (or more)
individuals possessing different life histories, personalities, interpersonal or
attachment styles, ways of organizing experience, expectations, and orientations to life. While this is often a rewarding and enriching experience (for
both parties) that also leads to good therapeutic work, it can also easily
lead to misunderstanding, tension, and conflict. Thus, it is appropriate to
discuss some of the patient and therapist variables that may make for stronger or weaker alliances. Most empirical work has involved looking at these
variables in relative isolation. What is missing most in the existing research
literature (perhaps indicating a future direction for research) is the *inter-
connected* character of these variables vis-à-vis the alliance—for instance,

TABLE 17.1. Patient and Therapist Variables Related to the Strength of the Therapeutic Alliance

	Positive predictors (or strong alliance)	Negative predictors (or weak alliance)
Patient variables		
Preconceptions and expectations	• Expectations for improvement	
Interpersonal functioning	• History of positive interpersonal relationships • Friendly and affiliative style • Comfortable relinquishing control	• Interpersonal chaos • Hostility • Low levels of affiliation • Avoidant, anxious, fearful of closeness
Attachment security	• Secure attachment style	• Insecure attachment style
Personality	• Open, agreeable, extraverted, conscientious • Motivational readiness to change	• DSM Clusters A and B personality disorders • Excessive friendliness
Patient object relations	• Good object relations • Stable concept of self • Ability to differentiate self and other • Internalization of therapist	• Poor object relations
Therapist variables		
Therapeutic techniques and skill	• Solid technical ability • Effective delivery of fundamental therapeutic techniques	• Misdiagnosis and poor case conceptualization • Overstructuring or understructuring therapy • Excessive use of techniques
Personal characteristics	• Professional demeanor • Interested, confident, and alert • Trustworthy, courteous, and honest • Warm, friendly, and empathic • Flexible	• Disinterested • Critical • Demanding, pushy, or unsupportive • Defensive
Responsiveness	• Appropriate responsiveness to patient and context • Sensitivity to interpersonal process • Adjustment of therapeutic activity and its timing.	
Observation skills	• Ability to observe patient • Self-awareness • Ability to regulate negative affect, to tolerate distress	

how these patient variables impact upon the therapeutic alliance and other therapeutic processes, which in turn impact upon these initial predisposing factors. There appears to be a rich interplay and fluidity among these constructs, a priori.

Patient Variables

Patient Expectations

An important set of variables related to the development of a strong alliance involves patient preconceptions and expectations. Specifically, patient expectations for improvement have been found to be associated with the quality of the therapeutic alliance (Messer & Wolitsky, Chapter 6, this volume). Further, positive expectations for improvement have been found to be associated not only with expansion of the alliance (Messer & Wolitsky, Chapter 6; and Watson & Kaloogerakos, Chapter 10, this volume) but also with a better overall outcome in psychotherapy.

Patient Interpersonal Functioning

Patients' interpersonal functioning, broadly construed, has also been associated with the alliance. The literature implies that patients with a history of positive interpersonal relationships who generally view individuals as helpful and trustworthy are better able to forge strong alliances than their opposite counterpart (Messer & Wolitsky, Chapter 6, this volume). Further, overall levels of interpersonal distress appear to be relevant, with those patients experiencing more interpersonal chaos or problems less likely to have strong alliances (Messer & Wolitsky, Chapter 6; Piper & Ogrodniczuk, Chapter 13; and Watson & Kaloogerakos, Chapter 10, this volume). However, caution must be exercised when considering these factors, especially this last point, as there is also some evidence that patients who begin psychotherapy with interpersonal chaos and poor alliances *can* certainly improve over the course of treatment (Benjamin & Critchfield, Chapter 7, this volume). As will be described in a subsequent section, such alliance gains may be associated with technical skills and/or competence.

There are also specific findings from the general interpersonal psychotherapy literature that could serve as warning signs. For example, it seems prudent to attend especially closely to alliances with patients presenting with hostile dominant interpersonal styles, as they have been found to have weaker alliances (Benjamin & Critchfield, Chapter 7; and Messer & Wolitsky, Chapter 6, this volume). Patient hostility, in particular—whether self-directed or directed toward the therapist—is generally detrimental to the alliance (Benjamin & Critchfield, Chapter 7; and Messer & Wolitsky, Chapter 6, this volume). The types of intrasession power struggles or therapist defensiveness that may grow out of the latter scenario (i.e., patient hostility directed at the therapist) certainly may contribute to alliance weakness. Similarly, patients with low levels of affiliation toward others experience difficulty in establishing alliances, even if they wish to have them. In contrast, patients who are friendly and more comfortable with relinquishing nominal control (i.e., to the therapist) are able to forge a stronger alliance. Further, patients who often "wall off" or distance themselves from the therapist are also be at risk of establishing poor alliances. Thus, all things being equal, friendly and affiliative patients who are willing to engage the interpersonal processes that are a central feature of psychotherapy are more likely to manifest strong alliances in session than those who are more anxious, avoidant, uncomfortable with interpersonal interchanges, and fearful of interpersonal closeness (Benjamin & Critchfield, Chapter 7; Messer & Wolitsky, Chapter 6; and Watson & Kalogerakos, Chapter 10, this volume).

Patient Attachment Style

Attachment style is also a commonly-assessed psychological construct with a general relevance for psychotherapy and a specific relevance for interpersonal behavior. Although the literature in this area appears to be complex, the weight of the evidence implies that patients with secure attachments are more likely to form strong alliances than insecurely attached individuals (Watson & Kalogerakos, Chapter 10, this volume). Further, one study found that the course of the alliance (i.e., predictable types of alliance fluctuations) over time may be related to attachment style, with preoccupied and secure styles assuming U-shaped patterns whereas those with dismissing styles may be relatively consistent in the beginning and middle of treatment with a decline toward the end (Stiles & Goldsmith, Chapter 3, this volume). Replications and extensions of these findings are needed.

Patient Personality

Building on the preceding section, patient personality factors have also been reliably implicated in the alliance literature, and therapists should be mindful of the clinical manifestations of these traits. At the level of diagnosis, there is evidence that patient *DSM* Cluster A (paranoid) and Cluster B (histrionic, narcissistic, antisocial) personality disorders strongly predict poor early alliance (Muran et al., 1994).

At the level of personality traits, the factors of Openness, Agreeableness, and Extraversion are associated with stronger alliances (Benjamin & Critchfield, Chapter 7, this volume). For example, individuals possessing high levels of Openness to new experiences would presumably be excited by the unique demands and challenges that psychotherapy entails. Further, it seems reasonable to assume that the cooperativeness and friendliness of patients high in Agreeableness would likely assist in the formation of alliances. However, excessive friendliness may sometimes be indicative of alliance problems in a particular subset of patients (Tsai, Kohlenberg, & Kanter, Chapter 9, this volume). In other words, the *function* being served by the friendliness must always be thoughtfully considered. Also, patients with high levels of Extraversion experience positive emotions and find connections with others to be energizing and positive experiences, factors likely conducive to the alliance. And finally, it appears that there is some indirect evidence that Conscientiousness may be relevant to the alliance as well, as patients high in this trait are very goal-driven and prone to desire the generation of goals and tasks with the therapist. Indeed, patients displaying motivation and motivational readiness to change evidence stronger alliances in both individual and group therapy (Messer & Wolitsky, Chapter 6; and Piper & Ogrodniczuk, Chapter 13, this volume).

Patients' Object Relations

Another set of factors relevant to practice guidelines arises primarily from the psychoanalytic tradition, namely, patients' object relations. Specifically, patients with good object relations, a stable conception of themselves, and an ability to differentiate between self and other are all associated with stronger alliances (Messer & Wolitsky, Chapter 6, this volume). This more general finding assumes additional importance when combined with an empirical finding implying that it may be particularly important to improve the alliances of patients with poor object relations to achieve a good outcome (Messer & Wolitsky, Chapter 6, this volume). Limited evidence also exists that "internalizing" the therapist and his or her behaviors is positively associated with the alliance (Benjamin & Critchfield, Chapter 7, this volume). However, this seems to be a concept that need not be exclusively relegated to dynamic therapists alone, as cognitive therapists, for example, hope that their patients will eventually internalize the therapeutic process and its "teachings" (Barber & DeRubeis, 1989) for the purpose of becoming their own cognitive therapist.

Therapist Factors

As discussed by Muran, Safran, and Eubanks-Carter (Chapter 16, this volume), therapist individual differences have also been found to predict alliance. There are any number of important variables to consider, and some of these may be relevant owing to the fact that they may be potential obstacles for therapists to overcome. Some of these behaviors/characteristics appear to be conducive to therapist training or remediation, whereas others are more associated with the personal characteristics and type of person that a therapist is. However, as will be discussed in a subsequent section, there has indeed been progress in training therapists in alliance-fostering techniques. Finally, several of the characteristics described below might serve a more directly positive function as "regulative ideals" intended to orient general therapist behavior and prompt personal improvement.

Therapist Technical Skills

One needs to keep in mind that the therapeutic alliance is not an intervention but rather could be seen as an "outcome" of an intervention as well as a way of facilitating the delivery of interventions (Barber, Khalsa, & Sharpless, Chapter 2, this volume). Thus, there is a complex interactive or dialectical process between techniques and alliance. Empirically there appears to be a consensus building in this volume that good techniques are associated with a good alliance. In other words, the technical aspects of therapy—and not solely the nonspecific factors often described in the literature (e.g., warmth and empathy)—make substantive contributions to the alliance. Switching to the negative side, both misdiagnoses and poor case conceptualizations have been associated with poor alliances. In fact, it has often been recommended that ruptures and weak alliances might best be considered to be useful opportunities to reflect upon (and possibly reconsider) clinical formulations (Castonguay, Constantino, McAleavey, & Goldfried, Chapter 8, this volume), and we would agree.

Interventions have also been implicated in the alliance. At the level of what could be termed "basic" or "fundamental" therapeutic techniques, facilitating the expression of affect, making accurate interpretations, working on a patient's relationship problems, exploring interpersonal themes, noting past therapy successes, and reducing patient self-hatred have all been found to predict a stronger alliance (Benjamin & Critchfield, Chapter 7; Crits-Christoph, Crits-Christoph, & Gibbons, Chapter 15; Hill, Chapter 4; and Messer & Wolitsky, Chapter 6, this volume). However, it is important to note that the competence and judgment that underlie both the choice of and manner in which interventions are implemented may be as important as the interventions themselves (e.g., Sharpless & Barber, 2009). For instance, specific techniques have also been shown to have negative repercussions on the alliance. Both overstructuring and understructuring therapy predicts a negative alliance, as does the excessive use of either therapist silence or self-disclosure. Further, evidence from the behavioral therapy literature found that excessive use of techniques was associated with patients liking the therapist less and viewing them as less competent (Castonguay et al., Chapter 8, this volume). Therefore, a therapist's judgment, nuance, and clinical acumen appear to interact with technical knowledge and the fostering of a strong therapeutic alliance. This pattern is likely a reflection of general therapeutic training and clinical experience and therefore may not be readily reversible through quick training fixes or remediation.

We would like to make a more general comment about the relationship between techniques and the alliance. Precisely, the way they are related is not yet clear, and at least two relationships appear possible. First, they could be highly correlated yet conceptually distinct. Second, they could be so inextricably tied together that differentiating between the two is neither practically nor theoretically meaningful. More empirical work is required to determine which of these possibilities is more reflective of reality.

Therapist Personality

Empirical evidence also exists that implicates certain therapist personality traits in the creation of the alliance. This finding likely comes as no surprise to readers who are clinicians, as the active and technical work conducted in any orientation of therapy is ineluctably filtered through the person (and personality) of the therapist. Indeed, the empirical findings appear to be face valid and dovetail nicely with what clinical intuition would predict. For example, it appears that many of the traits associated with a "professional" demeanor are important. Specifically, therapists who are interested, confident, and alert engender stronger alliances. In contrast, those who appear disinterested, distant, bored, tense, distracted, uncertain in their ability to help the patient, or frequently change their intervention strategies are less capable in this regard (Benjamin & Critchfield, Chapter 7; Escudero, Heatherington, & Friedlander, Chapter 12; Hill, Chapter 4; Messer & Wolitsky, Chapter 6; and Watson & Kalogerakos, Chapter 10, this volume). Further, strong alliances have been associated with what could be termed "respectful" traits or behaviors. For example, therapists who are trustworthy, courteous, and honest in their dealings with patients are more likely to evince good alliances than those who are critical, demanding, pushy, and defensive (Benjamin & Critchfield, Chapter 7; Castonguay et al., Chapter 8; Hill, Chapter 4; Messer & Wolitsky, Chapter 6; and Watson & Kalogerakos, Chapter 10, this volume). Similarly, traits associated with what most people would consider "being human" are also important. For instance, warmth, friendliness, empathy, and being "down-to-earth" are qualities that foster feelings of comfort in patients, leading to a good alliance. In contrast, unsupportive behaviors are not associated with such therapeutic benefits (Castonguay et al., Chapter 8; Escudero et al., Chapter 12; Hill, Chapter 4; Messer & Wolitsky, Chapter 6; and Watson & Kalogerakos, Chapter 10, this volume). Finally, therapist flexibility also appears to have a role in the forging of therapeutic alliances and may be more generally associated with therapist competence, as discussed above (Messer & Wolitsky, Chapter 6, this volume). Interestingly, many of the traits mentioned appear to be part of a therapist's way of "being in the world." In contrast to the relative ease of increasing a technical skill, it may be quite hard to rectify perceived deficiencies in these alliance-facilitating traits. We would hope that all beginning therapists possess these interpersonal strengths and aspect of "human-ness," but clearly individuals greatly vary in their personal attributes. However, personal motivation combined with close supervision can go a long way toward remedying most, if not all, of these identified deficits.

Therapist Responsiveness to Patient and Context

The alliance has also been associated with what is often described as a therapist's "responsiveness" to patients (Hatcher, Chapter 1; and Stiles & Goldsmith, Chapter 3, this volume); however, we should note that the best particular manner in which a therapist should be responsive remains elusive and is difficult to specify in advance, as it may reflect the more "artistic" and "non-rule-governed" aspects of psychotherapy. Regardless, there does appear to be a general consensus that certain populations (e.g., persons with severe personality disorder, those distrustful of psychological treatments) may require different levels of therapeutic activity to foster a working alliance. Closely allied with the discussion of the competent application of therapeutic techniques (as described above), studies show that therapists should be especially attentive to various aspects of a patient's presentation at particular points in time (Hill, Chapter 4, this volume). This regimen seems essential to recognizing and resolving ruptures (Muran, Safran, & Eubanks-Carter, Chapter 16, this volume). The evidence regarding increased adherence to orientation-specific techniques in the face of alliance ruptures and poorer outcome supports this approach (Castonguay et al., Chapter 8; and Muran et al., Chapter 16, this volume). Taken further, evidence exists that the adjustment of technical interventions to the appropriate level of a patient's defensive functioning is a factor associated with building a strong alliance (Messer & Wolitsky, Chapter 6, this volume). Taken to a more abstract level, the act of bridging the gulf between a patient and therapist's unique experiences and understandings appears to be another core prerequisite of therapy in general, and the alliance in particular.

Therapist Observational Skills

A therapist's ability to observe appears to also possess relevance for the alliance. There seems to be a consensus that therapists should continually monitor both the content of what is said as well as the manner in which it is said (and, likely, that which is not said at all, as nonutterances can also be very telling, particularly from the psychoanalytic point of view). Although therapists are often aware when therapy is going smoothly (i.e., when the alliance is strong), some evidence exists that therapists are often unaware of patient dissatisfaction and that this failing can lead to poor alliances, ruptures, or premature terminations (Hill, Chapter 4, this volume; Muran & Safran, Chapter 5; and Muran et al., Chapter 16, this volume). This attentiveness appears to be a fairly general therapeutic skill that could readily be improved with supervision. We would recommend that trainees' supervisors model active listening skills and utilize trainees' audio or video recordings of sessions to make these ideas more easily understood. Further, therapist self-awareness and capabilities for self-observation appear to be as important, if not more important, than a therapist's ability to observe their patients. As one example, evidence seems to be accumulating that expressions of therapist hostility are detrimental to the alliance (Barber et al., Chapter 2; and Benjamin & Critchfield, Chapter 7, this volume). Thus, therapists must be able to both observe their own nontherapeutic reactions to patient's material and neither fall prey to enactments of the patient's maladaptive patterns nor act out their own unresolved issues (Benjamin & Critchfield, Chapter 7, this volume). As noted by Muran et al. (Chapter 16, this volume), therapist self-awareness may also have bearing on therapists' ability to regulate their own negative affects and negotiate rupture events with their patients.

ALLIANCE PEDAGOGY

From our perspective, a number of the observations made above can be implemented into a training program oriented toward teaching alliance skills. Evidence is slowly building up that alliance-generating and alliance rupture resolution skills can be improved through instruction, and earlier chapters (e.g., Binder & Henry, Chapter 14; Crits-Christoph et al., Chapter 15; and Muran et al., Chapter 16, this volume) have outlined several training programs in detail. We will not repeat their details here but will briefly note some of their more interesting findings. Principally, it is important to note that manuals currently exist that detail alliance management techniques, and several of these have demonstrated empirical support for their efficacy and utility. The ready availability of these tools will certainly make the dissemination of techniques easier. However, we should also note that no consensus yet exists on the best or most effective course of training on these specific techniques. It may well be the case that these techniques vary in their efficacy, depending on orientation. We also find it interesting that, although alliance skills can be increased through instruction, the capacity for alliance building varies greatly among therapists who received the same training (Crits-Christoph et al., Chapter 15, this volume). Given that alliance training likely has different foci based on both the developmental level of the therapist (e.g., the instruction given to a first-year doctoral student is likely different from that given to a seasoned protocol therapist) and each therapists' particular strengths and weaknesses, the variability in results is perhaps not surprising. Thus, there likely must be a responsiveness of the alliance supervisor to the particular clinical skills of the trainee if everyone's instruction is to be optimal.

More generally, there is an openness in this field of instruction, and we encourage further exploration by one all to reach the shared overarching goal of better fostering alliances with our patients. In the remaining text we therefore provide five tentative recommendations and future directions derived from both the foregoing chapters and our own experiences with supervision. First, we recommend that therapists become familiar with at least one of the manuals focused on alliance ruptures (preferably one possessing empirical support, as in Muran & Safran, Chapter 5, this volume). The development of readily usable "templates" for alliance rupture resolution procedures would be a valuable addition to the clinical armamentarium of any therapist. Second, we recommend that therapists review their patients' alliances with them regularly, especially with those who may present with significant alliance "warning signs," as detailed above and summarized in Table 17.1. Although revisiting goals and tasks is generally considered to be a good clinical practice with all patients, those patients exhibiting more brittle alliances deserve a more frequent and studied review. Third—and highly relevant to evaluations of trainees and other therapists (e.g., protocol therapists)—the ability to generate and manage alliances should be a key area highlighted in any rigorous 360-degree assessment of clinical skills. As noted throughout this volume, a multitude of measures and means of assessing the alliance are readily available, and these could be implemented in any practicum setting regardless of resources. Fourth, demonstration of good and bad alliance models (via videotape, role plays, or novel virtual reality technologies) in didactics would be a useful adjunct to standard supervision and the review of relevant manuals. Finally a perusal of the list of therapist qualities described above and in Table 17.1 would seem to imply that training models used in rupture resolution require therapists who, among other things, are self-aware, interpersonally sensitive, and able to regulate their affects to best effect (e.g., Muran et al., Chapter 16, this volume).

FUTURE DIRECTIONS

The research on the therapeutic alliance has benefited from a large amount of effort, most likely the most concentrated effort we have seen in the expansive field of psychotherapy research. At this point, we have strong evidence demonstrating that a strong early alliance is critical to overall change and patient retention, although there may be some further relation to early treatment gains, which requires more investigation. There is also evidence regarding the predictive quality of certain patient and therapist variables on the strength of the alliance, many of which have been outlined in this chapter. In addition, we have a growing body of evidence demonstrating the prevalence and predictive validity of ruptures and rupture–repair patterns. Finally, there are a few promising studies suggesting that therapists can be trained to improve their abilities to manage the therapeutic alliance. Of course, much more research is needed, and—as it is often the case in science—the empirical efforts thus far have stimulated a number of additional questions. In the coming years, these are some of the questions that we think will be of greatest interest to practitioners and researchers alike:

1. What is the best definition of the therapeutic alliance? More specifically, what are the boundaries of the concept? How is the alliance distinguishable from other facets of the therapeutic relationship (e.g., Hatcher, Chapter 2; and Horvath, Symonds, & Villanueva, Chapter 11, this volume)? Likewise, it would be helpful to formulate better definitions of alliance rupture. How can it be better demarcated? For example, what is its relevance to transference–countertransference and the notion of enactment?

2. How is the alliance created during therapy, and how early in therapy does it happen? Is it created from the "first encounter," in whatever sense of the term (e.g., initial phone contact; viewing the therapist's picture on a website)? Likewise, what constitutes the first rupture? Can it be present from the beginning?

3. Is the alliance a function of the patient, a therapist contribution, or both? Likewise, is rupture a function of the patient or therapist contributions or both (Barber, 2009)?

4. Are all ruptures equally important? Should some favor more clinical attention and intervention than others? Further, when, optimally, should ruptures first be addressed? Are there times when they are better ignored or minimized? Are there differences between early-phase and late-phase ruptures?

5. What is the relationship between therapeutic techniques and the alliance in the various types of therapy (Barber, 2009)?

6. Is the alliance as important in cognitive-behavioral therapy as it is in dynamic, interpersonal, and humanistic therapies (Barber, 2009)? Do alliance ruptures occur as often in CBT as they occur in more interpersonally oriented treatments?

7. Is the alliance equally important for the treatment of patients with different diagnoses? For example, is the alliance comparatively more important in treating personality disorders?

8. There seems to be some association between a patient's object relations and interpersonal functioning and the development of the therapeutic alliance. Yet, there is a need for more investigation of these patients' and therapists' characteristics, the alliance, therapists' interventions, and outcome. Is there an "optimal" match for patient and therapist that helps to assure a strong alliance?

9. More broadly, is the therapeutic alliance a meaningful concept for the physician–patient relationship more broadly? Does a strong alliance in *other* medical practices improve outcome and patient satisfaction?

10. How can we further amplify the ability of a therapist to develop a therapeutic alliance with a wide variety of patients and to resolve alliance ruptures as they occur? Can we identify the key skills needed for these types of complex interactions?

In conclusion, endeavoring to answer questions as significant as those outlined above requires the application of two approaches to knowledge that work in tandem. It will entail a combination of advanced conceptual analysis of the alliance construct as well as the implementation of novel and complex empirical designs. These efforts will not only be likely to advance alliance research, but may also serve to advance the field of psychotherapy research as a whole.

REFERENCES

Accreditation Council for Graduate Medical Education. (2002). General competencies. Retrieved on December 18, 2009, from *www.acgme.org/acWebsite/irc/irc_competencies.pdf*.

Barber, J. P. (2009). Towards a working through of some core conflicts in psychotherapy research. *Psychotherapy Research, 19*, 1–12.

Barber, J. P., & DeRubeis, R. (1989). On second thought: Where the action is in cognitive therapy for depression. *Cognitive Therapy and Research, 13*, 441–457.

Breuer, J., & Freud, S. (1955). Studies on hysteria. In J. Strachey (Ed. & Trans.), *The Standard Edition of the Complete Psychological Works of Sigmund Freud* (Vol. 2). London: Hogarth Press. (Original work published 1893–1895)

Cohen, J. J. (2006). Professionalism in medical education, an American perspective: From evidence to accountability. *Medical Education, 40*, 607–617.

Foulds, N. A., Grus, C. L., Hatcher, R. L., Kaslow, N. J., Hutchings, P. S., Madson, M. B., et al. (2009). Competency benchmarks: A model for understanding and measuring competence in professional psychology across training levels. *Training and Education in Professional Psychology, 3*(4, Suppl.), S5–S26.

Jones, W. H. S. (1868). *Hippocrates' collected works.* Cambridge, MA: Harvard University Press.

Kenkel, M. B., & Peterson, R. L. (Eds.). (2009). *Competency-based education for professional psychology.* Washington, DC: American Psychological Association.

Mead, N., & Bower, P. (2000). Patient-centeredness: A conceptual framework and review of the empirical literature. *Social Science and Medicine, 51,* 1087–1100.

Muran, J. C., Segal, Z. V., Samstag, L. W., & Crawford, C. E. (1994). *Journal of Consulting and Clinical Psychology, 62*(1), 185–190.

Sharpless, B. A., & Barber, J. P. (2009). A conceptual and empirical review of the meaning, measurement, development, and teaching of intervention competence in clinical psychology. *Clinical Psychology Review, 29*(1), 47–56.

Suchman, A. L., & Matthews, D. A. (1988). What makes the doctor–patient relationship therapeutic?: Exploring the connectional dimensions of medical care. *Annals of Internal Medicine, 108,* 125–130.

Index

Group cohesion, 264. *See also* Group alliance
alliance concept comparison, 265
evidence, 266–267
definition difficulties, 264
outcome prediction, 267–269
Group Cohesion Questionnaire, 267
Group therapy, 263–282
alliance versus cohesion, outcome, 267–269
clinical example, rupture, 274–277
cohesion, 264
expectancy, 269–270
independent constructs evidence, 266–267
mediating effects, 269–270
pattern of alliance, 270–271
practice guidelines, 271–273
strong alliance strategies, 273–274
Growth collaborator concept, 139, 141, 145
Guidance
acceptance balance, 202–203
and client resistance, 203–204
in experiential psychotherapy, 202–204

H

"Helping alliance," 99
Helping Alliance Questionnaire
epistemology, 45
linear increase study, 47
Helping Alliance Questionnaire–II, 267
High–low–high (U-shaped) patterns
alliance developmental course, 48–49
clusters, 50
Hispanic families, unbalanced alliances, 246
Homework, in promoting change, families, 251
Hostage relationship, family therapy, 257
Hostile anger
qualitative study, 68–69
training in coping with, 71
working with, 68–69
Hostility. *See also* Self-directed hostility
alliance detriment, 344–345
in therapist, Vanderbilt studies, 287–294
in therapy, alliance effects, 134

Humanistic psychotherapy, 191–205
alliance research, 198–205
client factor, 200–202
subjective experience studies, 198–200
Carl Rogers' theory, 191–192
empathy function, 193–194
guidance and acceptance balance, 202–204
nondirective approach, 192–196
ruptures, 199–200
therapist's process, managing of, 204–205

I

Idealizing transferences, 55
Identification, as copy process, 137–139, 138n13
Immediacy, training in, 71
Immigrant families, challenge, 255
Impasses
in family therapy, 252–254
qualitative studies, 67–68
reasons for, 67–68
shift intervention, 253–254
In-session behaviors
clinical relevance, 176–178
functional analysis, 177–178
and functional analytic psychotherapy, 176–177
client improvements, 176–177
client problems, 176
"In-to-out parallels," 183–184
in vivo interventions
in clinically-relevant behaviors, 185–186, 185f
relationship focus of, 164
Indirect self-report method, 86–87
description of, 86
rupture data comparison, 84t
rupture–repair studies, 86–87
Individuation, and termination process, 329
"Inert knowledge," and training, 299–300
"Intact" alliances, couples, 218–219
Integrative cognitive therapy (ICT)
randomized controlled trial, 82
rupture resolution, 82, 163
Integrative Psychotherapy Alliance Scales, 245
Internal working alliance, models, 12

Moderators of outcome, 33–35
  definition, 33–34
  as measurement challenge, 35
Motivation
  alliance effect, 113
  in rupture resolution, 253
Motivational enhancement therapy
    (MET)
  in alliance-fostering training, 305
  techniques, 306
Multidimensional family therapy
    (MDFT)
  adolescent challenges, 255–256
  outcome research, 243
Multi-problem families, alliance
    predictors, 244
Mutual affirmation, bond enhancement,
    310
Mutuality, in therapy relationship, 100

N

Natural reinforcement
  in change process, 175–176
  versus contrived, 175
Naturalistic observation paradigm
  observer-based methods, 83–86
  in rupture research, 75, 82–87
  self-report method in, 83
Negative complementarity
  and outcome, 134
  Vanderbilt I study, 134
Negative process
  managing of, 285–301
  Vanderbilt I study, 287–292
  Vanderbilt II study, 289–299
Negative psychotherapy experiences,
    63–73
  angry clients, 68–70
  evidence for occurrence of, 63
  impasses, cases of, 67–68
  misunderstandings, cases of, 65–67
  qualitative studies, 63–72
  training in coping with, 71
Negotiation
  in therapeutic alliance, 321–322
  in working alliance, 12
NIMH Collaborative Depression Study,
    34, 36, 37, 117
Nondirective approach
  Carl Rogers' emphasis, 192–196
  congruence condition, 194

empathy condition, 193–194
research,195
unconditional positive regard in, 193
Nonspecfic factors, in therapeutic alliance,
    152–153

O

Object relations theory
  and patient's alliance, 346
  positive relationship promotion, 117
  relationship factors in, 106, 117
  therapeutic alliance view, 100–101
Observational measures
  advantages, 246
  in clinical process, 246
  family therapy, 246–249
Observational skills, therapist, 349–350
Observer-based methods, 83–86
  in rupture research, 83–86
  versus self-report, 83–85, 84t
"Out-to-in parallels," 183–184
Outcome, 29–43
  alliance as mediator, 35–36
  alliance as moderator, 33–35
    measurement challenge, 35
  alliance as predictor, 29–40
    temporal factor, 30–33, 33t, 39
    therapy interventions interaction,
      36–37
    validity, 29–40
  alliance-fostering techniques, 313–314
  alliance primary role, 38–40
    equivocal data on, 40
    therapist attributes, 38
  alliance training effect, 38–39
  couple therapy, 214–223
    gender effects, 217–218
    individual therapy comparison,
      214
    measurement challenge, 214–216
    split alliances, 216–217
  family therapy research, 243–245
  group therapy, 267–269
    alliance versus cohesion, 267–268
  and later alliance, 53
  linear alliance increase, 51–52
  measurement, 30–33, 39
  psychodynamic research, 114–117
  therapy interactions, 36–37
  and third session alliance, 52–53
  U-shaped alliance course, 52